AJPH
A PUBLICATION OF THE
AMERICAN PUBLIC HEALTH ASSOCIATION

AMERICAN JOURNAL of PUBLIC HEALTH
JULY 2026
Issue 7

Ultraprocessed Foods and Corporate Influence

- UPF Consumption and Health in the United States
- Tobacco-Owned UPF Companies
- Science-Based Policy Actions
- Structural Changes to Prevent UPF Harm

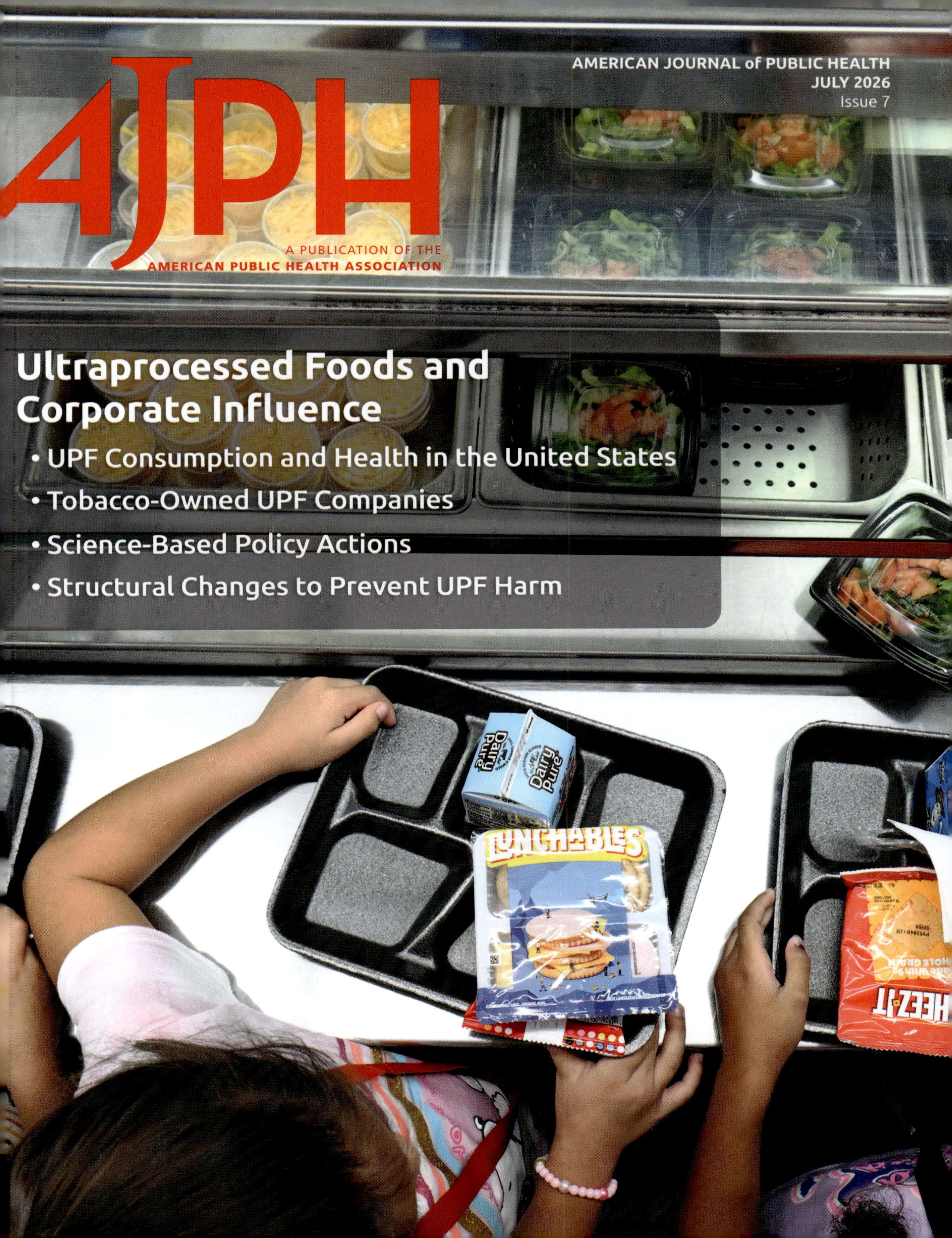

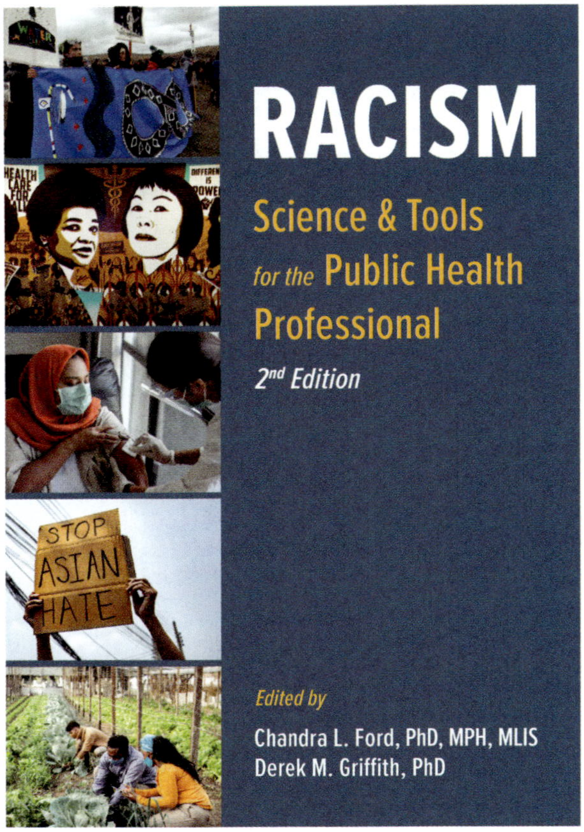

Racism: Science and Tools for the Public Health Professional, 2nd edition

Chandra L. Ford, PhD, MPH, MLIS, and Derek M. Griffith, PhD

ISBN 978-0-87553-352-0, 600 PP., 2025, SOFTCOVER

Racism: Science and Tools for the Public Health Professional, 2nd edition enables public health professionals to address the health impacts of racism. This vital title also responds to the watershed events of the past five years: the COVID-19 pandemic and its intersection with overt forms of racism across all socioecological levels, the 2020 murder of George Floyd by Minneapolis police and the unprecedented domestic and global movements toward racial justice that transpired, and other major global events.

APHABOOKSTORE.ORG

APHA PRESS

AN IMPRINT OF AMERICAN PUBLIC HEALTH ASSOCIATION

AMERICAN PUBLIC HEALTH ASSOCIATION
For science. For action. For health.

AJPH®, published monthly, is the official Journal of the American Public Health Association®, 800 I St NW, Washington, DC 20001-3710; (202) 777- APHA; TDD (202) 777-2500. APHA is a nongovernmental professional society founded in 1872, representing all disciplines and specialties in public health.

The *American Journal of Public Health*® (*AJPH*) (print ISSN: 0090-0036; electronic ISSN: 1541- 0048), first published in 1911, is the official journal of the American Public Health Association® (APHA). The oldest and largest organization of public health professionals in the world, APHA represents approximately 30 000 members from more than 50 occupations of public health.

Submissions: Visit www.editorialmanager.com/ajph for online manuscript preparation and submission guidelines. Contributions of original unpublished research, social science analyses, scholarly essays, critical commentaries, departments, and letters to the editor are welcome. Questions? Write ajph.submissions@apha.org or call APHA at (202) 777-2469.

Print plus online subscriptions: Institutional price (print copy with online access) for a single institution and all authorized users, regardless of geographic location varies by size of organization; multiple campuses not permitted without special arrangement. To order, write apha.subscriptions@apha.org.

Online-only subscriptions: Institutional price for one US federal institution and its authorized users is $1,015–$1,510. To order, write apha.subscriptions@apha.org. For academic, non-US federal consortia, or multisite subscriptions, contact apha.subscriptions@apha.org or visit http://research.ebsco.com for pricing information.

Print-only subscriptions: Institutional price is US $970, $1,065 international.

Back print issues: A limited number of print issues are for sale. Single copies are US $80, $90 international (air delivery). Shipping and handling fees will apply; prepay only. To order, write apha.subscriptions@apha.org.

Reprints: For prices and ordering information on 50 or more reprints, check the Reprints section at www.ajph.org. To order smaller quantities of reprints (rush delivery), use the "Purchase Article" link on the article site itself.

Electronic access: Online articles more than 10 years old are available free for personal use at www.ajph.org. Recent articles are available through pay-per-view: single PDF article for $24, single issue access for 24 hours for $33, or entire site access for 24 hours for $38.

Postal information: Periodicals postage paid at Washington, DC, and additional mailing offices. Postmaster: Send address changes to American Journal of Public Health, 800 I St NW, Washington, DC 20001-3710.

Address changes: Send to AJPH, Membership Department (members) or AJPH Subscriptions (subscribers), APHA, 800 I St NW, Washington, DC 20001-3710. Or write to membership.mail@apha.org (members) or apha.subscriptions@apha.org (subscribers).

Indexes: Publications that index or abstract articles from *AJPH* include the following: Ageline, Assia (Applied Social Science Index and Abstracts), Biological Abstracts, Chemical Abstracts, CINAHL, Criminal Justice Abstracts, EMBASE, EMCare, Environmental Abstracts, e-psyche, ERIC, ETOH (Alcohol and Alcohol Problems Science Database), Excerpta Medica, Food Science and Technology, General Science Index, Grateful Med, Hospital Literature Index, Human Resources Abstracts, International Pharmaceutical Abstracts (IPA), Medline, Physical Education Index, Pollution Abstracts, Psychological Abstracts, PsychINFO, Safety Science Abstracts, Sage Family Studies Abstracts, Sage Human Resources Abstracts, Science Citation Index, SCOPUS, SIIC Data Bases, Social Work Research and Abstracts, and Statistical Reference Index (SRI)/LexisNexis.

AJPH

A PUBLICATION OF THE
AMERICAN PUBLIC HEALTH ASSOCIATION

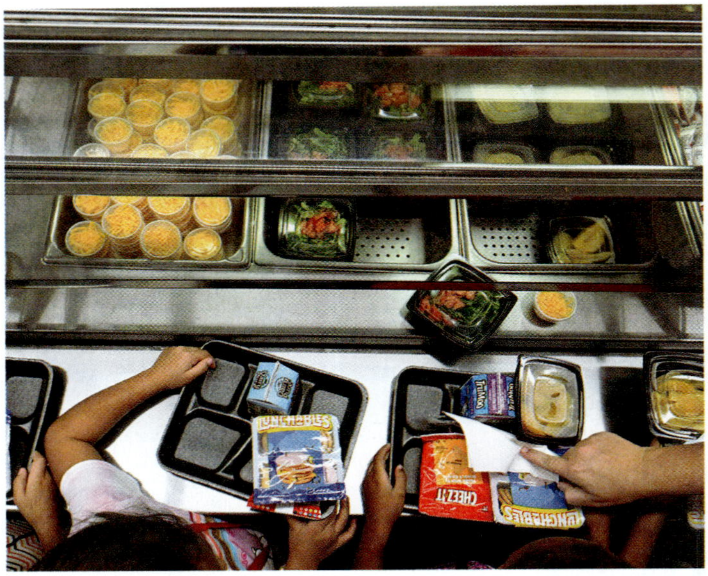

COVER: Students get boxes of Lunchables for lunch at Pembroke Elementary School on Thursday, September 07, 2023, in Pembroke, NC. The school has been serving Lunchables as a lunch choice for students this school year.

Cover concept and selection by Aleisha Kropf. Photo by Matt McClain/ The Washington Post via Getty Images. Printed with permission.

APHA
AMERICAN PUBLIC HEALTH ASSOCIATION
For science. For action. For health.

Promoting public health research, policy, practice, and education is the *AJPH* mission. As we widen our scope to embrace global issues, we also sharpen our focus to support the needs of public health practitioners. We invite contributions of original unpublished research, opinion and commentary, and letters to the editor.

The *Journal* is printed on acid-free recycled paper.

OPEN ACCESS | ONLINE ONLY | PODCAST | DATA SUPPLEMENT AVAILABLE

EDITOR'S CHOICE

869 Beyond Personal Responsibility: Lessons From the Tobacco War for Regulating Ultraprocessed Food
N. Chartres

OPINIONS, PRACTICE, & EDUCATION

EDITORIALS FROM THE ACADEMICS

871 Preventing Ultraprocessed Youths From Becoming Ultraprocessed Adults
D. M. Hoelscher and N. Ranjit

VACCINE ACCESS

874 In a Rapidly Evolving Public Health Landscape, Governors Are Investing in Durable Health Infrastructure
A. Botticella and K. Anupindi

EDITORIALS

877 Call to Action: Antihunger and Public Health Communities Must Find Common Ground to Advance a More Just and Nutritious Food System in the United States
J. Johnson, T. Beckelman, A. Gibson, J. Berg, and P. Lurie

881 Consumer Risk in the Compounded GLP-1 Boom: Why Compounded GLP-1s Demand Urgent Public Health Action
A. Agarwal, A. A. Agarwal, and F. C. Stanford

884 Slow Suicide: Listening to Community, Broadening Our Paradigms
S. R. Solomon and T. W. Glasgow

887 Approaches to Approximating National Public Health Data
B. R. Spoer, L. E. Thorpe, and M. N. Gourevitch

890 On Adoption Interest Among Transgender Individuals: Conceptual Ambiguity, Methodological Weakness, and Interpretive Overreach
C. H. Burt

891 Ogunbajo et al. Respond
A. Ogunbajo, T. DeAtley, A. Breslow, K. Gamarel, D. Operario, T. Kershaw, and A. Restar

PRACTICE EVALUATIONS

893 Evaluating the Impact of Singapore's Nutri-Grade Beverage Labels on Prepackaged Beverage Purchases and Product Nutrient Composition: A Before–After Study, 2019–2024
S. Shin and Y. N. Tan

ULTRAPROCESSED FOOD

898 Ultraprocessed Food and Corporate Influence: Evidence, Regulation, and Policy Pathways to Address Chronic Disease in the United States
N. Chartres

903 Ultraprocessed Food, Food Insecurity, and Improving the Food Environment for All in the United States
J. N. Gracia

906 Litigation as a Necessary Tool to Challenge Food Industry's Toxic Practices
J. L. Pomeranz and K. D. Brownell

909 Beyond the Body: The Ultraprocessed Food Industry's Environmental Toll
L. S. Taillie, N. Chartres, K. Anastasiou, and J. Yates

912 The Politics of Ultraprocessed Foods: Dietary Guidelines for Americans
M. Nestle

915 Food Environment Policies to Address the Market Power of Ultraprocessed Food Corporations
G. Scrinis

918 Practical and Equity Considerations for Ultraprocessed Foods Policies
J. A. Wolfson

RESEARCH & ANALYSIS

ULTRAPROCESSED FOOD

921 Ultraprocessed Foods in the Global Food System: The Role of US Tobacco Companies
T. L. Fazzino, S. Kong, G. Lee, and M. Stewart

932 What Do Nova and the Ultraprocessed Food Concept Offer to Policymakers? From Updating Dietary Guidance to Regulatory Action and Advancing Sustainable Food System Transitions
C. A. Monteiro, P. Baker, C. Corvalan, and B. M. Popkin

940 Tobacco Industry Contributions to the Development of Ultraprocessed Food in the United States, 1985–2007: A Case Study of Lunchables
L. A. Schmidt

950 Nutritional Characteristics of Foods With Addictive Potential: A Machine-Learning Approach
A. N. Gearhardt, Z. Hutelin, E. Nartey, M. L. Ahrens, M. E. Baugh, T. L. Fazzino, E. M. LaFata, K. R. Sonneville, and A. G. DiFeliceantonio

960 Public Awareness and Support for Governmental Intervention to Address Harms Associated With Consumption of Ultraprocessed Foods: A National Survey, United States, June 2025
J. Niederdeppe, C. L. Barry, S. E. Gollust, N. Porticella, K. D. Brownell, and A. N. Gearhardt

971 Associations Between Household Food Insecurity and Participation in Nutrition Assistance Programs, and Ultraprocessed Food Consumption and Diet Quality Among Pregnant Women in NHANES, 2001–2018
C. R. Fernández, S. H. Kahwaji, P. A. Koch, R. L. Wolf, E. Martínez-Steele, and J. W. Cadenhead

981 Ultraprocessed Foods and the Risk of Cognitive Impairment and Dementia in Older US Adults: 2013–2020 Health and Retirement Study
H. Lee, C. T. McEvoy, E. M. Steele, N. Khandpur, S. G. Heeringa, L. H. Ryan, K. M. Langa, J. A. Wolfson, and C. W. Leung

993 The Intersection of Diet Quality and Ultraprocessed Food Intake: Using Evidence-Based Categories to Characterize Differences in Cardiometabolic Profiles
E. Sheinberg, L. A. Schmidt, J. R. Mande, E. Martinez-Steele, D. K. Tobias, and C. W. Leung

1004 Changes in Neighborhood Foodscapes From 2003 to 2023 by Area Rurality in the United States
D. Wiese, M. M. Shams-White, Z. Zheng, K. A. Henry, M. L. McCullough, and F. Islami

1015 Ultraprocessed Food Versus Diet Quality in Relation to Cardiometabolic Health and All-Cause Mortality: NHANES 1999–2018
J. Hatta-Langedyk, L. Wang, B. Fan, P. Shi, and D. Mozaffarian

1025 Operationally Defining and Targeting Ultraprocessed Foods: Insights From US Policy Proposals
A. D'Angelo Campos, J. W. Krieger, C. E. Prestemon, B. A. Hollingsworth, and L. S. Taillie

OPEN-THEMED RESEARCH

1030 Protecting US Children From Lead Exposures: Applications of a Data-Mapping Blueprint for Focusing High-Impact Interventions
V. Zartarian, A. Walts, C. A. Gross-Davis, A. Poulakos, K. Triantafillou, K. R. Simoneau, N. Spalt, C. Durand, S. Sellars, M. Kromer, A. Burnett, R. Taylor, C. Neely, T. Speth, N. Kulikowski, V. H. Garrison, P. Han, R. Tornero-Velez, and L. W. Stanek

1038 Access to Abortion for US Military Service Members in 2024 After the *Dobbs v Jackson* Supreme Court Decision
C. Brander, K. Grindlay, C. Russell, E. Cardnell, and C. Gerdts

1044 Keeping Sight of Albay: Vitamin A Blindness, Randomized Controlled Trials, and Cold War Foreign Aid Policy
R. M. Sastry

Beyond Personal Responsibility: Lessons From the Tobacco War for Regulating Ultraprocessed Food

See also Ultraprocessed Food, pp. 898–1029.

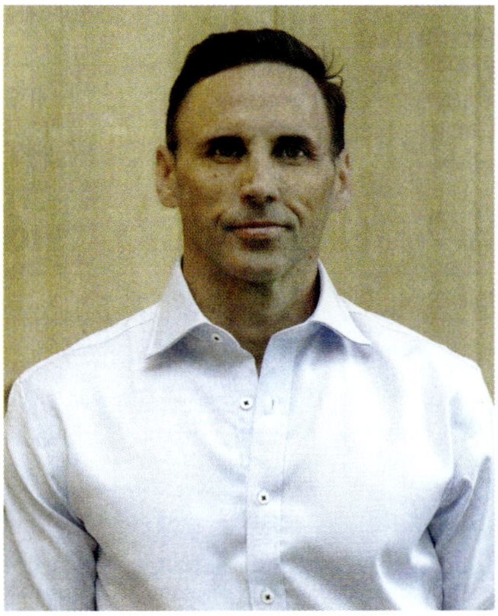

Nicholas Chartres, PhD, M Hum Nutr
The University of Sydney, Australia
The Center to End Corporate Harm, University of California, San Francisco
AJPH Associate Editor

When an anonymous box of internal tobacco industry documents from Brown & Williamson landed on the doorstep of Professor Stanton Glantz at the University of California, San Francisco, our understanding of what the tobacco industry knew about the harms of its products began to come to light. Despite increasing evidence to the contrary, tobacco executives had denied that their products were addictive and causally linked to cancer and heart disease.

Glantz's documents, now housed in the online University of California, San Francisco, Industry Documents Library, revealed that, as early as the 1960s, tobacco companies understood that cigarettes were addictive and viewed themselves as "in the business of selling nicotine, an addictive drug" and knew "at the best, the probabilities are that some combination of constituents of smoke will be found conducive to the onset of cancer or to create an environment in which cancer is more likely to occur" (https://bit.ly/4cpTKx3). For decades, the tobacco industry continued to deny this publicly and Americans continued consuming these products, assuming they were safe (https://bit.ly/4cEVLEt).

Things were about to change.

Now, research using these same internal industry documents has revealed the strategies tobacco companies have used to shape our diets and propensity for diet-related diseases. The evidence on the health harms of ultraprocessed food (UPF) is unequivocal, and there is extensive evidence that processed junk food has been reformulated to promote overconsumption and patterns of intake similar to those observed in nicotine dependence. The corporations that make these products are now, therefore, one of the leading vectors of disease in the United States (https://doi.org/10.1056/NEJMms2507028). We cannot continue to repeat the same mistakes with regulating UPF as we made with tobacco.

Things are about to change again.

In the early 1960s, the largest US tobacco companies, RJ Reynolds and Philip Morris, bought up major processed food and beverage companies. They entered the food industry with the goal of applying their proprietary research and technology for making cigarettes (e.g., artificial colors and flavors, processing and packaging technologies) to design food products that would be irresistible to consumers. By the mid-1980s, these acquisitions meant that the two largest tobacco companies owned and operated some of the largest food corporations, including Kraft General Foods, Del Monte, and Nabisco. These companies produced many of the most popular global snack food brands, including Lunchables, Oreo, Kentucky Fried Chicken, and Kraft Macaroni & Cheese. They reformulated UPFs to make them more appealing and hyperpalatable (using artificially high amounts of sodium, sugars, and fats), leading to uncontrollable cravings and overconsumption of these energy-dense products.

The UPF industry has tried to downplay the harm of their products, distracting the public by attributing obesity to a lack of physical activity and arguing that it is the individual's responsibility to control their intake. They have created "healthier" product lines focused on reformulation while still not addressing the cocktail of chemicals in their products. By reformulating products, the

AJPH July 2026, Vol. 116, No. 7

UPF industry has presented itself as part of the solution, thus staving off meaningful regulation of their deleterious products.

These are the same tactics the tobacco industry used in their fight to delay regulation (http://bit.ly/494Q8hl). However, public awareness is growing, and momentum is shifting in understanding these tactics.

The pivotal moment for tobacco reform in the United States came in November 1998 when the Master Settlement Agreement was entered between the attorneys general of 46 states, five US territories, the District of Columbia, and the four largest US tobacco companies. The premise of the lawsuits was that the tobacco companies had caused the mounting health crisis by profiting from tobacco products. Critically, the effective tobacco industry defense used in private suits of "personal responsibility" was inapplicable to the causes of action alleged by the states, as the plaintiffs sued under consumer protection and antitrust laws, not tort law (i.e., civil claims for harm caused by wrongful conduct, such as negligence). This collective state action led to the tobacco companies agreeing to pay the states at least $206 billion over the first 25 years for medical costs related to smoking, limit certain product marketing practices, and release millions of internal industry documents.

On December 2, 2025, the San Francisco City Attorney filed a lawsuit against the country's largest UPF manufacturers for continuing to market these addictive products despite the evidence of their serious health harms. The time has now come for multistate attorneys general actions against the UPF industry, which will ultimately lead to critical legislative and regulatory reform as in the Master Settlement Agreement. This collective action has the potential to pave the way for the US public to reclaim the health care costs of these products and to prevent damage to Americans.

The US public deserves the same level of protection from UPF corporations as from US tobacco companies. The links between the tobacco and UPF corporations, the empirical evidence on the tactics they have used to delay regulation, and the addictive nature of their products and the harm they cause are irrefutable. We are in the midst of the "New Tobacco War," and litigation could play a defining role in addressing these commercial determinants of health and thus protect all Americans, especially our children, who do not have the ability to protect themselves from these harms. AJPH

DOI: https://doi.org/10.2105/AJPH.2026.308596

ORCID iD:
Nicholas Chartres https://orcid.org/0000-0002-9659-6739

Preventing Ultraprocessed Youths From Becoming Ultraprocessed Adults

Deanna M. Hoelscher, PhD, and Nalini Ranjit, PhD

ABOUT THE AUTHORS

Both authors are with The University of Texas Health Science Center, Houston School of Public Health, Austin, TX.

See also Ultraprocessed Food, pp. 898–1029 and Editorials from the Academics, https://bit.ly/4uSeKDi.

Mechanisms linking the consumption of ultraprocessed food (UPF) to adverse health outcomes are evolving, but sufficient epidemiologic data show that UPF consumption elevates cardiovascular and metabolic risks in adults and children, warranting public health action.[1,2] Efforts to reduce UPF intake have focused primarily on adults, but a more effective strategy might be to direct public health and prevention efforts toward children and adolescents.[3] Because high UPF consumption adversely affects children's health, society should act in loco parentis to protect children from UPF.

There are compelling reasons to focus on children's UPF intake. First, taste preferences and consumption habits developed during childhood persist into adulthood,[4] so establishing dietary behaviors early can provide lifelong benefits. Second, society generally supports regulations that focus on children, given their age and developmental stage, whereas similar policy solutions can be seen as limiting adult liberty or freedom. Third, programs and policies can be implemented in school environments, which reach most of the youth population. Finally, both the nutrition education literature and evidence from child health campaigns (e.g., campaigns to prevent vaping or smoking), provide us with ready toolkits of strategies that can be implemented and disseminated to children.

So, what can be done? Effective public health efforts to reduce UPF intake should include strategies to identify this type of food, restrict the availability of UPF in school food environments, regulate the child media environment, increase the availability of unprocessed food, and implement effective, behaviorally based nutrition education programs.

IDENTIFYING ULTRAPROCESSED FOOD

UPF can be difficult to characterize and label, especially because the Food and Drug Administration has not yet arrived at a single definition. Confusion about the UPF definition leaves consumers unsure of which food is healthy. Although several current definitions exist, the most widely used categorization system for UPF is the Nova classification.[5] Briefly, Nova classifies food into four groups: Nova group 1 includes minimally processed food, and Nova group 4 includes food with extensive processing, including food additives.[5] The *Lancet* series on UPF further defines UPF as "branded, commercial formulations made from cheap ingredients extracted or derived from whole foods, combined with additives, and mostly containing little to no whole food."[1(p2668)] Food manufacturers capitalize on the lack of a clear definition, which can cause further confusion by labels such as "natural" and "organic." Two articles in this *AJPH* issue (i.e., Campos et al. [p. 1025] and Monteiro et al. [p. 932]) have addressed this issue by proposing potential classification systems based on Nova that could be operationalized through regulation and labeling. Well-defined classification systems that can be used for food labels can serve as effective educational tools for children; our research shows that adolescents who read the nutrition facts label report eating healthier diets.[6]

THE SCHOOL FOOD ENVIRONMENT

It can be difficult to restrict food in schools, given financial constraints and the potential sales revenues. For example, a 2007 Institute of Medicine (now National Academies of Sciences, Engineering, and Medicine) report, *Nutrition Standards for Foods Served in Schools* (https://doi.org/10.17226/11899), provided recommendations for the school food environment that served as the evidence base for the US Department of Agriculture's policy Smart Snacks in Schools. The original Institute of Medicine report encouraged fruit, vegetables, whole grains, and nonfat or low-fat milk or dairy products as primary snack choices, and established nutrient standards for secondary snack options. Although these

AJPH July 2026, Vol. 116, No. 7

standards improved the overall nutrient profile of food sold in schools, the result was brand-name products formulated to meet school guidelines. The reformulated food fosters brand loyalty and confusion among students, who may not be able to distinguish between a UPF altered to meet school standards and one sold in stores.

Schools and the US Department of Agriculture are not at fault here—school nutrition services are usually self-sustaining and do not have the funds or additional refrigeration for fresh food. Thus, efforts to restrict UPF in schools should include not only changes to food and nutrient standards but also funding for appropriate kitchen design, refrigerated vending machines, and related equipment. Several states have already begun to change school food policies to restrict UPF. For example, California recently passed a law (AB 1264)[7] in 2025 to remove UPF that contains high levels of fat, sodium, sugar, and food additives associated with adverse health outcomes.

THE MEDIA ENVIRONMENT

UPF is heavily marketed to children in a variety of ways. Advertisements during children's TV shows, school-based advertising, and the use of mascots and character licensing have been used to reach children. In the online era, these strategies have been supercharged by personalized digital advertisements, social media influencers, and advergaming, which are particularly appealing to youths.[8] Regulating the marketing of junk food to children in the current media environment, given the diversity of agents and strategies, is challenging. Currently, there are voluntary regulations to curb advertising aimed at children through the Children's Food and Beverage Advertising Initiative. Despite strengthening the initiative's requirements, voluntary efforts can be difficult to enforce. Incorporating lessons from countries (e.g., the United Kingdom) that have implemented stricter laws on food marketing to children can help guide US efforts.[9] Key takeaways from implementing the UK policy include coordinating public health organizations; relying on a strong, timely research base; countering industry trade groups' delay tactics; and recognizing the benefit of these laws for all children, but especially those in need.[9]

INCREASING THE AVAILABILITY OF WHOLE, UNPROCESSED FOOD

Families need to develop the knowledge and skills to plan, prepare, and serve whole food instead of UPF. The decline in cooking skills over the past decades has led to greater reliance on UPF, which often is ready to eat or requires minimal preparation. The focus on culinary nutrition aims to stem this tide by teaching children and adults to prepare nutritious meals. Classes that blend culinary arts with nutritional sciences increase self-efficacy in food planning and preparation and can be part of home economics or experiential nutrition classes, which are reappearing in schools. School gardens are another effort to encourage children to consume whole, unprocessed food. School gardens introduce students to food production and increase fruit and vegetable consumption, especially when paired with cooking activities.[10]

EFFECTIVE NUTRITION EDUCATION PROGRAMS

Multicomponent school health programs that target nutrition-related behaviors can improve children's dietary intake and reduce obesity.[11] One example is the Coordinated Approach to Child Health (CATCH) program,[12] which uses a social cognitive theory framework to address school and home environments, norms, social support, and increased self-efficacy for selecting healthier options. The CATCH program teaches children to recognize and classify food as go, slow, or whoa: go food is eaten every day and is less processed; slow food is eaten in smaller quantities; and whoa food, which includes UPF, is eaten occasionally. The Go, Slow, Whoa approach uses pictures and concepts that younger children understand better than classification systems based on the degree of processing.

Addressing children's UPF consumption requires a focused, multipronged public health approach. The recent focus on UPF can provide a needed boost to nutrition education efforts, but to be most effective, these programs must be paired with policies that address children's environments, including media. UPF is the latest threat to the health of our children and our future—we need to capitalize on our current window of opportunity so that our ultraprocessed children do not become ultraprocessed adults. AJPH

CORRESPONDENCE

Correspondence should be sent to Deanna M. Hoelscher, The University of Texas Health Science Center at Houston, School of Public Health, 1836 San Jacinto Blvd, Austin, TX 78701 (e-mail: Deanna.M.Hoelscher@uth.tmc.edu). Reprints can be ordered at https://www.ajph.org by clicking the "Reprints" link.

PUBLICATION INFORMATION

Full Citation: Hoelscher DM, Ranjit N. Preventing ultraprocessed youths from becoming ultraprocessed adults. *Am J Public Health*. 2026;116(7): 871–874.

Acceptance Date: April 12, 2026.

DOI: https://doi.org/10.2105/AJPH.2026.308587

ORCID iDs:
Deanna M. Hoelscher https://orcid.org/0000-0002-0910-5031

Nalini Ranjit https://orcid.org/0000-0002-1771-9084

CONTRIBUTORS

D. M. Hoelscher conceptualized and wrote the editorial. N. Ranjit revised it critically for important intellectual content. Both authors approved the final version for publication and agree to be accountable for all aspects of the work.

CONFLICTS OF INTEREST

The authors have no conflicts of interest to report.

REFERENCES

1. Monteiro CA, Louzada ML, Steele-Martinez E, et al. Ultra-processed foods and human health: the main thesis and the evidence. *Lancet*. 2025;406(10520):2667–2684. https://doi.org/10.1016/S0140-6736(25)01565-X
2. United Nations Children's Fund. Ultra-processed foods and children: state-of-the-art review. December 2, 2025. Available at: https://knowledge.unicef.org/child-nutrition-and-development/resource/ultra-processed-foods-and-children-state-art-review#:~:text=The%20review%20finds%20strong%20evidence,obesity%2C%20and%20dental%20caries.%20A. Accessed April 6, 2026.
3. Matji JN, Brero M. Protecting children from ultra-processed foods. *Lancet*. 2025;406(10520):2610–2612. https://doi.org/10.1016/S0140-6736(25)02257-3
4. De Cosmi V, Scaglioni S, Agostoni C. Early taste experiences and later food choices. *Nutrients*. 2017;9(2):107. https://doi.org/10.3390/nu9020107
5. Monteiro CA, Cannon G, Levy RB, et al. Ultra-processed foods: what they are and how to identify them. *Public Health Nutr*. 2019;22(5):936–941. https://doi.org/10.1017/S1368980018003762
6. Pfledderer CD, Ranjit N, Pérez A, et al. Using the nutrition facts label to make food choices is associated with healthier eating among 8th and 11th-grade students: an analysis of statewide representative data from the 2019–2020 Texas School Physical Activity and Nutrition Survey. *Nutrients*. 2024;16(2):311. https://doi.org/10.3390/nu16020311
7. Gabriel J. AB 1264: Pupil nutrition: restricted school foods and ultraprocessed foods of concern: prohibition (2025–2026). Available at: https://calmatters.digitaldemocracy.org/bills/ca_202520260ab1264. Accessed April 12, 2026.
8. Packer J, Croker H, Goddings AL, et al. Advertising and young people's critical reasoning abilities: systematic review and meta-analysis. *Pediatrics*. 2022;150(6):e2022057780. https://doi.org/10.1542/peds.2022-057780
9. Montgomery KC, Chester J. Regulating the digital obesogenic ecosystem: lessons learned from the 20-year effort to pass the United Kingdom's online ban on unhealthy food and beverage advertising. January 19, 2024. Available at: https://democraticmedia.org/reports/regulating-the-digital-obesogenic-ecosystem. Accessed April 6, 2026.
10. Landry MJ, van den Berg AE, Hoelscher DM, et al. Impact of a school-based gardening, cooking, nutrition intervention on diet intake and quality: the TX Sprouts randomized controlled trial. *Nutrients*. 2021;13(9):3081. https://doi.org/10.3390/nu13093081
11. Hoelscher DM, Brann LS, O'Brien S, Handu D, Rozga M. Prevention of pediatric overweight and obesity: position of the Academy of Nutrition and Dietetics based on an umbrella review of systematic reviews. *J Acad Nutr Diet*. 2022;122(2):410–423.e6. https://doi.org/10.1016/j.jand.2021.11.003
12. Hoelscher DM, Springer AE, Ranjit N, et al. Reductions in child obesity among disadvantaged school children with community involvement: the Travis County CATCH Trial. *Obesity (Silver Spring)*. 2010;18(suppl 1):S36–S44. https://doi.org/10.1038/oby.2009.430

In a Rapidly Evolving Public Health Landscape, Governors Are Investing in Durable Health Infrastructure

Angela Botticella, MPA, and Komala Anupindi, MPP

ABOUT THE AUTHORS

Angela Botticella is the managing director of the Governors Public Health Alliance at the time of publication. Komala Anupindi is the operations associate at the Governors Public Health Alliance at the time of publication.

See also Ultraprocessed Food, pp. 898–1029.

AJPH July 2026, Vol. 116, No. 7

In moments of national uncertainty, coordination itself is a public health intervention.

The United States is entering a new public health landscape—with rapidly changing realities at the federal level and state level that require strong leadership and coordinated responses.

Recent federal actions have illustrated this new tumultuous reality. The United States' withdrawal from the World Health Organization has disrupted long-standing global disease surveillance and early warning systems,[1] pushing more responsibility for preparedness and response to states and local health systems.

Similarly, changes to federal vaccine recommendations, advisory committee processes, and regulatory posture have created uncertainty for families, clinicians, and schools about how to proceed.[2] This new reality places the responsibility on governors and state health leaders to provide clarity and preserve public trust at a moment when federal leadership is falling short.

In response to these changing environments and the need for collaboration, governors came together to establish the Governors Public Health Alliance (PHA).

A NEW MODEL FOR STATE-LEVEL PUBLIC HEALTH COORDINATION

Launched[3] in October 2025, PHA is composed of the governors of California, Colorado, Connecticut, Delaware, Guam, Hawaii, Illinois, Maryland, Massachusetts, New Jersey, New York, North Carolina, Oregon, Rhode Island, and Washington, representing approximately one third of the US population. An initiative of GovAct, PHA is a nonpartisan coalition of governors working together to strengthen public health systems and protect communities from emerging health threats.

Although regional collaboratives and other information-sharing structures have emerged, PHA complements these efforts by supporting broader, nationwide coordination among governors. This is new infrastructure for governors to coordinate to protect public health, drawing on scientific evidence and navigating the realities of implementation.

While collaborations among state health officials have long existed, governors identified the need for a national, governor-led structure to coordinate strategy, share information, and act collectively when risks transcend state boundaries. It operates at the directive of participating governors' offices, which determine its governing structure. Each office has designated a lead in their office to interface with their peers in other offices and participate in briefings, information-sharing, and other opportunities.

As PHA has grown in size, capacity, and reach, it has emphasized nonpartisan engagement, creating space for collaboration among states that may be hesitant to work across political lines in the wake of the COVID-19 pandemic. This reticence underscores the need for a trusted structure to facilitate coordination on shared public health priorities.

By focusing on immediate, practical challenges such as outbreak preparedness, vaccine access, and coordinated public communication, PHA is helping to reestablish lines of engagement where traditional channels have frayed. These efforts create opportunities for states to share information, align approaches, and respond more effectively to emerging threats.

WHAT GOVERNORS HAVE DONE TOGETHER SO FAR

Governors launched PHA to meet this moment and have done so with decisive action. In January 2026, after the American Academy of Pediatrics (AAP) stressed the importance of maintaining routine childhood immunization, PHA publicly endorsed[4] and amplified this guidance. Member states aligned with the AAP's recommendations, reinforcing a shared commitment to evidence-based vaccine policy.

Governors supported by PHA are also taking steps to protect access to disease intelligence following the United States' withdrawal from the World Health Organization. PHA is coordinating with Boston University's Center on Emerging Infectious Diseases to leverage the Biothreats Emergence, Analysis and Communications Network (BEACON),[5] a network that tracks outbreaks and shares timely analysis to strengthen preparedness and cross-state response.

Last fall, PHA developed and distributed a Back-to-School Vaccine Toolkit in response to governors' requests for clear, accessible summaries and concrete options as federal guidance for routine immunizations evolved. The toolkit outlined changes in guidance, identified potential risks to access, and offered model actions states could take to preserve vaccine availability for children and families.

In January 2026, PHA released a complementary Vaccine Access Toolkit to support governors' offices in protecting long-term access and stability. Dozens of states have since taken action to safeguard vaccine access.

Building on this coordinated approach, governors also pursued legislative safeguards as federal vaccine policy shifted. In response to recent changes to federal vaccine recommendations and schedules, governors took action to preserve access to evidence-based childhood immunizations. To date, at least 27 states and Washington, DC, have declined to follow some or all of the revised federal vaccine schedule, with 23 states and Washington, DC, fully rejecting the changes and instead adopting guidance from the AAP.[6]

Across states, the common thread is that governors are working in close partnership with pediatricians, hospitals, insurers, and state health departments to ensure that science, not politics, continues to guide childhood vaccination policy and practice. And we hope to expand PHA's membership and work as we continue to build relationships and trust.

PREPARING FOR WHAT COMES NEXT

As 2026 unfolds, governors anticipate continued shifts in the national health landscape. At the same time, states will be responsible for managing a series of high-stakes, large-scale events.

The FIFA World Cup across North America and other major mass gatherings will bring millions of people together across state and national borders, placing heightened demands on disease surveillance, vaccination readiness, and clear public communication.

These pressures come as US engagement with global public health institutions continues to erode. International disease surveillance and early warning systems have long played a role in informing state and local response to emerging threats.[7] Any disruption to those information flows carries consequences that states must be prepared to manage.

States must be able to assess emerging evidence, coordinate with trusted medical societies, align guidance where appropriate, and mobilize resources quickly when risks emerge. PHA is focused on building durable capacity for that work.

FRAMEWORK FOR EVIDENCE-BASED PUBLIC HEALTH LEADERSHIP

Trust is built locally and over time. By creating a structure for cross-state coordination at the gubernatorial level, PHA offers a stabilizing force.

In addition, aligning with independent medical societies like the AAP, collaborating with the Vaccine Integrity Project at the University of Minnesota's Center for Infectious Disease Research and Policy to support transparent evidence reviews and scientific recommendations, and strengthening alternative disease surveillance coordination through initiatives such as BEACON anchors this new policy structure in evidence and expert consensus rather than shifting political winds.

Public health threats do not change based on who occupies the White House, and neither should the systems that protect people from preventable disease. PHA is working to ensure that public health policy remains grounded in evidence, not shifting political winds.

PHA represents one important effort to meet this moment with coordination, evidence, and a shared commitment to the health of the people governors serve. AJPH

CORRESPONDENCE

Correspondence should be sent to Komala Anupindi, 265 Putnam Ave, Cambridge, MA 02139 (e-mail: komala.anupindi@govsforhealth.org). Reprints can be ordered at https://www.ajph.org by clicking the "Reprints" link.

PUBLICATION INFORMATION

Full Citation: Botticella A, Anupindi K. In a rapidly evolving public health landscape, governors are investing in durable health infrastructure. *Am J Public Health*. 2026;116(7):874–876.

Acceptance Date: April 10, 2026.

DOI: https://doi.org/10.2105/AJPH.2026.308585

ORCID iD:

Komala Anupindi https://orcid.org/0009-0005-4674-4958

CONTRIBUTORS

Both authors contributed equally to this work.

ACKNOWLEDGMENTS

We thank our team at the GovAct for this article.

This article is part of a curated collection of editorial perspectives on vaccine accessibility, equity, and public health impact. Check out the rest of the collection here: https://bit.ly/4l98J12

CONFLICTS OF INTEREST

There are no conflicts of interest.

REFERENCES

1. Gostin LO, Koh HH, Williams M, et al. US withdrawal from WHO is unlawful and threatens global and US health and security. *Lancet.* 2020;116(7):293–876. https://doi.org/10.1016/S0140-6736(20)31527-0
2. National Foundation for Infectious Diseases. Experts sound alarm after ACIP members removed. June 10, 2025. Available at: https://www.nfid.org/experts-sound-alarm-after-acip-members-removed. Accessed April 15, 2026.
3. McKay B. Exclusive: Blue states are setting up a shadow public-health alliance to counter RFK Jr. *Wall Street Journal.* October 15, 2025. Available at: https://www.wsj.com/health/healthcare/rfk-jr-hhs-democratic-public-health-alliance-6a6a7e28. Accessed May 27, 2026.
4. Ernst D. AAP maintains routine vaccine recs in 2026 schedule despite CDC changes. *Vaccine Advisor.* January 28, 2026. Available at: https://www.vaccineadvisor.com/news/aap-maintains-routine-vaccine-recs-in-2026-schedule-despite-cdc-changes. Accessed May 27, 2026.
5. Boston University Center on Emerging Infectious Diseases. Biothreats Emergence, Analysis and Communications Network (BEACON). Available at: https://www.bu.edu/ceid/projects-partnerships/beacon. Accessed March 31, 2026.
6. Szabo L. States, health organizations reject new CDC vaccine guidance. Center for Infectious Disease Research and Policy. January 12, 2026. Available at: https://www.cidrap.umn.edu/public-health/states-health-organizations-reject-new-cdc-vaccine-guidance. Accessed May 27, 2026.
7. Cordes KM, Cookson ST, Boyd AT, et al. Real-time surveillance in emergencies using the early warning alert and response network. *Emerg Infect Dis.* 2017;23(13):S131–S137. https://doi.org/10.3201/eid2313.170446

Call to Action: Antihunger and Public Health Communities Must Find Common Ground to Advance a More Just and Nutritious Food System in the United States

Joelle Johnson, MPH, Toby Beckelman, MS, MPH, Angelica Gibson, Joel Berg, and Peter Lurie, MD, MPH

ABOUT THE AUTHORS

Joelle Johnson, Toby Beckelman, and Peter Lurie are with Center for Science in the Public Interest, Washington, DC. Angelica Gibson and Joel Berg are with Hunger Free America, New York, NY.

Most antihunger and public health advocates agree that all people in the United States, regardless of their circumstances, should have access to quality, affordable, convenient, and nutritious food. However, too often, public health and antihunger groups have been at odds, focusing on a few areas of disagreement rather than coalescing around jointly held beliefs and strategies to fix our broken food system. With power and resources highly concentrated in the food industry and large-scale corporate agriculture, public health and antihunger advocates must find common ground to forge a more powerful, better coordinated food justice movement. This united front has never been more necessary as advocates face the Trump administration and a Republican-controlled US Congress, both of which are actively dismantling science-based public health policy and research and have already slashed food assistance by $186 billion over 10 years, a significant toll on the 42 million people who rely on the Supplemental Nutrition Assistance Program (SNAP).[1]

Historically, the antihunger and public health communities have directed their attention to different aspects of the food system. Antihunger advocates tend to emphasize that tens of millions of people in the United States either cannot afford or cannot access nutritious food locally, that levels of government food assistance are limited, and that many working in the food system have low wages. Many public health advocates identify the central problem as a food industry that overwhelms our food environment with heavily processed and marketed cheap food products, often high in salt, sugar, and saturated fat, leading to the growing prevalence of obesity and its consequences. Of course, these two characterizations are not mutually exclusive.

The scale and sweep of the underlying problems in our food system are more significant than any single organization or movement can tackle alone and should be a clarion call for a concerted effort to protect and strengthen policies that promote food and nutrition security. Advocates agree that the three issues described subsequently are especially troubling aspects of the current US food system.

First, according to the US Department of Agriculture (USDA), the number of people in the United States who live in food-insecure households (households unable to afford an adequate and consistent supply of food) increased by 41%—from 34 million to 48 million—between 2021[2] and 2024.[3] The number of children living in food-insecure homes jumped by 56% (from 9 million[2] to 14 million[3]) over a similar period, in part because of the termination of COVID-19 pandemic era benefits. Widespread food insecurity in a land as wealthy and agriculturally abundant as the United States not only is morally appalling but greatly harms the nation's economic productivity,[4] educational performance,[5,6] military readiness,[7] and health.[8]

Second, most people in all income brackets in the United States struggle to achieve a healthy diet, consuming too much salt, sugar, and saturated fat and not enough fruits and vegetables.[9] Diet-related chronic diseases such as diabetes, heart disease, and cancer remain among the top causes of death and disability.[10] Together, dietary risks and high body mass indexes result in the loss of approximately twice as many lives and disability-adjusted life-years as tobacco.[11] Preventing and managing chronic disease can reduce health care costs and improve quality of life.

Finally, food security and health outcomes are greatly influenced by the

AJPH July 2026, Vol. 116, No. 7

social determinants of health, including structural racism and discrimination, unaffordable housing, limited access to quality health care, and insufficient employment opportunities that ensure a living wage.[12] These outcomes are reflected in wide disparities in food insecurity and chronic disease rates across race/ethnicity, income, and geographical regions.[3,13,14] The Trump administration may try to erase evidence of such disparities by banning certain terminology, removing online databases, discontinuing its annual study measuring the household food insecurity of Americans, and defunding any entities that highlight these disparities, but the reality is that they are real and persistent.

Despite shared framing of the problems in the food system, historical flash points have sometimes magnified tensions between antihunger and public health groups. These include an unfortunate trade-off confronted by food advocates in 2010 when federal lawmakers accelerated the end of an increase in SNAP benefits for families with low incomes and used the savings to offset the cost of improving the nutritional quality of school meals for families of all income levels. Similarly, the SNAP Nutrition Security Act of 2023 highlighted divisions on how to approach nutrition in SNAP, with the public health community supporting the establishment of nutrition security metrics (metrics that measure equitable access to health-promoting food) and antihunger advocates mostly opposed to data collection on SNAP purchases, fearing that such efforts would undercut the hunger-fighting mission of SNAP.

More recently, debates around restricting certain types of food purchases with SNAP benefits have driven a wedge between public health and antihunger advocates. Some public health advocates support such restrictions, arguing that SNAP should better align with the Dietary Guidelines for Americans, whereas antihunger advocates are concerned that these restrictions are paternalistic and would lead to increased stigma and thus less SNAP participation.

These polarizing debates often boil down to a single question: should public policy prioritize supporting the ability of people with limited incomes to obtain more food or to obtain healthier food? The reality is that people experiencing food insecurity want and deserve both. In any case, with the sheer existence of the US food safety net at risk in the current political environment, advocates simply cannot afford to be diverted by polarizing side debates.

As we face federal leaders bent on drastically cutting essential food and nutrition programs while dismantling vast swaths of the public health workforce , it is time that we set our differences aside and focus on what we can accomplish by working together to make meaningful progress toward a more just and nutritious food system.

FEDERAL ADVOCACY

Federal advocacy is a vital tool for opposing threats to national programs that support basic needs, whether through budget bills or the Farm Bill. The latter, historically the most significant piece of legislation affecting our food system, is reauthorized by Congress roughly every five years and funds SNAP, the largest food assistance program in the United States. It also has consequential effects on agriculture and food production more broadly, playing a key role in determining the relative prices and availability of healthy and less healthy food. The next Farm Bill will be another flash point in debates over food access and nutrition.

Together, advocates can fight to ensure that there are no further cuts to SNAP and to reverse the cuts that were instituted as part of the budget reconciliation bill passed by the US Senate and House of Representatives and signed by President Trump into law on July 4, 2025. We can also unite in opposing House Republicans' proposed cuts to the fruit and vegetable allotments of the Supplemental Nutrition Assistance Program for Women, Infants, and Children (WIC).

Another federal advocacy opportunity resides in the USDA's approval of state waivers to restrict use of SNAP funds to purchase candy and sugar-sweetened beverages. Purported concerns over the health of beneficiaries, as encapsulated in proposals to ban the purchase of these products, should not be a smokescreen for a benefit reduction or a tool to ensure tax cuts for the wealthy. We can all agree that any waivers should, in theory, be comprehensively evaluated; however, the publicly available evaluation plans for states granted such waivers are thin, and there is little evidence that removing sugar-sweetened beverages from the program would do much to improve diet quality for SNAP participants.[15,16] In addition, when asked about ways to make the program healthier, people with low incomes, and especially SNAP shoppers, have said that increasing the purchasing power of SNAP and increasing healthy food availability in their neighborhoods would do more to enable them to improve their diets than would restrictions on their purchases.[17–19]

Furthermore, restricting SNAP purchases does nothing to address the root causes of food insecurity. The arbitrary nature and lack of rigorous evaluation of the proposed state restrictions undermine policymakers' assertions that they are motivated to improve public health. That is why the Center for Science in the Public Interest and Hunger Free America support federal policies that would require the USDA to develop metrics and reporting for nutrition security and transparently report on SNAP food purchasing data. Advocates can use these data to push for evidence-based policies that would meaningfully improve diet and health.

Advocates should also come together to demand that any approved waivers to test SNAP purchasing restrictions include rigorous evaluations to assess their impact on diet, health, and program access and any unintended consequences. In addition, advocates can work together to urge the USDA to help SNAP retailers stock more nutritious food, remove restrictions on using SNAP benefits to purchase hot prepared foods, simplify the SNAP application process, and eliminate "benefit cliffs" through which people who are given raises or work more hours lose more in benefits than they gain in wages.

STATE AND LOCAL ADVOCACY

Much innovative energy resides at the state and local levels, where states have advanced initiatives such as universal school meals and easing of SNAP eligibility for college students and previously incarcerated individuals. Some states are pursuing strategies to improve food safety by eliminating harmful food dyes from school meals.[20] Antihunger and public health groups can work together to protect the progress made and prevent misguided policies that would further weaken states' abilities to provide for their residents. Outside of the traditional antihunger and public health realms, advocates can come together to support state and local Child Tax Credits that benefit families of varying income levels in an effort to address the root causes of food insecurity and poor health outcomes.

ADDRESSING COMMON TARGETS

In the 2024 election cycle, agribusinesses spent $178 million on federal lobbying[21] and donated $197 million to federal campaigns.[22] Public health and antihunger organizations generally do not donate to political campaigns and have limited lobbying resources. Yet, together, advocates can demand that food corporations provide consumers with more transparency through front-of-pack labeling, make healthier choices for kids in restaurants easier, and promote nutritious items in more prominent places in grocery stores.

CONCERTED COMMITMENTS TO HEALTH AND NUTRITION

In September 2022, for the first time in 50 years, the White House convened experts and stakeholders from across the country to address hunger and poor nutrition. The conference set an ambitious goal of ending hunger and increasing healthy eating and physical activity by 2030. Health systems, insurers, companies, nonprofits, philanthropic groups, academic institutions, and local elected officials made a total of 141 specific commitments to make necessary and lasting improvements to our food and health care systems, ranging from increasing food donations to reducing added sugars in school meals.[23] Although the recommendations outlined in the conference report seem unlikely to be adopted by the Trump administration, the goals and strategies that emerged provide a pathway for positive change and should not be discarded. Advocates can identify and reframe strategies from the report to align with current political feasibility. Antihunger and public health groups can work together to ensure that these commitments are honored, but private sector commitments should not distract from much-needed public policy changes.

CENTERING THE VOICES OF PEOPLE WITH LIVED EXPERIENCE

A number of antihunger organizations have done an excellent job developing ways to empower people who have experienced food insecurity to be top advisors and public spokespeople on these issues. Public health organizations can learn from this approach and bring these individuals to the table to help set policy priorities.

A SHARED RESEARCH AGENDA FOR FOOD AND NUTRITION SECURITY

There is much to learn about how best to ensure the equitable distribution of food and how to maximize its nutritive value. Yet the Trump administration has proposed a huge cut, nearly $18 billion, to the National Institutes of Health, endangering research across the country.[24] Health and Human Services Secretary Robert F. Kennedy Jr.'s focus on chronic disease is encouraging; however, doing so at the expense of infectious disease prevention and research efforts, as the secretary has proposed,[25] is extremely troubling, particularly if paired with cuts to social safety net programs or regulatory agencies. Collaborating on research priorities could ensure that both food and nutrition security perspectives are informing policies and programs. Defining and establishing metrics for nutrition security is an essential first step and would complement existing measurements of food security as well as serve as an important screening tool. In addition, there is a critical opportunity for advocates to push for continued annual data collection and reporting on food security, which provides a critical foundation for understanding the state of hunger in the United States and the effects of federal policy changes to food assistance programs.

Although antihunger and public health resources may be limited relative to the food industry and corporate agriculture, we can unlock unprecedented progress if we align on the key political priorities and opportunities identified here. The current attacks on public health require nothing less. We owe it to the public to set our differences aside and come together to drive change toward a more just and nutritious food system that includes a robust public safety net and increased access to healthy food. AJPH

CORRESPONDENCE

Correspondence should be sent to Peter Lurie, MD, MPH, Center for Science in the Public Interest, 1250 I St NW, Suite 500, Washington, DC 20005 (e-mail: plurie@cspi.org). Reprints can be ordered at https://www.ajph.org by clicking the "Reprints" link.

PUBLICATION INFORMATION

Full Citation: Johnson J, Beckelman T, Gibson A, Berg J, Lurie P. Call to action: Antihunger and public health communities must find common ground to advance a more just and nutritious food system in the United States. *Am J Public Health*. 2026;116(7):877–880.

Acceptance Date: November 29, 2025.

DOI: https://doi.org/10.2105/AJPH.2025.308378

ORCID iDs:
Joelle Johnson https://orcid.org/0000-0002-9431-1568

Toby Beckelman https://orcid.org/0009-0003-2501-6770

Peter Lurie https://orcid.org/0000-0001-7867-4951

CONTRIBUTORS

All of the authors contributed to the conception of the work as well as the drafting and final approval of the article.

ACKNOWLEDGMENTS

This article was funded by the From Now on Fund.

Note. The funder had no involvement in the preparation of the article for publication.

CONFLICTS OF INTEREST

Hunger Free America received $25 000 from the American Beverage Association Foundation in 2023 to create a nutrition education curriculum.

REFERENCES

1. Congressional Budget Office. Estimated budgetary effects of Public Law 119-21. Available at: https://www.cbo.gov/publication/61570. Accessed April 28, 2025.
2. Coleman-Jensen A, Gregory CA, Rabbitt MP, Singh A. Household food security in the United States in 2021. Available at: https://ers.usda.gov/sites/default/files/_laserfiche/publications/104656/ERR-309.pdf?v=51819. Accessed April 28, 2025.
3. Rabbit MP, Reed-Jones M, Hales LJ, Burke MP. Household food security in the United States in 2023. Available at: https://ers.usda.gov/sites/default/files/_laserfiche/publications/113623/ERR-358.pdf?v=63839. Accessed April 28, 2025.
4. Shepard DS, Setren E, Cooper D. Hunger in America: suffering we all pay for. Available at: https://cdn.americanprogress.org/wp-content/uploads/issues/2011/10/pdf/hunger_paper.pdf. Accessed April 28, 2025.
5. Alaimo K, Olson CM, Frongillo EA. Food insufficiency and American school-aged children's cognitive, academic, and psychosocial development. *Pediatrics*. 2001;108(1):44–53.
6. El Zein A, Shelnutt KP, Colby S, et al. Prevalence and correlates of food insecurity among U.S. college students: a multi-institutional study. *BMC Public Health*. 2019;19(1):660. doi:https://doi.org/10.1186/s12889-019-6943-6
7. Leibman A, Protas J. Hungry in the military: food insecurity among military families in the U.S. Available at: https://mazon.org/wp-content/uploads/MAZON-Military-Hunger-Report-April-2021.pdf. Accessed April 28, 2025.
8. Gregory CA, Coleman-Jensen A. Food insecurity, chronic disease, and health among working-age adults. Available at: https://www.ers.usda.gov/publications/pub-details?pubid=84466. Accessed April 28, 2025.
9. Food and Drug Administration. FDA's nutrition initiatives. Available at: https://www.fda.gov/food/nutrition-food-labeling-and-critical-foods/fdas-nutrition-initiatives. Accessed April 28, 2025.
10. National Center for Health Statistics. Leading causes of death. Available at: https://www.cdc.gov/nchs/fastats/leading-causes-of-death.htm. Accessed April 28, 2025.
11. Mokdad AH, Ballestros K, Echko M, et al. The state of US health, 1990–2016: burden of diseases, injuries, and risk factors among US states. *JAMA*. 2018;319(14):1444–1472. doi:https://doi.org/10.1001/jama.2018.0158
12. Drewnowski A. Food insecurity has economic root causes. *Nat Food*. 2022;3(8):555–556. doi:https://doi.org/10.1038/s43016-022-00577-w
13. Gundersen C, Ziliak JP. Food insecurity and health outcomes. *Health Aff (Millwood)*. 2015;34(11):1830–1839. doi:https://doi.org/10.1377/hlthaff.2015.0645
14. Benavidez GA, Zahnd WE, Hung P, Eberth JM. Chronic disease prevalence in the US: sociodemographic and geographic variations by zip code tabulation area. *Prev Chronic Dis*. 2024;21:E14. doi:https://doi.org/10.5888/pcd21.230267
15. Harnack L, Oakes JM, Elbel B, et al. Effects of subsidies and prohibitions on nutrition in a food benefit program: a randomized clinical trial. *JAMA Intern Med*. 2016;176(11):1610–1618. doi: https://doi.org/10.1001/jamainternmed.2016.5633.
16. Harnack LJ, Oakes JM, Elbel B, et al. Effects of inclusion of food purchase restrictions and incentives in a food benefit program on diet quality and food purchasing: results from a randomized trial. *J Acad Nutr Diet*. 2024;124(5):569–582.e3. doi:https://doi.org/10.1016/j.jand.2023.11.024
17. Wolfson JA, Leung CW, Moran A. Meeting the moment: policy changes to strengthen SNAP and improve health. Available at: https://www.milbank.org/quarterly/opinions/meeting-the-moment-policy-changes-to-strengthen-snap-and-improve-health. Accessed April 28, 2025.
18. Hunger Free America. Hunger Free America survey of low-income parents. Available at: https://www.hungerfreeamerica.org/en-us/survey/survey-of-low-income-parents. Accessed April 28, 2025.
19. Moscaritolo K. What Bronx residents with limited incomes say about how and why they choose the food they buy and eat. Available at: https://www.hungerfreeamerica.org/en-us/research/nutrition-survey-memo. Accessed April 28, 2025.
20. Rogers K. Over half of US states are trying to eliminate food dyes. Here's what you can do now. Available at: https://www.cnn.com/2025/03/29/health/food-dye-bans-states-wellness/index.html. Accessed April 28, 2025.
21. OpenSecrets. Agribusiness lobbying profile. Available at: https://www.opensecrets.org/federal-lobbying/sectors/summary?id=A. Accessed April 28, 2025.
22. OpenSecrets. Agribusiness top contributors. Available at: https://www.opensecrets.org/industries/contrib?cycle=2024&ind=A. Accessed April 28, 2025.
23. US Department of Health and Human Services. White House challenge to end hunger and build healthy communities: commitments. Available at: https://odphp.health.gov/sites/default/files/2024-02/White%20House%20Challenge%20Commitments.pdf. Accessed April 28, 2025.
24. US Department of Health and Human Services. Fiscal year 2026 budget in brief. Available at: https://www.hhs.gov/sites/default/files/fy-2026-budget-in-brief.pdf. Accessed August 27, 2025.
25. Heidt A, Ledford H. Vaccine sceptic RFK Jr is now a powerful force in US science: what will he do? Available at: https://www.nature.com/articles/d41586-025-00439-y. Accessed April 28, 2025.

Consumer Risk in the Compounded GLP-1 Boom: Why Compounded GLP-1s Demand Urgent Public Health Action

Aakshi Agarwal, BA, Ank A. Agarwal, BA, and Fatima Cody Stanford, MD, MPH, MPA, MBA

ABOUT THE AUTHORS

Aakshi Agarwal is a second-year law student at Duke University School of Law in Durham, NC. Ank A. Agarwal is a fifth-year MD, PhD, student at Stanford University School of Medicine in Stanford, CA. Fatima Cody Stanford is an associate professor of medicine and pediatrics at Harvard Medical School, and practices and teaches at Massachusetts General Hospital/Harvard Medical School, Boston.

As consumer excitement for glucagon-like peptide 1 (GLP-1) medications for obesity treatment surges, startups have capitalized by selling compounded GLP-1s directly to consumers at attractive discounts. However, compounded drugs are distinct from branded GLP-1s and compromise consumer safety. Rapid proliferation of compounded GLP-1s is a growing public health concern, marked by preventable adverse events, consumer deception, and widening inequities in safe treatment access.

Compounded drugs are not subject to the US Food and Drug Administration's (FDA's) rigorous safety and effectiveness review, and compounding companies often fail to disclose that their products are compounded.[1] As national shortages of semaglutide and tirzepatide have resolved, the continued sale and marketing of compounded GLP-1s by 503A pharmacies demand urgent regulatory attention.

RISE OF COMPOUNDED DRUGS

In 1997, Congress passed the Food and Drug Administration Modernization Act, authorizing 503A pharmacies to create patient-specific versions of medications when FDA-approved drugs cannot meet a patient's medical needs, but not to produce drugs in large quantities.[1] While 503A pharmacies were historically state-regulated, a fungal meningitis outbreak propelled Congress to heighten scrutiny with the Compounding Quality Act.[1]

The Compounding Quality Act also created 503B facilities, which are authorized to produce compounded drugs at scale that are "essentially a copy" of approved drugs on the FDA's drug shortage list, as opposed to the patient-specific focus of 503A pharmacies.[1] When GLP-1s were added to the shortage list in 2022, 503B pharmacies were temporarily permitted to compound them.[2]

The 503B pharmacies are subject to current good manufacturing practice requirements and required to report to the FDA. However, they are exempt from federal requirements for labeling with adequate directions for use, premarket drug approval, and track-and-trace.[1] Compounded drugs are also not FDA-evaluated for safety, efficacy, or quality before marketing, unlike branded products.[1] The 503A pharmacies are additionally regulated by state boards of pharmacies, with varying degrees of oversight.[1]

SAFETY RISKS

By July 2025, the FDA received more than 1100 adverse event reports associated with compounded GLP-1s—a figure the FDA believes is an undercount as 503A pharmacies are not required to report such events.[1,3] The absence of mandatory reporting further undermines public health surveillance.

Many may involve dosing errors, including overdoses five- to 20-fold higher than intended, with outcomes including severe vomiting, acute pancreatitis, and hospitalization.[3,4] Because compounded versions are commonly dispensed in multidose vials with nonstandardized instructions, prescribers and patients can miscalculate dosing.[4]

By contrast, FDA-approved products come in prefilled, single-use pens with preset doses.[3,4] The FDA's Adverse Event Reporting System shows 21 incorrect dose reports for Wegovy and 54 for Mounjaro taken alone in 2025.[5] Pharmaceutical companies are mandated to submit adverse event reports.

Compounding pharmacies also sell GLP-1s with active ingredients differing from those in approved drugs, exposing consumers to unknown risks.[3]

AJPH July 2026, Vol. 116, No. 7

Counterfeit compounded GLP-1s containing contaminants, unknown drugs, or excess active ingredients have entered the supply chain.[3]

MISLEADING PATIENT MARKETING

While the FDA requires "prescription drug promotion" to be "truthful, nonmisleading and accurate," compounded GLP-1s are frequently advertised without disclosure of compounding status and sold without prescriptions.[6,7] When GLP-1s are sold without prescriptions or provider consultation, consumers may not understand the risks, including that GLP-1s require indefinite use and discontinuation leads to weight rebound. Misleading marketing also prevents patients from making informed health decisions and erodes trust in physician-guided prescribing.

THE FUTURE OUTLOOK: COORDINATED PUBLIC HEALTH RESPONSE

The FDA declared tirzepatide (2024) and semaglutide (2025) shortages resolved and announced phased plans to restrict their compounding by 503B facilities.[1,2] The Outsourcing Facilities Association sued the FDA, but the court upheld the FDA's authority to remove GLP-1s from the shortage list.[2]

In response, some companies intend to continue offering GLP-1 drugs at scale by shifting to 503A status and offering "personalized" doses, including by compounding with vitamin B12.[8,9] However, this is legally tenuous, as 503A compounding is only permitted for individual patients with specific medical needs that branded products cannot meet.[1]

Moreover, public health risks will intensify as oral GLP-1s enter the market.[9] Pills are more attractive than injectables, particularly to adolescents, but enable direct-to-consumer and black-market distribution. Consumer confusion may increase as former compounding companies, such as Ro, are distributing branded oral GLP-1s.[10]

In response, federal agencies, clinicians, and Congress must execute a coordinated public health response. Given limited resources and similar regulatory exploitation with medical cannabis, federal enforcement is a critical first step.

The FDA should first prioritize enforcement against companies that continue to market online, using digital monitoring teams to send warning letters and coordinating with the Department of Justice, state attorneys general, and pharmacy boards to expedite referrals and license actions. The FDA can also immediately expand its advertisement oversight to include compounded drugs in collaboration with the Federal Trade Commission. Lastly, the FDA can impose requirements for compounding pharmacies to disclose suppliers and collaborate with federal agencies to intercept ingredient shipments.

Congress should also allocate funding to sustain these activities and tighten loopholes in the Compounding Quality Act that enable large-scale production under the guise of personalized medicine. While federal legislation will take time, states can immediately strengthen oversight of 503A pharmacies through regular inspections and reporting requirements.

However, given current constraints on enforcement and legislation, a broader coalition is essential. Providers, public health officials, professional associations, consumer advocacy groups, and media should publicize verified cases of harm and composite adverse event data from compounded GLP-1s. Pharmaceutical companies can complement by pursuing litigation against compounders. Overall, public attention can generate grassroots pressure for legislative and regulatory response.

Providers should also proactively educate patients about the risks associated with compounding, inquire about patients' sources of medication, and verify the legitimacy of those sources. Clinicians should also report adverse events to the FDA. Professional societies can reinforce these duties by issuing guidelines for prescribing and counseling.

Lastly, to minimize dosing and instruction-related errors when a patient may legitimately need a compounded GLP-1, professional pharmacy associations should develop standardized labeling, concentration ranges, and device reference standards.

ACCESS AND AFFORDABILITY CONCERNS

However, stricter enforcement could limit access. Compounded GLP-1s have provided affordable access to patients who are unable to obtain brand-name GLP-1s because of costs, copays, or formulary restrictions. The White House is collaborating with pharmaceutical manufacturers to lower prices for GLP-1s for Medicare and Medicaid beneficiaries, government purchasers, and direct-to-consumer buyers.[11] The announced $350-per-month direct-to-consumer price—expected to decrease to $245 for Medicare and Medicaid beneficiaries—may lower financial barriers, but is unlikely to eliminate economic incentives that encourage patients to opt for compounded GLP-1s. Pharmaceutical companies have also introduced lower-cost options to compete with compounders.[12] This may unintentionally exacerbate price competition, prompting a "race to the bottom" in which compounding pharmacies cut production costs, thereby heightening risks of contamination or counterfeit ingredients. Low-income populations would also be more disposed to using these cheaper, unsafe products.

As enforcement tightens, patients using GLP-1s for off-label treatment of obesity may face renewed access barriers or turn to unregulated sellers, worsening the safety issues enforcement aims to solve. To mitigate inequities, regulators and manufacturers should expand patient-assistance programs and accelerate development of lower-cost biosimilar options.

CONCLUSION

The rise of compounded GLP-1s has exposed gaps in patient safety, consumer protection, and public health oversight. Ongoing compounding of GLP-1s erodes trust in pharmaceutical standards and public health. Swift, coordinated action from the FDA, Congress, and clinicians is essential to ensure access to safe, approved treatments. AJPH

CORRESPONDENCE

Correspondence should be sent to Fatima C. Stanford, MD, MPH, MPA, MBA, Massachusetts General Hospital Weight Center, 50 Staniford St, 4th Floor, Boston, MA 02114 (e-mail: fstanford@mgh.harvard.edu). Reprints can be ordered at https://www.ajph.org by clicking the "Reprints" link.

PUBLICATION INFORMATION

Full Citation: Agarwal A, Agarwal AA, Stanford FC. Consumer risk in the compounded GLP-1 boom: why compounded GLP-1s demand urgent public health action. *Am J Public Health*. 2026;116(7): 881–883.

Acceptance Date: February 17, 2026.

DOI: https://doi.org/10.2105/AJPH.2026.308514

ORCID iDs:

Aakshi Agarwal https://orcid.org/0009-0008-9022-9787

Ank A. Agarwal https://orcid.org/0000-0002-8307-4931

Fatima Cody Stanford https://orcid.org/0000-0003-4616-533X

CONTRIBUTORS

A. Agarwal originated the idea for the article, conducted the initial research, and drafted the first full version of the article. A. A. Agarwal and A. Agarwal jointly expanded, revised, and substantively edited the article, including additional literature review, regulatory analysis, and policy development. F. C. Stanford provided senior supervision, critical revisions, and overall guidance on framing, interpretation, and argumentation. All authors reviewed and approved the final article and agree to be accountable for all aspects of the work.

ACKNOWLEDGMENTS

Funding was received from National Institutes of Health grants NIDDK P30 DK040561, U24 DK132733, and UE5 DK137285 (FCS).

CONFLICTS OF INTEREST

The authors report no conflicts of interest.

REFERENCES

1. Sheikh HZ. Drug Compounding: FDA Authority and Possible Issues for Congress. Congressional Research Service. 2018. Available at: https://www.congress.gov/crs-product/R45069. Accessed October 17, 2025.
2. US Food and Drug Administration. FDA clarifies policies for compounders as national GLP-1 supply begins to stabilize. September 19, 2025. Available at: https://www.fda.gov/drugs/drug-safety-and-availability/fda-clarifies-policies-compounders-national-glp-1-supply-begins-stabilize. Accessed October 17, 2025.
3. US Food and Drug Administration. FDA's concerns with unapproved GLP-1 drugs used for weight loss. September 25, 2025. Available at: https://www.fda.gov/drugs/postmarket-drug-safety-information-patients-and-providers/fdas-concerns-unapproved-glp-1-drugs-used-weight-loss. Accessed October 17, 2025.
4. US Food and Drug Administration. FDA alerts health care providers, compounders and patients of dosing errors associated with compounded injectable semaglutide products. July 26, 2024. Available at: https://www.fda.gov/drugs/human-drug-compounding/fda-alerts-health-care-providers-compounders-and-patients-dosing-errors-associated-compounded. Accessed October 17, 2025.
5. US Food and Drug Administration. FDA Adverse Event Reporting System (FAERS) Public Dashboard. December 7, 2023. Available at: https://www.fda.gov/drugs/fdas-adverse-event-reporting-system-faers/fda-adverse-event-reporting-system-faers-public-dashboard. Accessed February 10, 2026.
6. Winkler R, O'Brien SA. How dozens of websites sell knock-off drugs, no prescription required. *Wall Stret Journal*. August 16, 2023. Available at: https://www.wsj.com/health/healthcare/ozempic-mounjaro-no-prescription-websites-726b3928. Accessed October 17, 2025.
7. US Food and Drug Administration. Compounding and the FDA: questions and answers. September 16, 2025. Available at: https://www.fda.gov/drugs/human-drug-compounding/compounding-and-fda-questions-and-answers. Accessed October 17, 2025.
8. Advisory Board. Companies find ways around end of GLP-1 shortage. Daily Briefing. Available at: https://www.advisory.com/daily-briefing/2025/05/27/glp-1-compounders. Accessed October 17, 2025.
9. Loftus P. Novo Nordisk escalates fight against Hims & Hers. *Wall Street Journal*. February 9, 2026. Available at: https://www.wsj.com/health/pharma/novo-nordisk-escalates-fight-against-hims-hers-69c15e2b. Accessed February 9, 2026.
10. Ro. Guide to oral GLP-1 medications for weight loss and diabetes. Available at: https://ro.co/weight-loss/oral-glp-1. Accessed February 9, 2026.
11. Academy of Managed Care Pharmacy. Federal update: Trump administration announces deal to bring most-favored-nation pricing to GLP-1s. November 12, 2025. Available at: https://www.amcp.org/letters-statements-analysis/federal-update-trump-administration-announces-deal-bring-most-favored-nation-pricing-glp-1s. Accessed November 26, 2025.
12. NovoCare. Get your GLP-1 medications delivered with NovoCare® pharmacy. Available at: https://www.novocare.com/pharmacy.html. Accessed February 12, 2026.

Slow Suicide: Listening to Community, Broadening Our Paradigms

Sara R. Solomon, DrPH, and Tyrique W. Glasgow

ABOUT THE AUTHORS

Sara R. Solomon is with the Penn Injury Science Center, University of Pennsylvania, Philadelphia. Tyrique W. Glasgow is with the Young Chances Foundation, Philadelphia, PA.

"We laugh at it because we have to be strong. Dying is not an option," said one focus group participant when asked about suicide. In many Black communities, open talk of suicide is shrouded by cultural silence and stoicism.[1] In some Black communities, people describe something else—a "slow suicide," a gradual self-destruction born of living under relentless hardship.

This concept, emerging from community voices, urges public health to expand its definition of suicide beyond singular, isolated acts. It also demands recognition of the structural violence and historical trauma that make mere survival a daily act of resilience. This call to broaden our lens comes at a crucial time: the suicide rate among Black adolescents has surged 144% in recent years, as systemic inequities continue to block access to mental health care.[2] To save lives, we must reckon with how survival itself can become a slow dying under conditions of injustice—and reimagine prevention accordingly.

RETHINKING "SUICIDE" THROUGH A COMMUNITY-GROUNDED LENS

The Centers for Disease Control and Prevention defines suicide as "death caused by self-directed injurious behavior with an intent to die as a result of the behavior."[2] This definition is rooted in Eurocentric and biomedical paradigms of individual pathology, shaped by centuries of moral, religious, and legal frameworks that positioned suicide as a sin, a crime, or a mental disorder.[3,4] In Western thought, suicide has often been viewed as a personal failing rather than a societal outcome—an outlook that continues to inform the language, measures, and models used in contemporary public health.

In many Black communities, the language of suicide is heavily stigmatized, and overt expressions of suicidal ideation are rare.[1] Cultural and religious beliefs often frame suicide as morally or spiritually taboo, whereas narratives of resilience reinforce expectations to "push through" or "keep going" despite pain. This framing frequently obscures the broader social and structural conditions—systemic racism, poverty, trauma—that shape suffering and drive self-destructive behaviors. Moreover, it fails to account for the ways suicide is expressed, interpreted, and communicated in nondominant cultural contexts.

COMMUNITY PERSPECTIVES ON SLOW SUICIDE

In our work with Black communities in southwest Philadelphia, Pennsylvania, the word "suicide" evoked visceral reactions. "When I hear the word suicide, I just think of sadness," one person shared. Some described it as an escape: "You just want to get out from feeling all this pain." Others framed it as extreme: "You took a permanent answer for a nonpermanent situation."

The concept of "slow suicide," however, deeply resonated. Participants defined it as a pattern of self-destructive behavior—like smoking, substance use, gambling, or neglecting one's health—that gradually wears down the body or spirit. The key distinction, they noted, was intent. "The plan is not to go," one participant clarified. "We're just chilling. . . . We're not intentionally making it happen." Another added: "I don't want to die now, but I'm doing this knowing I might not make it past sixty." These insights challenge dominant definitions of suicide by naming harm as both a symptom of suffering and a survival strategy within unjust environments.

Although these narratives may not be flagged as suicidal ideation by clinical systems, they reflect a profound erosion of hope, connection, and will to live. Substance use, emotional numbing, risky behavior, and social withdrawal can function as vehicles of slow suicide. Yet these often go unrecognized by formal systems, leaving individuals unsupported until their distress escalates to crisis, or ends in death not classified as suicide.

Community residents stressed that slow suicide cannot be separated from trauma or the lack of safe outlets for emotional expression. "Some people don't have outlets," one said. "You're forced to keep it all in." Unaddressed pain, they emphasized, manifests physically and psychologically: "That's where the cancers come from, the depression. That didn't just happen." They highlighted body language and mood

AJPH July 2026, Vol. 116, No. 7

changes as signs of inner turmoil, and described reassurance and connection as essential lifelines: "If somebody knows I'm here at three in the morning, that might make them strong enough to reach out." Practical solutions emerged—counseling in schools, faith-based gatherings, mentoring, and simply "being around people you love." But these were tempered by structural barriers: "Where can you access a therapist in your neighborhood right now?" The silence that followed said everything.

RESEARCH AND INTERVENTION FRAMEWORKS

Public health definitions shape surveillance, funding priorities, and the design of interventions. When suicide is defined only as an acute act rooted in individual intent, we miss the chronic, cumulative, community-recognized pathways to premature death. Naming slow suicide is not about pathologizing hardship—it is about making visible what communities have long named, rendering it measurable, and designing interventions that prevent the outcomes they live with every day.

To develop effective and equitable prevention strategies, we propose the term "slow suicide" to describe the chronic self-harming behaviors that emerge in contexts of sustained violence, racism, and historical trauma. This concept builds on Lauren Berlant's "slow death"—the attritional toll of structural marginalization—and extends it to show how some people withdraw from life not with one action, but through patterns of disinvestment in their own health, safety, and future.[5] Unlike "deaths of despair," which emphasize economic dislocation among White working-class populations,[6] slow suicide emerges from Black communities' descriptions of how structural racism and chronic hardship gradually wear down life.

Slow suicide, as illustrated in Figure 1, sits at the intersection of structural conditions, individual coping behaviors, and community counterforces. Structural stressors—such as racism, poverty, and violence—create chronic distress. In response, individuals may engage in coping behaviors (withdrawal, substance use, neglect of health) that ease pain but degrade well-being over time. Counterforces—community, care, faith, connection—can shift the trajectory from slow suicide toward survival and collective resilience. The continuum at the model's base reflects how survival is not a fixed state but a dynamic negotiation within social and structural constraints.

EXPANDING SUICIDE PREVENTION TO SUSTAIN LIFE

Public health must listen to the language and logic of community—not just clinical definitions. Expanding the suicide prevention paradigm means recognizing the slow, everyday processes through which despair accumulates and hope erodes in marginalized communities. This community-named phenomenon resonates with patterns observed in other oppressed groups worldwide—such as the Guarani-Kaiowá in Brazil—where suicide has also been interpreted as an outcome of structural violence rather than individual pathology.[7]

If we truly hear the voices of those living under structural violence, then prevention must move upstream—to housing, safety, school supports, economic dignity, and spaces of belonging. It must also move laterally—to faith communities, peer mentors, barbershops, and block captains—as trusted sources of healing and intervention.

Naming slow suicide affirms what Black communities already know: not all suicides are sudden, and not all suffering speaks in clinical terms. To prevent these deaths, we must treat lived experience as expertise. We must fund what fosters life. And we must build a suicide prevention field that doesn't just react to crisis, but sustains the

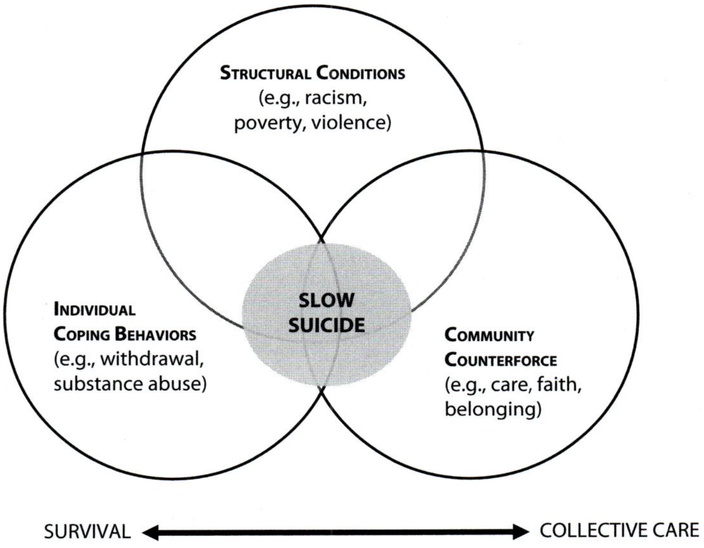

FIGURE 1— Conceptional Framework of Slow Suicide

AJPH July 2026, Vol. 116, No. 7

everyday conditions where life, connection, and joy can take root. AJPH

CORRESPONDENCE

Correspondence should be sent to Sara R. Solomon, 3600 Civic Center Blvd, Floor 6, Room 300, Philadelphia, PA 19104 (e-mail: sarasol@upenn.edu). Reprints can be ordered at https://www.ajph.org by clicking the "Reprints" link.

PUBLICATION INFORMATION

Full Citation: Solomon SR, Glasgow TW. Slow suicide: listening to community, broadening our paradigms. *Am J Public Health*. 2026;116(7): 884–886.

Acceptance Date: December 15, 2025.

DOI: https://doi.org/10.2105/AJPH.2026.308434

ORCID iD:

Sara R. Solomon https://orcid.org/0000-0001-6905-4988

CONTRIBUTORS

Both S. R. Solomon and T. W. Glasgow are accountable for all aspects of this work and made substantial contributions. S. R. Solomon drafted the work with input and final approval from T. W. Glasgow. T. W. Glasgow conceptualized the term Slow Suicide.

ACKNOWLEDGMENTS

We acknowledge the residents of South Philadelphia for their substantial contributions during the focus groups, and the Young Chances Foundation for hosting the sessions, serving as a vital part of the community, and helping to shape the content of this article. We also thank Max Mohink for his assistance in supporting the content development, including proofreading and locating relevant literature.

CONFLICTS OF INTEREST

There are no conflicts of interest to report.

HUMAN PARTICIPANT PROTECTION

This study was approved by the Young Chances Foundation community research review board. Approval from the University of Pennsylvania institutional review board is in progress for future related work.

REFERENCES

1. Rivera KJ, Zhang JY, Mohr DC, Wescott AB, Pederson AB. A narrative review of mental illness stigma reduction interventions among African Americans in the United States. *J Ment Health Clin Psychol*. 2021;5(2):20–31. https://doi.org/10.29245/2578-2959/2021/2.1235
2. Centers for Disease Control and Prevention. Facts about suicide. March 26, 2025. Available at: https://www.cdc.gov/suicide/facts/index.html. Accessed November 9, 2025.
3. Alvarez A. *The Savage God: A Study of Suicide*. London, UK: Weidenfeld and Nicolson; 1972.
4. Mishara BL, Weisstub DN. Ethical and legal issues in suicide research. *Int J Law Psychiatry*. 2005;28(1): 23–41. https://doi.org/10.1016/j.ijlp.2004.12.006
5. Berlant L. *Cruel Optimism*. Durham, NC: Duke University Press; 2011.
6. Case A, Deaton A. Rising morbidity and mortality in midlife among White non-Hispanic Americans in the 21st century. *Proc Natl Acad Sci U S A*. 2015; 112(49):15078–15083. https://doi.org/10.1073/pnas.1518393112
7. De Souza MLP, Orellana JDY. Suicide mortality in São Gabriel da Cachoeira, a predominantly indigenous Brazilian municipality. *Braz J Psychiatry*. 2012;34(1):34–37. https://doi.org/10.1590/S1516-44462012000100007

Approaches to Approximating National Public Health Data

Ben R. Spoer, PhD, MPH, Lorna E. Thorpe, PhD, and Marc N. Gourevitch, MD, MPH

ABOUT THE AUTHORS

The authors are with the Department of Population Health, New York University Grossman School of Medicine, New York, NY.

As federal sources of public health data come under threat because of reductions in funding and staff, public health professionals are considering strategies to partially compensate for the loss of these long-relied-on resources.[1] We are exploring some of these strategies as leaders of a nationwide public health data dashboard initiative. Although intriguing approaches are emerging, major challenges remain regarding data availability, standardization, and validation. Erosions of access to federal data sets or data set quality will be difficult to compensate for.

We currently depend on federal data sources for the public dashboards we produce, which cover more than 1200 US cities and all 435 congressional districts (Box 1).[2,3] Nearly three quarters of the measures displayed on these free and widely used Web sites—the City Health Dashboard and the Congressional District Health Dashboard—are drawn from the US Census Bureau's American Community Survey (ACS); the National Vital Statistics System, which is part of the Centers for Disease Control and Prevention (CDC); and PLACES, the CDC's Behavioral Risk Factor Surveillance System (BRFSS)–based initiative.

The ACS is an ongoing survey conducted by the Census Bureau that provides geographically and demographically granular data for the entire country. ACS measures offer an essential context for locally specific health data, and the survey's demographic data provide denominator values for many public health metrics. The National Vital Statistics System collates birth and death records provided by states to the CDC and uses those records to produce national mortality and natality statistics. At the CDC, the BRFSS aggregates state-collected data on numerous public health domains and PLACES generates geographically granular estimates with national coverage.[4]

The future of these data sources, and many others, is uncertain after reductions in federal funding and staff. Here we describe our early-stage efforts to obtain related data if federal data sets are not maintained or updated or are otherwise compromised.

AGGREGATING AND HARMONIZING STATE DATA SETS

One potential approach is to identify data sets produced, maintained, and released by states and then undertake the aggregation, analysis, and validation functions that have been the province of federal agencies.

Unless independent agreements were signed with each state, this approach would be limited to jurisdictions that release data publicly. Some, but not all, states make their vital record data and BRFSS survey results publicly available, and there is substantial variation in the type and format of data released by these states. Considerable resources would be required to aggregate and harmonize data across heterogeneous sources. Also, many federal data resources, including public-facing National Vital Statistics System mortality and natality data sets, are developed with granular data not released to the public because of confidentiality or other concerns. Generating the national data sets we are familiar with may not be possible if only data that states approve for public release are used, and privacy standards should not be compromised to release more granular data. We are currently creating an inventory of publicly available state-released databases and will attempt to harmonize them in collaboration with other data-oriented organizations. Regional alliances among states, cities, and other entities are pursuing related approaches.[5]

DOWNSCALING COUNTY- OR STATE-LEVEL DATA

Numerous federal agencies have developed methods to model geographically granular metric estimates from larger geographies using demographic and other data from smaller geographies (e.g., the PLACES initiative). Nonfederal researchers could develop and apply such methods to nationally harmonized county- and state-level data sets to generate similar estimates. The federal

AJPH July 2026, Vol. 116, No. 7

BOX 1— Characteristics of Three Federal Data Sources Relevant to Public Health Data Dashboards: United States

Data Source	Data Collection Source	Data Analysis Source	Collection Method	Use in Public Health Data Dashboards
US Census Bureau American Community Survey	US Census Bureau	US Census Bureau	Mailed survey	Supplies population data that form the denominator for many metric calculations and that can be used to calculate metrics
CDC National Vital Statistics System	State and local medical examiners	CDC National Center for Health Statistics	Birth and death records voluntarily reported by states to the CDC	Calculating natality- and mortality-related metrics
CDC PLACES project	State departments of health	CDC Division of Population Health[a]	Phone survey	Providing geographically granular estimates of numerous health behavior and outcome metrics

Note. CDC = Centers for Disease Control and Prevention.
[a]Name before the winter 2025 CDC reduction in force.

data landscape includes many interdependencies, however, that could challenge this approach. The PLACES downscaling method, for example, is dependent on access to county-level BRFSS data as well as geographically granular demographic ACS data. If ACS data were to become unreliable or unavailable, downscaling analyses would become more difficult.

In addition, if results from other national health surveys (e.g., the National Health Interview Survey) become unreliable or unavailable, validation of downscaled estimates will be more challenging owing to the loss of "gold standard" comparators, and benchmarking and adjustment of other data sets will become more difficult as well. This is especially important given that the accuracy and precision of imputed estimates vary by location and direct estimation of these measures may not be feasible. We are reviewing downscaling methods for potential adoption.

ARTIFICIAL INTELLIGENCE–GENERATED IMPUTATION

Artificial intelligence (AI) models can address various thorny data challenges, including prediction and imputation of missing data. Neural network-based foundation models trained on vast amounts of data might fill in for missing federal data set updates as well as impute absent data if federal data collection is incomplete.[6] AI-based modeling approaches may require less person power to maintain than aggregating state data or downscaling. However, as with downscaling approaches, external data required to validate AI models can prove difficult to identify, a challenge that will intensify if federal data sets become less reliable. We are working with partner organizations to better understand AI's potential to impute population health data.

ELECTRONIC HEALTH RECORD–BASED APPROACHES

Networks of electronic health records (EHRs) can be used to estimate the burden and incidence of important health measures. Nearly 90% of health systems in the United States use EHRs, yet networks vary significantly in terms of patients represented and how data are collected. Large, multisystem EHR networks increasingly offer large samples, timely data capture, and a wealth of standardized clinical, diagnostic, and prescribed medication data, including longitudinal clinical information.

However, data collected by EHR networks are convenience samples with inherent biases, requiring rigorous bias adjustment and validation. Patients in EHRs are more likely to be older, female, and of higher socioeconomic status and to have higher rates of chronic diseases than the general population.[7] Iterative development of condition definitions (known as rule-based phenotyping) and statistical adjustment approaches are needed to develop EHR-based prevalence estimates. Moreover, not all conditions are well measured in EHRs, and bias adjustment methods are more likely to be effective when EHR networks have achieved a certain level of penetration within a community. We are currently investigating biases in EHR data and developing bias-adjustment methods.

CONCLUSION

Each of the four approaches described here holds promise, although they would at best only partially compensate for diminishment of federal data sets. Nonetheless, the substantial development and validation work required to determine their utility should be undertaken with rigor and speed. Aggregating, harmonizing, and downscaling population-representative data sets hold promise, especially if reliable smaller-geography information is available. AI approaches offer the prospect of estimating social and demographic data, but their value in estimating health trends remains uncertain. EHR data are well suited for estimating the prevalence of select health conditions, particularly if they are well measured in EHRs and appropriate bias adjustment is undertaken. In the case of all of these approaches, validation, often relying at least in part on ACS data, will remain a central challenge.

Others have commented on the bedrock importance of resilient public health data infrastructure, whether in identifying outbreaks or in measuring progress in reducing the burden of chronic disease. The American people have a right to the public health data collected from them, and continued modernization of public health data infrastructure must be embraced as part and parcel of the current administration's focus on combating chronic disease.[8] We emphasize that alternative approaches to developing public health data sets are not likely to yield quick or easy replacements of the federal data sources on which public health professionals rely. We must play both sides of this challenge: advocating fiercely for the preservation and constant strengthening of federal public health data systems while undertaking an intensive effort to explore alternative approaches to replacing them if they are diminished. AJPH

CORRESPONDENCE

Correspondence should be sent to Ben R. Spoer, PhD, MPH, 180 Madison Ave, 5-11, New York, NY 10016 (e-mail: benjamin.spoer2@nyulangone.org). Reprints can be ordered at https://www.ajph.org by clicking the "Reprints" link.

PUBLICATION INFORMATION

Full Citation: Spoer BR, Thorpe LE, Gourevitch MN. Approaches to approximating national public health data. *Am J Public Health*. 2026;116(7):887–889.

Acceptance Date: January 2, 2026.

DOI: https://doi.org/10.2105/AJPH.2026.308442

ORCID iDs:

Ben R. Spoer https://orcid.org/0000-0002-0311-7963

Lorna E. Thorpe https://orcid.org/0000-0002-5535-2674

Marc N. Gourevitch https://orcid.org/0000-0001-6865-2126

CONTRIBUTORS

The authors contributed equally to the article.

ACKNOWLEDGMENTS

This editorial was funded by the Robert Wood Johnson Foundation, grant numbers 81459 and 82755.

Note. The views expressed here do not necessarily reflect the views of the Robert Wood Johnson Foundation.

CONFLICTS OF INTEREST

The authors have no conflicts to declare.

REFERENCES

1. Freilich J, Price WN, Kesselheim AS. Disappearing data at the US federal government. *N Engl J Med.* 2025;392(24):e55.
2. NYU Langone Health. City Health Dashboard. Available at: https://www.cityhealthdashboard.com. Accessed October 3, 2025.
3. NYU Langone Health. Congressional District Health Dashboard. Available at: https://www.congressionaldistricthealthdashboard.org. Accessed October 3, 2025.
4. Centers for Disease Control and Prevention. PLACES: Local Data for Better Health. Available at: https://www.cdc.gov/places/index.html. Accessed February 20, 2026.
5. Goldstein J. New York and other states form health bloc as answer to Trump's policies. Available at: https://www.nytimes.com/2025/09/18/nyregion/northeast-public-health-collaborative-trump.html. Accessed October 3, 2025.
6. Agarwal M, Sun M, Kamath C, et al. General geospatial inference with a population dynamics foundation model. Available at: https://arxiv.org/pdf/2411.07207. Accessed October 3, 2025.
7. Romo ML, Chan PY, Lurie-Moroni E, et al. Characterizing adults receiving primary medical care in New York City: implications for using electronic health records for chronic disease surveillance. *Prev Chronic Dis.* 2016;13:E56.
8. Zhang AD, Turbow SD, Weerahandi HM, Anderson TS. Enhancing health survey infrastructure for chronic disease. *JAMA.* 2025;333(23):2049–2050.

On Adoption Interest Among Transgender Individuals: Conceptual Ambiguity, Methodological Weakness, and Interpretive Overreach

Callie H. Burt, PhD

ABOUT THE AUTHOR

Callie H. Burt is a professor in the Department of Criminal Justice and Criminology and faculty affiliate of the Center for Research on Interpersonal Violence (CRIV) at Georgia State University, Atlanta.

AJPH July 2026, Vol. 116, No. 7

In their recent article, Ogunbajo et al.[1] report associations between "gender affirmation" and interest in adoption among transgender adults in Washington State, from which they draw a series of health care and policy implications. Unfortunately, the analytic strategy and interpretations exceed what the data can support.

The multinomial regression results are largely uninterpretable because of sparse joint distributions across multiple predictors and outcome categories. Two related features drive this. First, extreme cell sparsity is induced by cross-classifying multiple highly imbalanced categorical predictors (e.g., residential geography, employment, education, gender identity) with a three-category outcome, yielding many cells with very small counts and some plausibly empty. Second, the "interested in adoption" category is overwhelmingly dominated by a narrow subgroup. For example, approximately 97% of respondents in this category are transgender women; 97% report receiving hormones (if wanted); 98% report gender-affirming surgery (if wanted); and 99% are employed. Together, these features leave too few informative comparisons to support meaningful regression estimates.

A second concern is how gender-affirming care is operationalized, which creates construct validity and selection problems. Medical and legal affirmation variables are restricted to respondents whose "gender goals" included the relevant interventions, conditioning on a selected subgroup and redefining the estimand. These variables also plausibly proxy socioeconomic advantage. The operationalization therefore conflates affirmation with access (e.g., insurance, income, time, legal assistance), leaving the proposed mechanism empirically ambiguous.

A third concern is interpretive overreach. The outcome is a single attitudinal item ("Are you interested in adopting a child?"), *not* readiness, feasibility, eligibility, or engagement in adoption processes. Yet the conclusion states "important public health implications," including that the findings "underscore the need for coordinated efforts across health care, legal, and social service sectors to create more inclusive and supportive pathways to family formation." Adoption interest alone cannot establish unmet need, systemic exclusion, or readiness for family formation, and cannot justify interventions absent evidence on barriers encountered or transitions from interest to action.

Finally, additional modeling choices further undermine interpretability. The measure labeled "internalized transphobia" is a single item ("glad to be trans"), which does not capture the construct. Simultaneously including both overall family support and the proportion of supportive family members also conditions on overlapping information in a conceptually incoherent way (e.g., the effect of proportion of supportive family members net of level of family support).

In short, the analysis does not support the public health implications advanced. AJPH

CORRESPONDENCE

Correspondence should be sent to Callie Burt, 55 Park Place, STE 535, Atlanta, GA 30303 (e-mail: cburt@gsu.edu). Reprints can be ordered at https://www.ajph.org by clicking the "Reprints" link.

PUBLICATION INFORMATION

Full Citation: Burt CH. On adoption interest among transgender individuals: conceptual ambiguity, methodological weakness, and interpretive overreach. *Am J Public Health*. 2026; 116(7):890.

Acceptance Date: February 12, 2026.

DOI: https://doi.org/10.2105/AJPH.2026.308496

ORCID iD:
Callie H. Burt https://orcid.org/0000-0001-7191-9602

CONFLICTS OF INTEREST

The author has no conflicts of interest to declare.

REFERENCE

1. Ogunbajo A, DeAtley T, Breslow A, et al. Association between gender affirmation and adoption interest among a large sample of transgender, nonbinary, and gender-diverse populations in Washington State, 2023. *Am J Public Health*. 2026;116(2):229–239. https://doi.org/10.2105/AJPH.2025.308312

Ogunbajo et al. Respond

Adedotun Ogunbajo, PhD, MPH, Terea DeAtley, PhD, MPH, Aaron Breslow, PhD, Kristi Gamarel, PhD, Don Operario, PhD, Trace Kershaw, PhD, and Arjee Restar, PhD, MPH

ABOUT THE AUTHORS

Adedotun Ogunbajo is with the RAND Corporation, Arlington, VA. Terea DeAtley is with the Department of Family and Preventive Medicine, University of Utah School of Medicine, Salt Lake City. Aaron Breslow is with the Department of Psychiatry and Behavioral Sciences, Albert Einstein College of Medicine, Bronx, NY. Kristi Gamarel is with the University of Michigan School of Public Health, Ann Arbor. Don Operario is with the Department of Behavioral, Social, and Health Education Sciences, Emory University Rollins School of Public Health, Atlanta, GA. Trace Kershaw and Arjee Restar are with the Department of Social and Behavioral Sciences, Yale University School of Public Health, New Haven, CT.

We appreciate the opportunity to respond to Burt's commentary on our article examining gender affirmation and adoption interest among transgender populations.[1] Although constructive scholarly critique advances science, it must be grounded in methodological accuracy. Unfortunately, the commentator substantially mischaracterizes our analytic approach, reflecting either a fundamental misunderstanding of multinomial logistic regression or selective reading that prioritizes a predetermined narrative over methodological precision. This can contribute to the misinterpretation of transgender health research at a time when precise and accurate scientific communication, particularly in areas with legal and judicial implications, is paramount.[2,3] We welcome the opportunity to clarify these points and advance dialogue on this understudied topic. Our intent in this response is to clarify the analytic approach and interpretation of the data, rather than to comment on the commentator's perspectives.

The commentator claims our "interested in adoption" response category is "overwhelmingly dominated by a narrow set of characteristics." This interpretation reflects a reading of Table 1 that differs from how the data are structured, as the table presents column percentages (distributions within each outcome category), not row percentages (outcome distributions across subgroups). For example, although 96.6% of those interested were transgender women, this group accounted for only 82.2% of the total sample. This interpretation also overlooks an important finding: 65.6% of transgender women expressed interest compared with 14.7% of transgender men and 6.0% of nonbinary individuals, variations our multinomial regression was designed to examine.[4] Peer reviewers raised this point, noting that some transgender men's reproductive anatomy may allow pregnancy options affecting adoption considerations, which we addressed in our discussion.

The commentary emphasizes gender identity and medical gender affirmation while placing less emphasis on substantial heterogeneity across other characteristics. Our Table 1 demonstrates meaningful variation across all three outcome categories, even by column percentages, including race/ethnicity (42.5% of interested participants were people of color vs 40.0% not interested), residential geography (23.0% interested lived in small towns vs 23.0% not interested), educational attainment (60.2% interested had completed high school or less vs 37.3% not interested), and medical affirmation status (34.6% not interested had received hormone therapy vs 97.3% interested). Focusing on selected characteristics without equal attention to this heterogeneity may inadvertently obscure the diversity present within transgender populations.[5]

The commentary further says that medical and legal affirmation variables were "restricted to respondents whose 'gender goals' included the relevant interventions," framing this as a methodological weakness. This concern is inconsistent with established practices in transgender health survey research: assessing receipt of gender-affirming care is meaningful only among individuals who desire such care, and asking whether someone received hormone therapy when they never wanted it would be methodologically inappropriate and inconsistent with participant-centered survey design. Our analysis accounts for this restriction.

Another interpretive difference involves the application of causal inference standards to explicitly descriptive research. Our study examined factors associated with adoption interest—a distinction we clearly articulated when we stated that the "cross-sectional design prevents causal inference."[1(pe9)] Our interpretations carefully followed this framing, highlighting the need for further data exploration in this area. We employed associational language throughout; however, the commentary's critiques are grounded in causal inference logic, standards that differ from those typically applied to associative research describing patterns in understudied topics.

The commentary also questions whether interest in adoption justifies discussions of service development. Descriptive epidemiology has long informed public health practice; characterizing population health outcomes and behavioral patterns fundamentally precedes the development of interventions. Our recommendations (e.g., provider training, reducing economic barriers, and inclusive services) are standard practice-oriented implications that characterize population health scholarship.

In transgender health research, interpretive differences occur within broader social and policy contexts. Judicial and legislative debates have documented how partial readings of evidence and rhetorical strategies are mobilized to challenge access to care and legal protections.[2,3] Scholars therefore bear the responsibility to represent methods and findings accurately and to interpret them within the scope of the research design, especially in contested policy domains.

We have previously emphasized the importance of positionality and transparency in transgender health scholarship.[6] We are an interdisciplinary team of researchers with decades of experience in sexual and gender health research, interested in how transgender people define their family formation goals. Disclosure of expertise, methodological grounding, and relationship to the evidence base strengthens scientific discourse and is an important component of rigorous critique in this field. Transparency clarifies how different interpretations may emerge and supports productive scientific exchange.

Our findings are straightforward and demonstrate what the data show: adoption interest varied across subgroups, with some transgender individuals expressing interest, others not, and some uncertain. More research is warranted in this area of scholarship. Misrepresenting or cherry-picking our research findings can reinforce misinformation that unfairly undermines transgender people's right to start families. We remain committed to rigorous, transparent, and community-engaged research that supports evidence-based public health practice and affirms transgender people's rights to define their own families and futures. AJPH

CORRESPONDENCE

Correspondence should be sent to Adedotun Ogunbajo, 1200 S Hayes St, Arlington, VA 22202 (e-mail: dotunogunbajo@gmail.com). Reprints can be ordered at https://www.ajph.org by clicking the "Reprints" link.

PUBLICATION INFORMATION

Full Citation: Ogunbajo A, DeAtley T, Breslow A, et al. Ogunbajo et al. respond. *Am J Public Health*. 2026;116(7):891–892.

Acceptance Date: March 20, 2026.

DOI: https://doi.org/10.2105/AJPH.2026.308552

ORCID iDs:
Adedotun Ogunbajo https://orcid.org/0000-0002-3074-6431

Terea DeAtley https://orcid.org/0000-0002-2234-1629

Aaron Breslow https://orcid.org/0000-0003-2894-7485

Kristi Gamarel https://orcid.org/0000-0001-9405-7515

Arjee Restar https://orcid.org/0000-0003-2992-8198

CONTRIBUTORS

All authors contributed equally to the development of this work.

ACKNOWLEDGMENTS

This study was funded by the University of Washington Center for AIDS Research (grant AI027757) and the University of Washington Behavioral Research Center for HIV (grant P30MH123248).

Note. The contents of this article are solely the responsibility of the authors and do not necessarily represent the official views of the funders.

CONFLICTS OF INTEREST

The authors have no conflicts of interest to declare.

HUMAN PARTICIPANT PROTECTION

The Human Subject Division of the University of Washington's institutional review board approved all study procedures (no. STUDY00015878). All enrolled participants provided electronic informed consent and consent for publication.

REFERENCES

1. Ogunbajo A, DeAtley T, Breslow A, et al. Association between gender affirmation and adoption interest among a large sample of transgender, nonbinary, and gender-diverse populations in Washington State, 2023. *Am J Public Health.* 2026; 116(2):229–239. https://doi.org/10.2105/AJPH.2025.308312
2. Coldwater K. Decoding the misinformation–legislation pipeline: an analysis of Florida Medicaid and the current state of transgender healthcare. *J Med Libr Assoc.* 2023;111(4):750–761. https://doi.org/10.5195/jmla.2023.1724
3. Wuest J, Last BS. Agents of scientific uncertainty: conflicts over evidence and expertise in gender-affirming care bans for minors. *Soc Sci Med.* 2024; 344:116533. https://doi.org/10.1016/j.socscimed.2023.116533
4. Petrucci CJ. A primer for social worker researchers on how to conduct a multinomial logistic regression. *J Soc Serv Res.* 2009;35(2):193–205. https://doi.org/10.1080/01488370802678983
5. Razum O, Namer Y. Trans people and the myth of homogeneous societies. *Lancet.* 2018;391(10119): 430. https://doi.org/10.1016/S0140-6736(18)30149-1
6. Restar AJ. Why confronting positionality matters to advancing trans research and discourse. *Lancet Reg Health Am.* 2023;24:100568. https://doi.org/10.1016/j.lana.2023.100568

Evaluating the Impact of Singapore's Nutri-Grade Beverage Labels on Prepackaged Beverage Purchases and Product Nutrient Composition: A Before–After Study, 2019–2024

Soye Shin, PhD, and Yan Ning Tan, BA

In December 2022, Singapore implemented mandatory Nutri-Grade front-of-pack labels for beverages. Using household scanner data (April 2019–March 2024), we evaluated changes in sugar purchases and product formulation. Households reduced sugar purchases by 3.1 grams per day (−18%), and purchases of unhealthy beverages fell 44%. Reformulation and reassortment lowered sugar content by 1.16 grams per 100 milliliters (−21%) but increased sweetener and lactose use. Higher-income and nutritionally literate households showed larger reductions. Findings support mandatory labeling but highlight equity concerns and supplier substitution risks. (*Am J Public Health*. 2026;116(7):893–897. https://doi.org/10.2105/AJPH.2026.308476)

To address Singapore's burden of noncommunicable diseases,[1,2] the government implemented the Nutri-Grade (NG) policy on December 30, 2022, mandating front-of-pack nutritional labeling for all prepackaged nonalcoholic beverages.[3]

INTERVENTION AND IMPLEMENTATION

Under this policy, beverages are assigned a color-coded grade from A (healthiest) to D (least healthy), based primarily on free sugar content, and further downgraded if saturated fat thresholds are exceeded (Appendix Figure A, available as a supplement to the online version of this article at http://www.ajph.org). Products graded C or D must display NG labels, and D-graded beverages are prohibited from advertising.

This mandatory labeling scheme builds on the existing voluntary Healthier Choice Symbol program. A two-year transition period (late 2020–2022) was provided to enable supplier reformulation before full enforcement. The rollout of NG labeling created a natural policy window to evaluate both consumer purchasing shifts and industry reformulation or product assortment changes.

PLACE, TIME, AND PERSONS

This evaluation was conducted in Singapore, using NielsenIQ HomeScan data from a nationally representative panel of 1000 households (Appendix I Table A, available as a supplement to the online version of this article at http://www.ajph.org). We analyzed purchases of prepackaged beverages in two time periods: prepolicy (April 2019–March 2020) and postpolicy (April 2023–March 2024). Analyses focused on the 799 households with purchase data in both periods. To examine variation in responses, additional data on primary shoppers' educational attainment and nutritional knowledge were collected through an add-on survey in March 2023. Nutritional content data for 1949 beverage products was compiled from government nutrient databases, manufacturer and retailer websites, and in-store audits conducted by the research team.

PURPOSE

The study aimed to evaluate the real-world effectiveness of Singapore's NG beverage labeling policy using a pre–post quasi-experimental design. Unlike most prior studies, which focused on short-term or laboratory-based effects,[4,5] this study examined both sustained consumer behavior and industry responses, including reformulation and product reassortment. This study addressed two unresolved gaps: first, there is limited policy-scale evidence on mandatory, nutrient-specific front-of-pack labels in Asian contexts; and second, few evaluations jointly quantify consumer purchasing changes and producer adaptation over time under a mandatory labeling regime.[6] By leveraging longitudinal scanner data and fixed-effects regression models, the study provided rare, policy-relevant evidence from an Asian context on the population-level impact of mandatory nutrient-specific labeling. We hypothesized that, relative to a counterfactual projected from prepolicy trend, NG implementation would reduce household sugar purchased and shift purchases toward healthier beverages (grades A and B), and that manufacturers would respond via reformulation and reassortment to lower free sugar and saturated fat across products.

EVALUATION AND ADVERSE EFFECTS

For the demand-side analysis, the primary outcome was the daily average total sugar (in grams [g]) purchased per household. This was calculated by aggregating the sugar content of beverages purchased at the household-month level and dividing it by the number of days in each calendar month. Secondary outcomes included the daily average saturated fat (g) purchased per household, as well as the daily average volume (in milliliters [mL]) of healthier (grades A and B) and less healthy (grades C and D) beverages purchased.

For the supply-side analysis, key outcomes included the monthly average free sugar (g) and saturated fat (g) content per 100 mL of beverages purchased. Additionally, we examined changes in the proportion of purchased beverages containing sweeteners and changes in lactose content (g) per 100 mL.

Statistical Analysis

We employed fixed-effects linear regression with a binary variable for the policy period and its interaction with a linear time trend. This estimates post-policy outcomes relative to a counterfactual projected from prepolicy trends. For household-level outcomes, fixed effects absorb time-invariant household characteristics. Only time-varying covariates, including a household size categorical variable (1–2, 3, 4, or ≥ 5 members) and an indicator for income (≥ Singapore $7001), were included in the model. Heterogeneous effects on the primary outcome were examined by stratifying models by (1) high household income (≥ Singapore $7001) versus otherwise, (2) minority race/ethnicity (Malay, Indian, others) versus Chinese, (3) high education (university and above) versus otherwise, and (4) high nutritional knowledge (median score and above) versus below median. For supply-side responses, fixed-effects estimation was conducted separately for standalone producer effects (changes among unique products) and net effects (results weighted by purchase quantities). The same analyses were conducted for all beverages combined and, separately, for dairy beverages. Additionally, to minimize overlap with early COVID-19 policies, we reestimated models using a stricter prepolicy period (April 2019–January 2020), with unchanged results (Appendix II).

Consumer Behavior

The NG policy shifted demand toward healthier beverages and reduced household sugar purchases (Figure 1). Compared with a counterfactual scenario without the policy, the NG policy was associated with a 3.11 g per day reduction in household total sugar purchases (−18%; 95% confidence interval [CI] = −4.99, −1.23) and no statistically significant reduction in saturated fat (−6%; 95% CI = −0.53, 0.25). The sugar reduction was both immediate and sustained over 12 months. Purchases of less healthy beverages (grades C and D) declined by 90 mL per day (−44%; 95% CI = −117.00, −63.75) and purchases of healthier beverages (grades A and B) increased by 79 mL per day (+82%; 95% CI = 59.05, 99.10), aligning with Singapore's guidance to prefer water and lower or no-sugar beverages.[7] This pattern suggests that consumers did not simply replace unhealthy beverages with healthier ones but may have increased their overall consumption of healthier beverages, potentially diluting health benefits if overall energy intake also rose.

Heterogeneity

Relative to the counterfactual, policy effects were larger among higher-income, Chinese households than among minority households, where changes were small or statistically insignificant (Appendix I Table B). Effects differed by nutritional knowledge rather than education, highlighting the need for targeted strategies to strengthen

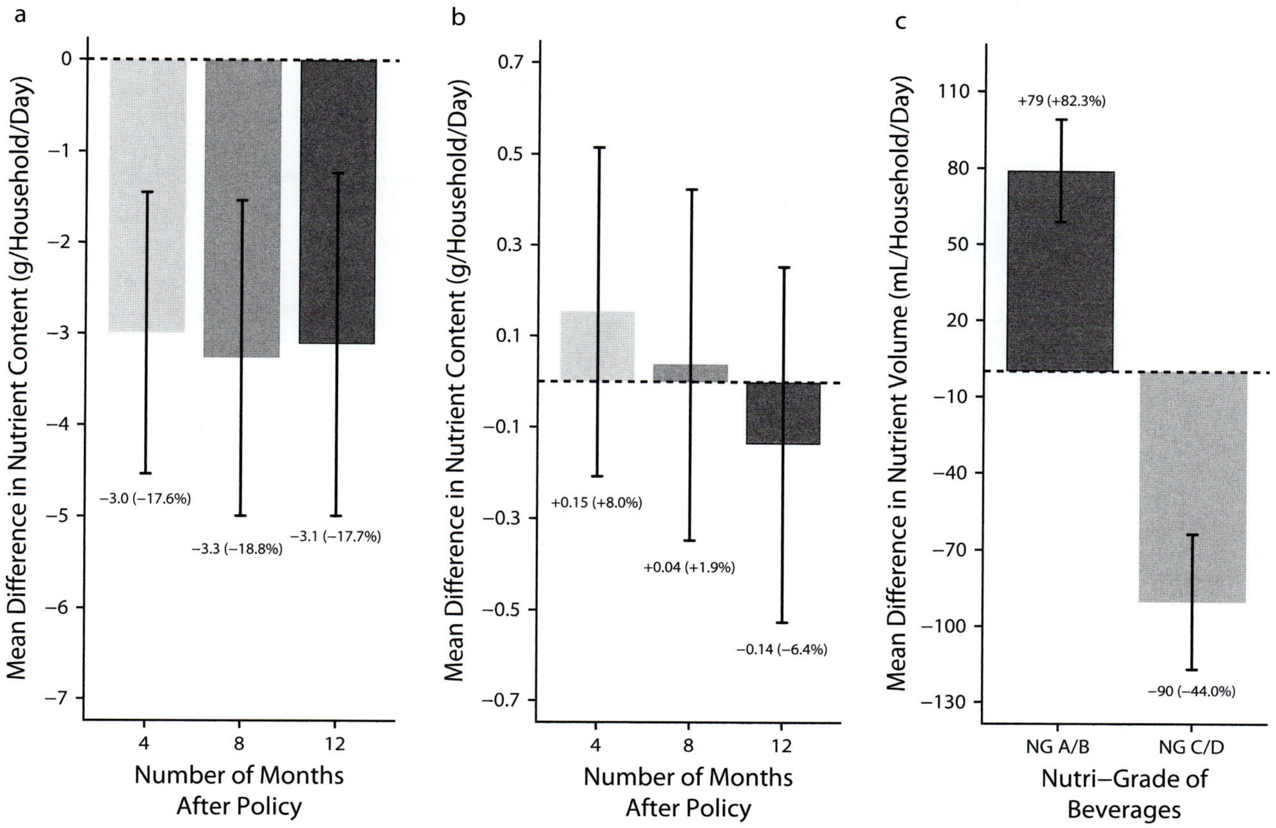

FIGURE 1— Mean Differences (and Percent Changes) in Nutrient Content and Volume of Household Purchases Between Postpolicy Purchases and Counterfactual Scenario Postpolicy Prepackaged Beverage Purchases for (a) Sugar, (b) Saturated Fat, and (c) Beverages: Singapore, April 2019–March 2024

Note. Overall model-estimated differences are derived from fixed-effects models comparing postpolicy nutrient content or volume of purchases to counterfactual postpolicy nutrient content or volume of purchases based on prepolicy trends. Purchase data were provided by Nielsen HomeScan data. Error bars indicate 95% confidence intervals. The x-axis of the left and middle graphs shows the number of months after Nutri-Grade (NG) policy implementation. On the x-axis of the right graph, NG A/B represents healthier beverages with a grade of A or B, and NG C/D represents less healthy beverages with a grade of C or D. The y-axis represents the amount of nutrient (in grams) or volume of beverage purchases (in milliliters) per household per day.

nutrition literacy beyond Singapore's "My Healthy Plate/Nutri-Grade" guidelines and school-based initiatives.[7,8]

Supplier Reformulation and Reassortment

Manufacturers reduced free sugar and saturated fat but increased sweetener use and lactose, with evidence of threshold-targeting. Analysis of unique products across time periods showed that the average free sugar content declined by 1.16 g per 100 mL (−21%; 95% CI = −1.17, −1.16) and saturated fat by 0.10 g per 100 mL (−19%; 95% CI = −0.10, −0.09; Figure 2). Meanwhile, the share of products containing sweetener rose by 6% (95% CI = 0.061, 0.062), and lactose content increased by 0.15 g per 100 mL (34%; 95% CI = 0.152, 0.154), suggesting that manufacturers substituted free sugar with alternative sweet-tasting compounds to avoid label penalties. Products clustering just below NG thresholds (e.g., 5 g and 10 g free sugar) further indicate strategic reformulation (Appendix I Figure B). Dairy beverages showed particularly large reductions in sugar (−30%; 95% CI = −1.69, −1.67) and a modest decline in saturated fat (−9.6%; 95% CI = −0.12, −0.11), but also sharp increases in lactose (+78%; 95% CI = 1.22, 1.23).

Net Effects Weighted by Volume Purchases

Purchase-weighted changes amplified sugar reductions but not saturated fat (Appendix I Figure C: free sugar, −1.5 g per 100 mL [−30%]; saturated fat, −0.1 g per 100 mL [−12%]). Among dairy beverages, free sugar fell 2.7 g per 100 mL (−63%), but saturated fat rose 0.1 g per 100 mL (+8%) and lactose rose 2.6 g per100 mL (+199%). This reflects persistent demand for

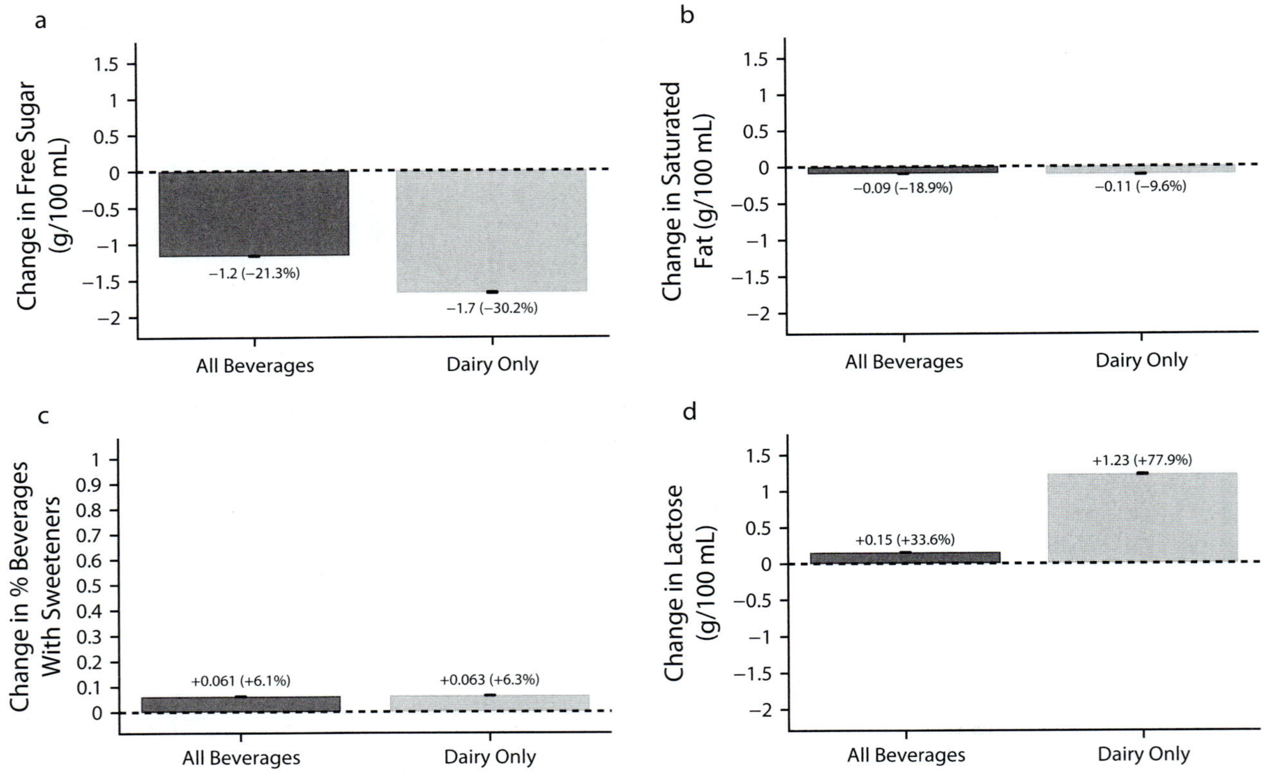

FIGURE 2— Mean Differences (and Percentage Changes) in Nutrient Profile Between All Unique Beverages: Singapore, April 2019–March 2024

Note. Overall model-estimated differences are derived from fixed-effects models comparing the 12-month postpolicy nutrient profile of all unique beverages to the counterfactual postpolicy nutrient profile of all unique beverage purchases based on prepolicy trends. Purchase data were provided by Nielsen HomeScan data. Error bars indicate 95% confidence intervals.

full-fat fresh milk (because of its taste and creaminess,[9] although it is not recommended for those older than two years[10]), which limited saturated fat impact. These findings underscore that consumer preferences ultimately shape the reach and effectiveness of labeling policies.[11]

Adverse Effects

Despite its overall effectiveness, the policy revealed several unintended consequences:

- Threshold-targeting near NG cutoffs[6];
- Increased use of sweeteners and lactose[12]: because grades penalize free sugar but not nonsugar sweeteners, suppliers can improve grades by replacing sugar with sweeteners—consistent with the observed rise in sweetener use;
- Equity concerns (smaller or null effects in some groups).[13]

SUSTAINABILITY

A mandatory, nutrient-specific label can sustain demand- and supply-side adjustments while preserving autonomy. Preparation and public communication facilitated compliance, and continued point-of-purchase exposure reinforced behavior change. In Singapore, NG was paired with public communications and a ban on grade D advertising across online and offline media. Sustaining impact will require tightening marketing restrictions on unhealthy foods, deploying targeted equity measures, and conducting regular, evidence-informed monitoring of product composition.

PUBLIC HEALTH SIGNIFICANCE

Relative to a counterfactual projected from prepolicy trends, NG produced measurable, policy-scale changes in both purchasing and product composition, addressing our core research question in a real-world setting. Two limitations merit note: our data capture household beverage purchases for home consumption (out-of-home purchases are not observed), and fixed-effects estimates do not fully control for unobserved time-varying factors that may influence purchasing behaviors. Even with these limitations, our findings indicate that mandatory labeling can meaningfully reduce sugar purchased through both consumer behavior changes and industry reformulation. Importantly, this study highlights the complexity of food-industry adaptation, including unintended consequences such as manufacturers' substitution of free sugar with sweeteners. Many front-of-pack labels—including Nutri-Grade and Nutri-Score—do not constrain nonsugar sweeteners. Labels should either build sweetener controls into the algorithm (e.g., disclosure plus penalties or thresholds, or overall "sweetness" caps) or be paired with complementary restrictions and active monitoring. The observed disparities in consumer response also underscore the importance of tailoring public health policies to reduce, rather than reinforce, existing inequities in diet-related disease risk.[14] For settings weighing front-of-pack labels (e.g., the United States), sugar gains alongside substitution call for adopt-if-robust designs—explicit sweetener controls with equity-focused oversight and evaluation. Taken together—and consistent with the World Health Organization's Global Action Plan for noncommunicable diseases (2013–2030)[15]—Singapore's experience with NG suggests that well-designed labeling policies, when supported by equity-focused measures, regulatory oversight, and ongoing evaluation of sustained responses, can play a critical role in improving nutritional environments while preserving consumer autonomy. AJPH

ABOUT THE AUTHORS

At the time of the study, Soye Shin and Yan Ning Tan were with the Program in Health Services Research and Population Health, Duke-NUS Medical School, Singapore.

CORRESPONDENCE

Correspondence should be sent to Soye Shin, Duke-NUS Medical School, 8 College Road, Singapore 169857 (e-mail: syshin@duke-nus.edu.sg). Reprints can be ordered at https://www.ajph.org by clicking the "Reprints" link.

PUBLICATION INFORMATION

Full Citation: Shin S, Tan YN. Evaluating the impact of Singapore's Nutri-Grade beverage labels on prepackaged beverage purchases and product nutrient composition: a before–after study, 2019–2024. *Am J Public Health*. 2026;116(7):893–897.

Acceptance Date: February 4, 2026.

DOI: https://doi.org/10.2105/AJPH.2026.308476

ORCID iDs:

Soye Shin https://orcid.org/0000-0002-8856-8236

Yan Ning Tan https://orcid.org/0009-0001-9653-5485

CONTRIBUTORS

S. Shin conceptualized the study, wrote the original draft, contributed to the review and editing of the manuscript, and was responsible for methodology, investigation, validation, project administration, and funding acquisition. Y. N. Tan wrote the original draft, contributed to the review and editing of the manuscript, and managed the visualization, investigation, formal analysis, and validation for the study.

ACKNOWLEDGMENTS

We thank the Singapore Health Promotion Board for supporting the data for this study.

CONFLICTS OF INTEREST

The authors have no conflicts of interest to disclose.

HUMAN PARTICIPANT PROTECTION

This study obtained institutional review board exemption from the National University of Singapore as it used secondary de-identified data.

REFERENCES

1. Health Promotion Board, Singapore. National Nutrition Survey 2022. 2022. Available at: https://www.hpb.gov.sg/workplace/useful-information-for-organisations/national-reports-and-surveys. Accessed April 9, 2026.
2. Ministry of Health and Health Promotion Board, Singapore. National Population Health Survey 2022. 2023. Available at: https://www.moh.gov.sg/others/resources-and-statistics/nphs-2022. Accessed April 9, 2026.
3. Ministry of Health, Singapore. Rollout of Nutri-Grade mark on 30 December 2022. 2022. Available at: https://www.moh.gov.sg/newsroom/rollout-of-nutri-grade-mark-on-30-december-2022/. Accessed April 9, 2026.
4. Braesco V, Drewnowski A. Are front-of-pack nutrition labels influencing food choices and purchases, diet quality, and modeled health outcomes? A narrative review of four systems. *Nutrients.* 2023;15(1):205. https://doi.org/10.3390/nu15010205
5. Shrestha A, Cullerton K, White KM, Mays J, Sendall M. Impact of front-of-pack nutrition labelling in consumer understanding and use across socio-economic status: a systematic review. *Appetite.* 2023;187:106587. https://doi.org/10.1016/j.appet.2023.106587
6. Alé-Chilet J, Moshary S. Beyond consumer switching: supply responses to food packaging and advertising regulations. *Mark Sci.* 2022;41(2):243–270. https://doi.org/10.1287/mksc.2021.1315
7. Health Hub. Nutritious foods for a healthy diet. Available at: https://www.healthhub.sg/programmes/nutrition-hub/eat-more. Accessed April 9, 2026.
8. Singapore Health Promotion Board. Healthy meals in schools programme. Available at: https://www.hpb.gov.sg/schools/school-programmes/healthy-meals-in-schools-programme. Accessed April 9, 2026.
9. Wang W, Sun B, Deng J, Ai N. Addressing flavor challenges in reduced-fat dairy products: a review from the perspective of flavor compounds and their improvement strategies. *Food Res Int.* 2024;188:114478. https://doi.org/10.1016/j.foodres.2024.114478
10. Health Hub. Should I switch my baby to low-fat milk? 2022. Available at: https://www.healthhub.sg/well-being-and-lifestyle/food-diet-and-nutrition/should-i-switch-baby-to-low-fat-milk. Accessed April 9, 2026.
11. Caltabiano ML, Shellshear J. Palatability versus healthiness as determinants of food preferences in young adults: a comparison of nomothetic and idiographic analytic approaches. *Aust N Z J Public Health.* 1998;22(5):547–551. https://doi.org/10.1111/j.1467-842x.1998.tb01436.x
12. Rebolledo N, Bercholz M, Adair L, Corvalán C, Ng SW, Taillie LS. Sweetener purchases in Chile before and after implementing a policy for food labeling, marketing, and sales in schools. *Curr Dev Nutr.* 2023;7(2):100016. https://doi.org/10.1016/j.cdnut.2022.100016
13. Greenthal E, Sorscher S. Can food labeling policy advance health equity? *Update*, fall 2021. Food & Drug Law Institute, Washington, DC. 2021. Available at: https://www.fdli.org/2021/09/can-food-labeling-policy-advance-health-equity. Accessed April 9, 2026.
14. Park SH, Nicolaou M, Dickens BSL, Yang Q, Tan KW, van Dam RM. Ethnicity, neighborhood and individual socioeconomic status, and obesity: The Singapore Multiethnic Cohort. *Obesity (Silver Spring).* 2020;28(12):2405–2413. https://doi.org/10.1002/oby.22995
15. World Health Organization. *Global Action Plan for the Prevention and Control of Noncommunicable Diseases 2013–2020.* Geneva, Switzerland: World Health Organization; 2013.

Ultraprocessed Food and Corporate Influence: Evidence, Regulation, and Policy Pathways to Address Chronic Disease in the United States

Nicholas Chartres, PhD, MHumNutr

ABOUT THE AUTHOR

Nicholas Chartres is with the School of Pharmacy, Faculty of Medicine & Health, University of Sydney, Australia, and the Center to End Corporate Harm, University of California, San Francisco. He is also an AJPH Associate Editor.

AJPH July 2026, Vol. 116, No. 7

See also Ultraprocessed Food, pp. 898–1029.

Ultraprocessed food (UPF) is the largest proportion of food in the US diet, and researchers have established from rigorous systematic reviews of observational studies and randomized controlled trials that its regular consumption has numerous adverse health effects.[1,2] Recent estimates link UPF consumption to approximately 2.3 million deaths globally.[3] Additionally, the production of UPF creates a devastating environmental footprint, with UPF corporations such as Coca-Cola, PepsiCo, and Nestlé, as some of the top global plastic polluters.[4]

Previous studies of internal food industry documents have exposed that consolidation of the UPF industry accelerated during the 1980s, when major tobacco companies acquired and operated some of the world's largest food corporations. Tobacco-owned food companies pioneered reformulations of UPF to make it more appealing to consumers, especially children,[5] and selectively disseminated hyperpalatable food into the US food system.[6] Other companies copied these strategies once hyperpalatable food proved profitable.[6] UPF now constitutes approximately 60% of the food purchased in the United States, and consumption of these products has increased most notably among youths and populations of lower income and education.[7–9] The San Francisco City, California, attorney has now sued some of the country's largest UPF manufacturers for continuing to market addictive and harmful products to maximize profits even after they learned they were making people sick (bit.ly/4wzEl5f).

Concurrently, a growing body of evidence has demonstrated the role the UPF industry has played in trying to influence what the public and policymakers know about the harms of these products. Major UPF corporations, including through their trade organizations, have funded nutrition research aimed at diverting attention from product-related harms[10] and have also provided funding to academic institutions,[11] scientific conferences,[12]

Continued on page 899...

HISTORY CORNER

5 YEARS AGO

Portion Sizes of Ultraprocessed Foods in the United States, 2002 to 2021

By 2002, many single-serve portions had enlarged 2- to 5-fold since they were introduced. Large portions have effects beyond calories; they encourage people to eat more and to underestimate how much they are eating. . . . In 2021, we examined the sizes of specific ultraprocessed food items sold as single servings that we have tracked since 2002: packaged products (candy bars, soda, and beer) and fast foods (hamburgers, french fries, and fountain soda). We selected this product sample from among those that are major contributors of calories in US diets, ranked highest in sales, associated in observational studies with weight gain and poor health, and marketed as single servings. We obtained portion-size information from package labels and from company Web sites, as described previously. We compared current portions with their sizes when first introduced and measured again in 2002. . . . [F]ood companies are still selling chocolate bars, bottled and canned soda and beer, hamburgers, french fries, and fountain sodas in larger portions than when first introduced. While some companies have reduced their portions by small amounts, most continue to sell the larger sizes; we observed little change from sizes offered in 2002.

From *AJPH*, December 2021, p. 2223.

leading nutrition scientists—including those involved in developing the *Dietary Guidelines for Americans*[13]—and influential professional organizations.[14]

As the burden of disease from consuming these UPF products continues to rise, it is critical that the public health community and scientists continue to study the health impacts on low-income communities, examine which subgroups are most affected and why, and identify the most appropriate public health strategies to effectively and equitably protect the public's health.

The UPF-featured section of this *AJPH* issue responds to the urgent need for evidence with five studies examining UPF consumption and health in the US foodscape, two studies analyzing the role of tobacco-owned food companies in shaping the UPF-dominated food system in the United States today, four studies bolstering the case for immediate policy action based on the best available science, and six editorials discussing the structural changes needed to combat the harms of UPF and the UPF industry.

This featured section of the *AJPH* issue therefore contributes something new: It views the problem of UPF in the United States through a public health lens, namely, as a commercial determinant of health. The featured section shows how, like other commercial determinants, UPF causes health inequities, is linked to other commercial harms, and is linked to the power and profit motive of corporate actors; it also shows how public health strategies honed during the tobacco war could be used to mitigate the harm of UPF.

HEALTH IN THE US FOODSCAPE

The first four articles examine associations between UPF consumption, as defined by the Nova food classification system, and cardiometabolic outcomes, dementia, household food insecurity, participation in nutrition assistance programs, and diet quality. Hatta-Langedyk et al. (p. 1015) conducted a cross-sectional study analyzing 47 999 adults (20–85 years) in the National Health and Nutrition Examination Survey (NHANES; 1999–2018) and found that increased energy intake from UPF is associated with higher body mass index, average blood sugar, diastolic blood pressure and greater prevalence of metabolic syndrome, diabetes, cancer, and all-cause mortality. Stronger associations were identified among lower income adults, and results remained significant even when adjusting for nutritional quality.

In a second cross-sectional study, which analyzed 15 760 US adults (≥ 20 years) in NHANES (2009–2018), Sheinberg et al. (p. 993) found that individuals with very low-quality diets per the Healthy Eating Index and high UPF consumption had the least favorable metabolic profiles, including the highest mean body mass index and fasting glucose. However, overall diet quality was found to be a strong predictor of cardiometabolic health, even with varying levels of UPF consumption.

Fernández et al. (p. 971) also measured Healthy Eating Index scores and UPF consumption. Among 1286 US pregnant women in NHANES (2001–2018), they found that food insecurity, but not UPF consumption, was linked to lower prenatal Healthy Eating Index scores. UPF consumption did not differ by Special Supplemental Nutrition Program for Women, Infants, and Children or Supplemental Nutrition Assistance Program (SNAP) participation status.

Continued on page 900...

HISTORY CORNER

16 YEARS AGO

Life and Health Insurance Industry Investments in Fast Food

[F]ast food consumption is linked to obesity and cardiovascular disease, 2 leading causes of preventable death. The industry markets heavily to children and often builds restaurants within walking distance of schools. . . . Major insurers own $1.88 billion of stock in the 5 leading fast-food companies, representing 2.2% of total market capitalization of these companies on June 11, 2009. . . . [I]nsurance companies have 2 ethical options. The first is to divest themselves of holdings in fast food companies as well as other industries that have a clearly negative public health impact. . . . A second option is that insurers could mitigate the harms of fast food by leveraging their positions as owners of fast food companies to force the adoption of practices consistent with widely accepted public health principles. Such moves could include encouraging companies to improve the nutritional quality of their products, reduce calorie density, serve smaller portions, and change marketing practices. To maximize their impact, insurers might turn over their proxy votes to an independent nonprofit organization that could pool votes in a way that effects meaningful change.

From *AJPH*, June 2010, pp. 1029–1030.

Finally, Lee et al. (p. 981) found that increased UPF consumption was associated with a higher risk of dementia (hazard ratio [HR] = 1.58; 95% confidence interval [CI] = 1.003, 2.480), cognitive impairment with no dementia (HR = 1.46; 95% CI = 1.13, 1.88), and cognitive impairment with no dementia or dementia (HR = 1.47; 95% CI = 1.16, 1.87) in 5370 older US adults (> 50 years) in a longitudinal study (2013–2020). They found unprocessed or minimally processed food consumption protective and associated with lower risks of dementia, cognitive impairment with no dementia, and a "composite outcome of cognitive impairment, combining cognitive impairment with no dementia and dementia."

To understand changes in the US foodscape overall and by area rurality between 2003 and 2023, Wiese et al. (p. 1004) estimated the percentages of census tracts defined as food deserts (i.e., having no grocery stores) and food swamps (i.e., having mostly fast-food restaurants). They found that neighborhood food environments have continued to become less healthy, with increases in the percentage of food swamps and no substantial progress in reducing food deserts. They call for improved access to healthy food retailers in rural and socioeconomically disadvantaged areas and strategic planning of public transit networks.

TOBACCO-OWNED FOOD COMPANIES' ROLE IN SHAPING FOOD SYSTEMS

Two studies provide critical insights into how the tobacco industry helped the UPF industry scale up in the US and global food systems. Using internal company documents, Schmidt (p. 940) shows that Philip Morris acquired Kraft Foods Group to profitably apply cigarette research and development to develop new UPF products, including Lunchables for kids. To design Lunchables, Philip Morris's cigarette design strategy, called "consumer-driven product development," was used to optimize for consumer pleasure. Schmidt argues that governments should extend existing consumer protection laws and regulations that protect children from tobacco products to include UPF.

Fazzino et al. (p. 921) also analyzed internal company documents to reveal how US tobacco food companies disseminated UPF and hyperpalatable food globally. Tobacco companies did so by expanding their international food businesses using the same approach they had used to establish their international tobacco businesses. They used a suite of tactics to drive sales of food and tobacco products, including manipulating product sizes and developing high flavor, light products to retain health-conscious users.

IMMEDIATE POLICY ACTION BASED ON THE BEST AVAILABLE SCIENCE

Gearhardt et al. (p. 950) used machine learning and a nationally representative sample of US adults (n = 1664) to identify nutritional characteristics (signatures) associated with the perceived addictive potential of food. UPF frequently exceeds multiple addictive nutrient thresholds for food higher in carbohydrates, glycemic load, energy density, and fat simultaneously, which are rare in minimally processed food. The results provide a data-driven framework for identifying food most likely to promote compulsive intake

Continued on page 901...

HISTORY CORNER

17 YEARS AGO

Proximity of Fast-Food Restaurants to Schools and Adolescent Obesity

We found that students in California were heavier and more likely to be overweight or obese if their school was located within one half mile of a fast-food restaurant, after control for student demographic characteristics, school characteristics, and detailed controls for the type of community in which the school was located. This main finding still held when other definitions of nearby (i.e., other than within 0.5 mile) were used and was not observed for other types of business establishments also commonly found near schools. Finally, we show that nearness to fast food was unrelated to smoking. We also addressed the concern that fast-food proximity may simply be a proxy for other unobserved characteristics about locations that are independently correlated with weight status, such as the degree of economic development around a school. Overall, our patterns are consistent with the idea that fast food near schools affects students' eating habits, overweight, and obesity. . . . Our results suggest that it might be useful to consider policies such as providing adolescents with alternatives to fast-food restaurants. . . . A more drastic public policy measure would be for local governments to restrict commercial permits for fast-food restaurants within walking distance of a school.

From *AJPH*, March 2009, p. 509.

and inform reformulation, labeling, and marketing policies similar to how tobacco and alcohol policies target high-risk formulations.

Niederdeppe et al. (p. 960) polled a nationally representative sample of 2000 US adults and found that more than half had heard of UPF, yet only one third felt confident explaining what it is, highlighting the need for a clear and scientifically supported definition of UPF for health communication and regulation. Additionally, approximately 70% of people polled believed UPF is addictive, with approximately 73% of people supporting warning labels about its health risks. The authors found broad bipartisan support for addressing UPF harms via several public policy and legal strategies.

D'Angelo Campos et al. (p. 1025) found that there have been 43 federal and state policy proposals targeting UPF introduced in the United States between 2021 and 2025, with most from states. About one third defined UPF based on a narrow set of specific food additives, and some used entire classes of additives. Some provided Nova-like definitions but lacked comprehensive lists of targeted ingredients. A third did not provide any definition. Most policies targeted food served or sold in schools and proposed warning labels and restrictions on marketing. The authors highlight that using UPF definitions that largely depart from Nova cannot be considered evidence based, with uncertain health protections provided across states.

Monteiro et al. (p. 932) explain how the Nova food classification system concept can inform and improve dietary guidance, monitoring, and food regulation and why government policy responses have been inadequate despite growing evidence of harm and awareness of the issue. This includes the influence of the UPF industry's leading corporations undermining policy responses, including disseminating disinformation about Nova. Critically, they provide examples of how Nova can be operationalized in policymaking and how UPF-based policies can complement existing policies based on addressing dietary nutrient imbalances.

STRUCTURAL CHANGES NEEDED TO COMBAT HARMS

Six editorials are included in this featured section that are policy focused and describe the structural changes needed to combat UPF harm. Nestle (p. 912) argues that although the 2025 to 2030 *Dietary Guidelines for Americans* for the first time called for limiting highly processed food, it frames diet - almost entirely as a matter of personal responsibility, sidelining concerns about health equity and the social determinants of diet. The author highlights that the food industry's support of this framing is likely because its leaders know education is not enough to change dietary behavior. The author calls for a wide range of policy options, including taxes, marketing restrictions, and subsidies aimed at making healthier food more available, accessible, and affordable.

Wolfson (p. 918) supports this argument by proposing that UPF policies needed to reduce intake should also consider and address structural, societal, and behavioral determinants of UPF consumption. Specifically, they should build necessary culinary skills and self-efficacy for preparing minimally processed meals, shifting societal norms and expectations on the gender balance of household labor and raising incomes and SNAP benefits to ensure equitable access to minimally processed diets.

Using examples from urban (Chicago, IL) and rural (West Virginia) areas, Gracia (p. 903) demonstrates how structural and systemic barriers to healthy eating, including distance to a grocery store and food insecurity, are related to incidence rate of diabetes and obesity. The author argues that policies focused on UPF consumption should also ensure increased availability, accessibility, affordability, and palatability of minimally processed food in communities and settings such as schools to avoid the unintended consequences of increased food prices, worsened food insecurity, and exacerbated health disparities.

Smith Tallie et al. (p. 909) highlight how most UPF policies have predominately focused on human health outcomes owing to consumption and they overlook the environmental impacts of UPF, including pollution, biodiversity loss, and greenhouse gas emissions. They explain how the UPF system is inseparable from plastics, with corporations such as Coca-Cola and Unilever as the top global plastic polluters. They propose policy efforts, including warning labels on these products that document not only the health but the environmental harms of UPF.

Pomeranz and Brownell (p. 906) outline the need for lawsuits initiated by state attorneys general and city and county attorneys and plaintiffs' attorneys who have the power to hold industry accountable after decades of calls for industry reform have not been implemented. Lack of implementation is owing to the legislative and administrative branches of government continuing to protect corporate interests. They explain that the impact of litigation by attorneys general would be magnified if multistate attorney general actions were launched, ultimately leading to critical legislative and regulatory reforms, as in the Master Settlement Agreement.

Scrinis (p. 915) concludes by discussing the need for policies that go beyond food environment policies to restrict the consumption of UPF one product at a time. The author argues for policies to reduce the power and influence of UPF corporations by directly and differentially addressing the power, products, and practices of these corporations in these food environments. For example, applying front-of-packet labels, marketing restrictions, and taxes only of large corporations and not other producers and UPF retailers.

The findings of this UPF-featured section further establish the UPF industry as a leading vector of chronic disease in the United States, like the tobacco industry.[3] They collectively pave the way for governments to regulate UPF using a science-based definition, such as Nova. Critically, leading experts suggest that these interventions should not focus on education, individual behavior change, and personal responsibility alone but that governments should implement coordinated, structural policies that reshape the food environment, regulate corporate power, and promote minimally processed food. Therefore, governments are ethically responsible for implementing appropriate evidence-based interventions to mitigate harm modeled on successful tobacco control policies, including bans on advertising, warning labels, and taxes.

This UPF-featured section aims to spur continuous discourse on this topic, and *AJPH* welcomes more submissions to document the effects of UPF and propose promising interventions to improve dietary intake and reduce UPF consumption. AJPH

CORRESPONDENCE

Correspondence should be sent to Nicholas Chartres, The University of Sydney, School of Pharmacy, Science Rd, Camperdown, NSW 2006, Australia (e-mail: nicholas.chartres@sydney.edu.au). Reprints can be ordered at https://www.ajph.org by clicking the "Reprints" link.

PUBLICATION INFORMATION

Full Citation: Chartres N. Ultraprocessed food and corporate influence: evidence, regulation, and policy pathways to address chronic disease in the United States. *Am J Public Health*. 2026;116(7):898–902.

Acceptance Date: April 14, 2026.

DOI: https://doi.org/10.2105/AJPH.2026.308591

ORCID iD:

Nicholas Chartres https://orcid.org/0000-0002-9659-6739

CONFLICTS OF INTEREST

The author has no conflicts of interest to report.

REFERENCES

1. Lane MM, Gamage E, Du S, et al. Ultra-processed food exposure and adverse health outcomes: umbrella review of epidemiological meta-analyses. *BMJ*. 2024;384:e077310. https://doi.org/10.1136/bmj-2023-077310
2. Hall KD, Ayuketah A, Brychta R, et al. Ultra-processed diets cause excess calorie intake and weight gain: an inpatient randomized controlled trial of ad libitum food intake. *Cell Metab*. 2019;30(1):67–77.e3. https://doi.org/10.1016/j.cmet.2019.05.008
3. Chartres N, Apollonio DE, Bero LA, et al. Corporate vectors of chronic disease—using internal industry documents to craft counterstrategies. *N Engl J Med*. 2026;394(12):1231–1237. https://doi.org/10.1056/NEJMms2507028
4. Cowger W, Willis KA, Bullock S, et al. Global producer responsibility for plastic pollution. *Sci Adv*. 2024;10(17):eadj8275. https://doi.org/10.1126/sciadv.adj8275
5. Nguyen KH, Glantz SA, Palmer CN, Schmidt LA. Transferring racial/ethnic marketing strategies from tobacco to food corporations: Philip Morris and Kraft General Food. *Am J Public Health*. 2020;110(3):329–336. https://doi.org/10.2105/AJPH.2019.305482
6. Fazzino TL, Jun D, Chollet-Hinton L, Bjorlie K. US tobacco companies selectively disseminated hyper-palatable foods into the US food system: empirical evidence and current implications. *Addiction*. 2024;119(1):62–71. https://doi.org/10.1111/add.16332
7. Zhang Z, Jackson SL, Steele EM, Gillespie C, Yang Q. Relationship between ultraprocessed food intake and cardiovascular health among US adolescents: results from the National Health and Nutrition Examination Survey 2007–2018. *J Adolesc Health*. 2022;70(2):249–257. https://doi.org/10.1016/j.jadohealth.2021.09.031
8. Wolfson JA, Tucker AC, Leung CW, Rebholz CM, Garcia-Larsen V, Martinez-Steele E. Trends in adults' intake of un-processed/minimally processed and ultra-processed foods at home and away from home in the United States from 2003–2018. *J Nutr*. 2025;155(1):280–292. https://doi.org/10.1016/j.tjnut.2024.10.048
9. Dunford EK, Miles DR, Popkin BM. Exploring disparities in the proportion of ultra-processed foods and beverages purchased in grocery stores by US households in 2020. *Public Health Nutr*. 2025;28(1):e85. https://doi.org/10.1017/S1368980025000606
10. Fabbri A, Holland TJ, Bero LA. Food industry sponsorship of academic research: investigating commercial bias in the research agenda. *Public Health Nutr*. 2018;21(18):3422–3430. https://doi.org/10.1017/S1368980018002100
11. Serodio P, Ruskin G, McKee M, Stuckler D. Evaluating Coca-Cola's attempts to influence public health "in their own words": analysis of Coca-Cola emails with public health academics leading the Global Energy Balance Network. *Public Health Nutr*. 2020;23(14):2647–2653. https://doi.org/10.1017/S1368980020002098
12. Atli Gunnarsson J, Ruskin G, Stuckler D, Steele S. Big food and drink sponsorship of conferences and speakers: a case study of one multinational company's influence over knowledge dissemination and professional engagement. *Public Health Nutr*. 2023;26(5):1094–1111. https://doi.org/10.1017/S1368980022002506
13. Mahase E. US dietary committee is plagued with "high risk conflicts of interest," report finds. *BMJ*. 2023;383:p2313. https://doi.org/10.1136/bmj.p2313
14. Carriedo A, Pinsky I, Crosbie E, Ruskin G, Mialon M. The corporate capture of the nutrition profession in the USA: the case of the Academy of Nutrition and Dietetics. *Public Health Nutr*. 2022;25(12):3568–3582. https://doi.org/10.1017/S1368980022001835

Ultraprocessed Food, Food Insecurity, and Improving the Food Environment for All in the United States

J. Nadine Gracia, MD, MSCE

ABOUT THE AUTHOR

J. Nadine Gracia is the president and chief executive officer of Trust for America's Health, Washington, DC.

See also Ultraprocessed Food, pp. 898–1029.

Research has shown that consuming ultraprocessed food (UPF) is associated with a variety of adverse health outcomes. These findings have garnered significant attention, prompting news headlines, public concern, and policy action across the country and globe. In 2025, Trust for America's Health's longstanding annual report, *The State of Obesity: Better Policies for a Healthier America* (https://bit.ly/3RnnTVC), included a feature section on emerging science and policy considerations for UPF. Broader policies to improve the food environment—in addition to those focused on UPF—will be a key component of addressing the health impacts of poor nutrition. Thoughtful and considered approaches to these policies will be essential for improving the health of all Americans.

Ultraprocessed food is part of the larger food environment in the United States that influences dietary patterns. Beyond the high consumption of UPF, Americans consume about one third of their calories in food prepared away from home and do not consume enough fruits and vegetables.[1] These dietary patterns involve factors that go beyond individual choices. The availability, accessibility, affordability, and palatability of food in a community significantly influence dietary patterns, and these factors are affected by local, state, and federal policies.[2] With the growing attention on UPF, it is critical that policymakers take a comprehensive approach that considers how decades of underinvestment in the systems, community conditions, policies, and programs that influence health and nutrition drive food insecurity, UPF consumption, and poor health outcomes.

STRUCTURAL BARRIERS TO NUTRITION

Cost and convenience are major barriers to healthy eating. A 2023 Cleveland Clinic poll found that the most commonly reported barriers to a healthier diet were the expense of healthy food, a lack of time to prepare healthy meals, and unfamiliarity with healthy cooking methods.[3] Comparatively, UPF is less expensive, is shelf stable, is hyperpalatable, and requires limited or no preparation. Food insecurity and continued price inflation, including a 3.1% increase in food prices in 2025, may have exacerbated these issues: as purchasing power decreases and budgets tighten, prices and shelf life become increasingly important to individuals.[4]

Structural and systemic barriers to healthy eating are present in cities, towns, and rural areas across the country and often result in Americans eating more UPF. Chicago, Illinois, provides one example of policy and environmental factors shaping nutrition options, reinforcing consumption of UPF, and contributing to health disparities. Chicago's North and South Sides have disparate demographics, food access, and health outcomes. In South Side neighborhoods—with predominantly Black residents and decades of underinvestment—99% of residents in some neighborhoods live more than a half mile from a grocery store, more than 500 000 South Side residents experience food insecurity, and type 2 diabetes rates are 80% higher than in the city as a whole.[5–7]

Food insecurity is not limited to urban communities. West Virginia, where nearly half of residents live in rural areas, has one of the highest food insecurity rates (13%) in the nation. Food insecurity is even worse in the southern parts of the state. Mingo and McDowell Counties together have only five full-service grocery stores eligible for the Supplemental Nutrition Assistance Program and the Special Supplemental Nutrition Program for Women, Infants, and Children. These counties also have the state's lowest per capita income and significantly higher rates of overall food insecurity (23%) and youth food insecurity (30%) than the rest of the state.[8] These counties also have the state's highest prevalence of diabetes and relatively high rates of obesity.[9]

AJPH July 2026, Vol. 116, No. 7

POLICY RESPONSES TO ULTRAPROCESSED FOOD

Chicago and West Virginia also model promising approaches to reducing food insecurity inequities and improving the food environment. Both areas have widely adopted the Community Eligibility Provision (https://www.fns.usda.gov/cn/cep), allowing schools to offer free school meals to all students in communities with disproportionately low incomes. This reduces social stigma, improves children's access to healthy food, and reduces families' grocery bills. The Greater Chicago Food Depository and the Urban Growers Collective, Chicago nonprofit organizations, are engaging in community-driven solutions, such as meal delivery to older adults and individuals with disabilities and converting unused lots into urban farms, to improve access to healthy food options.

New UPF policies could have widespread implications, as more than half of the total daily calories consumed in the United States are from UPF. Although no federal statutes or regulations define or regulate UPF specifically, there has been recent movement. The US Department of Health and Human Services, the Food and Drug Administration, and the US Department of Agriculture issued a request for information in July 2025 to help develop a uniform definition of UPF, and the new *Dietary Guidelines for Americans*, issued in January 2026, recommend that Americans "limit highly processed food."[10(p4)] Other federal policies discussed are focused on restricting the purchase of UPF in nutrition assistance programs.

Efforts to address the food supply, such as regulating UPF and specific additives, have growing bipartisan support, and many new laws and regulations have been adopted at the state level. However, in the absence of a universal definition of UPF, these efforts have varied significantly in scope, further highlighting the broad, potential impact of a universal, science-based definition. Other countries have also instituted policies on UPF, including recommendations in their dietary guidelines, limits for school meals, nutrition package labeling, advertising regulations, and taxation on certain unhealthy UPF.

When developing new policies, it is vital to avoid negative consequences. Policies focused on reducing UPF consumption should ensure that alternative food options are available, affordable, safe, and healthy. Without this consideration, policies could increase food prices, worsen food or nutrition insecurity, lead to less healthy food substitutes, and exacerbate health disparities. For example, efforts to limit UPF in school meals must be accompanied by funding for kitchen equipment for storage and preparation of fresh alternatives. In addition, policy shifts are concurrent with significant cuts to food security programs. The One Big Beautiful Bill Act of 2025 cuts $187 billion from the Supplemental Nutrition Assistance Program over the next decade—a nearly 20% reduction from current funding levels—and shifts additional food and administrative costs to states.[11] The legislation also ended the Supplemental Nutrition Assistance Program-Education program, which provided evidence-based nutrition education.

Parallel to UPF policies and regulations, the public health community and policymakers must continue to build on existing efforts to increase the consumption of healthy, minimally processed food; reduce the consumption of food high in added sugar, sodium, and saturated fat; and ensure access to good nutrition for all. Policy achievements over the past decade include the Department of Agriculture adding a new fruit and vegetable benefit to the Special Supplemental Nutrition Program for Women, Infants, and Children food package and the Food and Drug Administration's redesign of the nutrition facts labels to include added sugars. States and localities have also worked to improve nutrition by increasing access to healthy food (e.g., universal healthy school meals in nine states) and discouraging the consumption of unhealthy food (e.g., sugar-sweetened beverage taxes in nine localities).

Improving nutritional and diet quality in the United States is critical to promoting the health and well-being of Americans, lowering rising health care costs, and reducing health disparities. Poor diet is responsible for 500 000 deaths and $1.1 trillion in additional health care spending and lost productivity costs annually.[12] It is a pivotal moment for advancing and sustaining efforts to improve the nutritional quality of the food supply, remove structural barriers to healthy eating, and work toward a healthier food environment. AJPH

CORRESPONDENCE

Correspondence should be sent to J. Nadine Gracia, Trust for America's Health, 1730 M St, NW, Suite 900, Washington, DC 20036 (e-mail: ngracia@tfah.org). Reprints can be ordered at https://www.ajph.org by clicking the "Reprints" link.

PUBLICATION INFORMATION

Full Citation: Gracia JN. Ultraprocessed food, food insecurity, and improving the food environment for all in the United States. *Am J Public Health*. 2026;116(7):903–905.

Acceptance Date: April 12, 2026.

DOI: https://doi.org/10.2105/AJPH.2026.308588

ORCID iDs:

J. Nadine Gracia https://orcid.org/0009-0009-5389-3715

ACKNOWLEDGMENTS

Special thanks to Molly Warren and Drew Wallace of Trust for America's Health.

CONFLICTS OF INTEREST

The author has no conflicts of interest to disclose.

REFERENCES

1. Wolfson JA, Tucker AC, Leung CW, Rebholz CM, Garcia-Larsen V, Martinez-Steele E. Trends in adults' intake of un-processed/minimally processed, and ultra-processed foods at home and away from home in the United States from 2003–2018. *J Nutr.* 2025;155(1):280–292. https://doi.org/10.1016/j.tjnut.2024.10.048
2. Javed Z, Valero-Elizondo J, Maqsood MH, et al. Social determinants of health and obesity: findings from a national study of US adults. *Obesity (Silver Spring).* 2022;30(2):491–502. https://doi.org/10.1002/oby.23336
3. Cleveland Clinic. Americans cite cost of healthy food as biggest barrier to a heart-healthy diet, according to Cleveland Clinic survey. February 1, 2023. Available at: https://newsroom.clevelandclinic.org/2023/02/01/americans-cite-cost-of-heathy-food-as-biggest-barrier-to-a-heart-healthy-diet-according-to-cleveland-clinic-survey. Accessed January 13, 2026.
4. Bureau of Labor Statistics. Consumer Price Index—April 2026. Available at: https://www.bls.gov/news.release/pdf/cpi.pdf. Accessed May 19, 2026.
5. Chicago Health Atlas. Low food access. Available at: https://chicagohealthatlas.org/indicators/LFA?topic=low-food-access. Accessed May 19, 2026.
6. American Diabetes Association. 2023 Annual report. 2024. Available at: https://diabetes.org/sites/default/files/2024-06/ADA_2023_Annual Report.pdf. Accessed May 19, 2026.
7. Chicago Department of Public Health. Healthy Chicago 2025 data compendium. October 22, 2019. Available at: https://www.chicago.gov/content/dam/city/depts/cdph/CDPH/Healthy_Chicago_2025_Data-Compendium_10222019.pdf. Accessed May 19, 2026.
8. Feeding America. Food insecurity among the child population in West Virginia. Available at: https://map.feedingamerica.org/county/2017/child/west-virginia. Accessed May 19, 2026.
9. County Health Rankings and Roadmaps. West Virginia health data: diabetes prevalence. Available at: https://www.countyhealthrankings.org/health-data/west-virginia?year=2025&measure=Diabetes+Prevalence*. Accessed May 19, 2026.
10. US Department of Agriculture. Dietary guidelines for Americans. January 2026. Available at: https://cdn.realfood.gov/DGA.pdf. Accessed May 22, 2026.
11. Center for Science in the Public Interest. The nation's largest food aid program about to see cuts. November 3, 2025. Available at: https://www.cspi.org/cspi-news/nations-largest-food-aid-program-about-see-cuts-heres-what-know. Accessed May 19, 2026.
12. Nutrition Policy Initiative at Tufts University. Food is medicine. August 2023. Available at: https://tuftsfoodismedicine.org/wp-content/uploads/2023/09/Tufts-Food-is-Medicine-Institute_2023-FIM-Fact-Sheet.pdf. Accessed September 1, 2025.

Litigation as a Necessary Tool to Challenge Food Industry's Toxic Practices

Jennifer L. Pomeranz, JD, MPH, and Kelly D. Brownell, PhD

ABOUT THE AUTHORS

Jennifer L. Pomeranz is with the School of Global Public Health, New York University, New York, NY. Kelly D. Brownell is with the Sanford School of Public Policy, Duke University, Durham, NC.

See also Ultraprocessed Food, pp. 898–1029.

The food environment produces disease at dispiriting rates. Heart disease, cancer, diabetes, obesity, dementia, and Alzheimer's have been linked to consumption of calorie-dense, nutrient-poor, highly processed foods designed in ways that override biology and maximize consumption.

In the face of this crisis is an arresting reality. Despite the proven harm from industry practices, legislative and administrative branches of government default to protecting corporate interests. Decades pass without meaningful action, and the damage to public health can be counted in the millions of lives lost. This reality has occurred with tobacco, automobiles, firearms, fossil fuels, and opioids.[1]

Food follows the same pattern, with government inaction predicted by the tobacco industry script used decades earlier: harms and addictive properties are denied, scientific uncertainty is manufactured through conflicted research, and political influence and revolving doors prevent government action.[2,3] After decades of calls for food industry reform, food industry marketing and processing tactics have raced ahead, unimpeded, and the food environment is worse, much worse.[4–6] What, then, can break the logjam?

Lawsuits initiated by a new and powerful set of actors—state attorneys general and city and county attorneys (collectively referred to as AGs) and plaintiffs' attorneys—are less influenced by industry and have the power to hold industry accountable. This in turn can change public opinion and open the door to beneficial legislative actions.

Food industry lawsuits have begun to emerge, but there is a much greater role for litigation. We provide an overview of litigation in the context of harm-causing products by private plaintiffs—an individual or group who has been harmed—and litigation by AGs to protect public interests. We discuss the emergence of food-related litigation and warn of the potential for preemption (when the federal or state government provides immunity to an industry from being sued).

LITIGATION IN THE CONTEXT OF HARM-CAUSING PRODUCTS

Private litigation has led to key public health victories; for example, successful lawsuits against the automobile industry for failure to include lifesaving airbags preceded federal law requiring them.[7] Although private plaintiffs can bring actions under state consumer protection laws and tort liability (e.g., failure to warn, fraud), they are limited in that most states require an actual injury.[8] Success may produce large settlements, but they may be easily absorbed by industry and infrequently lead to policy or industry changes. Still, when there are provable injuries, monetary damages at least shift the burden from the harmed party to the responsible party.

AGs have broad authorities and powers to protect the public interest that are unavailable to private plaintiffs and other government officials. Unlike private plaintiffs, AGs do not need to prove an injury because their authority is premised on vindicating the public interest.[8] States can recover damages when, for example, health care budgets strain under the cost of treating industry-produced diseases or when unfair or deceptive practices have been used.[9] AGs also have the unique parens patriae (meaning "parent of the country") authority to protect states' interests in the physical and economic health, safety, and welfare of their residents. This was the theory used in the tobacco litigation that led to the 1998 Master Settlement Agreement, under which tobacco companies agreed to limit certain predatory marketing and pay damages to the states.[2]

In the context of harm-causing products, private litigation historically arises first, reflecting a failure of legislators and regulators to address public health and safety issues. Plaintiffs' attorneys help identify and correct industry wrongdoing. Such lawsuits publicize the issue and encourage other injured people to come forward. In the case of tobacco and opioids, individual actions

AJPH July 2026, Vol. 116, No. 7

were initially met with little success (with a few exceptions),[1] but private action can be a necessary precursor to encourage AGs to use their authority and hold harm-causing industries accountable. The most prominent example is tobacco: an initial wave of private lawsuits arguing cigarettes caused harm were unsuccessful. Success occurred when state AGs acted collectively to sue the major tobacco manufacturers, resulting in the Master Settlement Agreement.[2]

FOOD LITIGATION

An initial wave of lawsuits with food has likewise shown mixed and limited success related to false or deceptive labeling claims, such as "natural" and "whole grain."[8] A lawsuit, *Pelman v McDonalds*, filed in 2002 on behalf of two adolescents who claimed that their regular consumption of McDonalds food caused diet-related diseases, was dismissed after years of litigation.[8]

A second wave of food-related litigation is now under way premised on the unique harms of ultraprocessed food (UPF).[4,6] As science evolved to show that UPF is engineered to be overconsumed and that regular consumption leads to long-term health harms,[4,6] comprehensive lawsuits have been filed against the major UPF manufacturers.[10,11] First, a private plaintiff in Pennsylvania sued the major international food companies arguing that he developed diet-related disease from ingesting UPF. The complaint claimed the defendants engineered foods to be addictive, used predatory marketing, and concealed health risks from consumers.[10] This case was dismissed for failure to identify the specific foods that led to harm but may be revised and refiled. However, a groundbreaking 2025 lawsuit was filed by the San Francisco City Attorney against UPF companies, alleging defendants engineered food that harmed consumers, hid the truth from the public, relentlessly promoted these dangerous products, and harmed the city's finances because of the resulting public health crisis.[11] The time is ripe for additional city, county, and state AGs to do the same.

If such concerted action occurs, additional remedies become possible. With the Master Settlement Agreement as precedent, the challenge will be to earmark funds for health-related actions rather than general state use.[2] Settlement funds can be deployed for healthy food initiatives such as produce procurement for schools, evidence-based nutrition programs, and countermarketing campaigns such as the Truth Campaign for tobacco. Moreover, AGs can seek to compel industry actions (e.g., front-of-package warnings, reformulation targets) or prohibit industry from acting (e.g., cease marketing to children, making misleading claims, adding industrial ingredients without independently proven safety and biological/metabolic testing).

PREEMPTION

As litigation increases, industry may respond by seeking immunity. In response to the *Pelman* lawsuit, the National Restaurant Association took a page from the firearm industry playbook and lobbied for federal and state preemption of lawsuits claiming that long-term food consumption is associated with diet-related disease.[12] Twenty-six states passed such preemption laws.[11] Federal and state preemption of firearm litigation had dire implications for public health—providing the firearm industry immunity and dismissing pending lawsuits. This was pivotal because lawsuits led to industry creation of "smart gun" technology: lifesaving innovation that immediately ceased when preemption passed.

Concerns exist that as UPFs—highly profitable products for manufacturers—are targeted, the food industry will again lobby for immunity. This concern is more than theoretical; a federal bill proposed in 2025 aimed to shield infant formula companies from liability following successful private failure-to-warn lawsuits. One can anticipate similar bills being proposed in response to burgeoning litigation against the food industry.

CONCLUSIONS

Food industry lawsuits show great promise in changing industry practices, holding industry accountable for harm, and improving the food environment. The impact would be magnified if multistate AG actions were launched. Such actions can also shed light on industry processing and marketing practices, shift public opinion, thwart preemption efforts, and ultimately help unlock meaningful legislative and regulatory reforms. AJPH

CORRESPONDENCE

Correspondence should be sent to Jennifer L. Pomeranz, School of Global Public Health, New York University, 708 Broadway, New York, NY 10003 (e-mail: jlp284@nyu.edu). Reprints can be ordered at https://www.ajph.org by clicking the "Reprints" link.

PUBLICATION INFORMATION

Full Citation: Pomeranz JL, Brownell KD. Litigation as a necessary tool to challenge food industry's toxic practices. *Am J Public Health*. 2026;116(7): 906–908.

Acceptance Date: March 13, 2026.

DOI: https://doi.org/10.2105/AJPH.2026.308539

ORCID iDs:
Jennifer L. Pomeranz https://orcid.org/0009-0008-6949-763X

Kelly D. Brownell https://orcid.org/0000-0003-4117-726X

CONTRIBUTORS

Both authors contributed to the conceptualization and writing of the editorial.

CONFLICTS OF INTEREST

J. L. Pomeranz reports payments for being an expert witness for plaintiffs in cases against infant formula companies and royalties from Oxford University Press and funding from the National Institutes of Health unrelated to the current work. K. D. Brownell has no conflicts of interest to report.

REFERENCES

1. Pomeranz JL, Merrill TG, Schroth KRJ. *Public Health Law in Practice*. New York, NY: Oxford University Press; 2023.
2. Brandt AM. *The Cigarette Century: The Rise, Fall and Deadly Persistence of the Product That Defined America*. New York, NY: Basic Books; 2009.
3. Brownell KD, Warner KE. The perils of ignoring history: Big Tobacco played dirty and millions died. How similar is Big Food? *Milbank Q*. 2009;87(1):259–294. https://doi.org/10.1111/j.1468-0009.2009.00555.x
4. Gearhardt AN, Brownell KD, Brandt AM. From tobacco to ultraprocessed food: how industry engineering fuels the epidemic of preventable disease. *Milbank Q*. 2026;104(1):76–115. https://doi.org/10.1111/1468-0009.70066
5. Pomeranz JL, Broad Leib EM, Mozaffarian D. Regulation of added substances in the food supply by the Food and Drug Administration Human Foods Program. *Am J Public Health*. 2024;114(10):1061–1070. https://doi.org/10.2105/AJPH.2024.307755
6. Monteiro CA, Louzada ML, Steele-Martinez E, et al. Ultra-processed foods and human health: the main thesis and the evidence. *Lancet*. 2025;406(10520):2667–2684. https://doi.org/10.1016/S0140-6736(25)01565-X
7. Teret SP. Litigating for the public's health. *Am J Public Health*. 1986;76(8):1027–1029. https://doi.org/10.2105/AJPH.76.8.1027
8. Pomeranz JL. Litigation to address misleading food label claims and the role of the state attorneys general. *Regent Univ Law Rev*. 2014;26:421–455.
9. Pomeranz JL, Brownell KD. Advancing public health obesity policy through state attorneys general. *Am J Public Health*. 2011;101(3):425–431. https://doi.org/10.2105/AJPH.2010.198697
10. *Martinez v Kraft Heinz Company, Inc. et al.*, complaint (E.D. Pa, filed December 10, 2024).
11. *People of the State of California v Kraft Heinz Company, Inc., et al.*, complaint (San Francisco Sup Ct, December 2, 2025).
12. Pomeranz JL, Zellers L, Bare M, Pertschuk M. State preemption of food and nutrition policies and litigation: undermining government's role in public health. *Am J Prev Med*. 2019;56(1):47–57. https://doi.org/10.1016/j.amepre.2018.07.027

Beyond the Body: The Ultraprocessed Food Industry's Environmental Toll

Lindsey Smith Taillie, PhD, MPH, Nicholas Chartres, PhD, Kim Anastasiou, PhD, and Joe Yates, MS

ABOUT THE AUTHORS

Lindsey Smith Taillie is with the Department of Nutrition, Gillings School of Global Public Health and Carolina Population Center, University of North Carolina at Chapel Hill. Nicholas Chartres is with the School of Pharmacy, Faculty of Medicine & Health, The University of Sydney, Australia, and The Center to End Corporate Harm, University of California, San Francisco. Kim Anastasiou is with the Charles Perkins Centre and Sydney School of Public Health, Faculty of Medicine and Health, University of Sydney, New South Wales, Australia. Joe Yates is with the Faculty of Epidemiology and Population Health, London School of Hygiene and Tropical Medicine, London, United Kingdom.

See also Ultraprocessed Food, pp. 898–1029.

Growing evidence documents the pathways through which the ultraprocessed food (UPF) industry engineers, prices, and aggressively markets its products for profit, creating poor-quality diets linked to chronic disease. In response, the public health community has focused on the consequences of UPF consumption for human health. However, such approaches overlook a central dimension: the production of UPFs creates an extensive environmental footprint, including pollution, biodiversity loss, and greenhouse gas emissions. These harms occur as a result of the substances used to make UPFs and because most UPFs are nonessential, requiring additional environmental resources beyond what is needed for human health. These harms trigger cascading ecological, health, social, and economic consequences. To promote sustainable, healthy food systems, research and policy efforts should adopt an integrated framework that addresses both the environmental and health costs of UPFs.

PLASTICS: A MAJOR ROLE

The modern UPF system is inseparable from plastics, forming a mutually reinforcing cycle in which plastic packaging enables UPF expansion and UPF production accelerates plastic pollution. Plastics, especially single-use plastics, enable the scale, speed, and profitability of UPF production. By providing low cost, lightweight, and effective barriers to oxygen, moisture, and light, plastics enable long shelf lives, centralized mass production, and global distribution. Single-use plastics further promote consumption through individual-use, portable, and microwavable packages while supporting aggressive on-pack branding. Because the environmental and waste management costs of plastics are externalized to municipalities and ecosystems, these materials effectively subsidize the UPF industry, allowing it to scale rapidly, underprice fresh foods, and normalize frequent consumption.[1]

UPF-linked plastic pollution is a major source of harm. UPF corporations such as Coca Cola, PepsiCo, Danone, and Unilever are top global plastic polluters.[2] Plastics are derived almost exclusively from fossil fuels, whose extraction and production create toxic emissions disproportionately affecting fence-line communities and indigenous people.[3] More than 16 000 chemicals have been found in plastics, with 25% known to be hazardous[4] and more than 10 000 chemicals lacking official hazard classifications. Pervasive UPF litter creates macroplastics that clog sanitation systems and micro- and nano-plastic particles that accumulate in soil, water, the atmosphere, humans, and animals.

To manage plastic waste, millions undertake open burning, generating greenhouse gas emissions and air pollution. Even formal waste management systems—recycling and landfills—are ineffective: only 9% of all plastic waste is recycled once and less than 1% is recycled twice,[5] with these processes generating toxic secondary materials.[6] After decades of promoting recycling, the UPF industry and its petrochemical partners now face growing public scrutiny and litigation for misleading claims that recycling single-use plastic bottles offsets environmental damage.[7]

ADDITIONAL ENVIRONMENTAL HARMS

UPFs cause environmental harm across their supply chain. UPF production relies on cheap commodity inputs and is partly responsible for driving demand for intensive agricultural practices including monocultures, heavy tillage, and industrial meat production systems, which are reliant on fossil fuels

AJPH July 2026, Vol. 116, No. 7

for machinery, fertilizers, and pesticides, contributing to soil degradation. Data from Australia, France, Ireland, Sweden, and the Netherlands indicate that UPFs are responsible for 17% to 39% of diet-related energy use; 36% to 45% of diet-related biodiversity loss; up to one third of diet-related greenhouse gas emissions, land use, and food waste; and up to one quarter of diet-related water use.[8]

Although not unique to UPFs, these impacts are largely avoidable because UPFs are not necessary for human functioning or health and many could be removed from diets without replacement. Engineered and marketed for overconsumption, UPFs increase avoidable food production using ecosystem resources otherwise not required.[8] UPFs are also linked to land degradation, agrobiodiversity loss, eutrophication, and acidification, and likely to desertification, reducing long-term farmland availability.[8,9] These harms are unequally distributed: the Global South produces much of the UPF commodity base (approximately 60% of global exports of oils, fats, and sugar),[10] creating local ecosystem damage while profits flow to transnational corporations.[11]

THE COST OF INACTION

Despite increasing calls to reduce the UPF industry's environmental harms, to date little progress has been made. Most countries participating in the ongoing negotiations after the United Nations resolution 5/14 to "End Plastic Pollution: Toward an International Legally Binding Instrument" favor a "global plastics pollution treaty" addressing pollution at every stage of the plastic life cycle. However, progress is being inhibited by oil-, gas- and plastic-producing countries and industry groups advocating for a treaty focused on waste management and recycling, an approach that magnifies the harm of plastics via recirculation of the toxic chemicals they are made from and the release of microplastics.[1] The UPF industry leverages recycling claims as a competitive advantage to drive consumer loyalty despite established evidence of the harms of both recycled and biobased food packaging.[12]

Other greenwashing strategies abound, such as Coca Cola's recently launched "reverse vending machine" program that provides Scottish university students with canteen food credits for returning used bottles and cans. Such corporate social responsibility tactics are effectively a public relations ploy that positions corporations as sustainability leaders while failing to reduce the environmental harms of UPFs; plastics cannot be recycled safely because of their chemical composition and contributions to microplastic exposure.[1,12]

These solutions are UPF strategies used by companies to frame themselves as "part of the solution" for health through voluntary initiatives (e.g., marketing restrictions, front-of-package labels, reformulation) that make their portfolios appear healthier, improve their public image, and help them evade more substantial governmental intervention despite such initiatives having little impact on exposure or consumption.[13] As with health, failure to enact governmental regulations will allow UPF companies to continue to use these tactics to mislead consumers about the true environmental and health costs while continually perpetuating harms.

TOWARD AN INTEGRATED POLICY FRAMEWORK

To hold the UPF industry accountable and promote health and environmental cobenefits, we recommend an integrated approach based on the precautionary principle, which requires that the UPF industry demonstrate product safety for health and assumes harm (rather than safety) in the absence of proof. Specific recommendations include the following:

1. The public health community must raise public awareness of the UPF industry's environmental exploitation and the cumulative burden of disease caused by UPF consumption and production.
2. Scientists and regulators must identify and assess all negative externalities of UPFs to inform the public and policymakers of the true costs while not delaying immediate health-protective action.
3. Governments must implement extended producer responsibility and other "polluter pays principle" policies to reduce harms caused by environmental harm via increased UPF industry liability and must impose taxes and fees based on the volume produced and the recyclability of products.
4. Governments must implement policies aimed at directly reducing the use of single-use plastics, including taxes on products that can be used to mitigate and prevent their environmental harms.
5. Governments must ban UPF companies from marketing the health or nutrient benefits of their products as well as making sustainability claims.
6. Governments must implement warning labels on products that document not only the health but the environmental harms of UPFs.

CONCLUSION

Treating UPFs as both a public health and an environmental threat is no longer optional. Safeguarding planetary health requires an integrated, upstream package of policies that confront the UPF industry's full health, social, and ecological costs. AJPH

CORRESPONDENCE

Correspondence should be sent to Lindsey Smith Taillie, PhD, MPH, Carolina Population Center, University of North Carolina at Chapel Hill, CB# 8120 Carolina Square, Suite 210, 123 W Franklin St, Chapel Hill, NC 27516 (e-mail: taillie@unc.edu). Reprints can be ordered at https://www.ajph.org by clicking the "Reprints" link.

PUBLICATION INFORMATION

Full Citation: Taillie LS, Chartres N, Anastasiou K, Yates J. Beyond the body: the ultraprocessed food industry's environmental toll. *Am J Public Health*. 2026;116(7):909–911.

Acceptance Date: February 26, 2026

DOI: https://doi.org/10.2105/AJPH.2026.308525

ORCID iD:

Kim Anastasiou https://orcid.org/0000-0002-3338-5117

CONTRIBUTORS

L. Smith Taillie and N. Chartres generated the idea for the editorial. L. Smith Taillie prepared the initial draft and outline and contributed to the final editing. All of the authors contributed to the writing and editing of the article.

CONFLICTS OF INTEREST

Nicholas Chartres has received income from educational modules on nutrition, including ultraprocessed foods.

REFERENCES

1. Yates J, Kadiyala S, Deeney M, et al. A toxic relationship: ultra-processed foods and plastics. *Global Health.* 2024;20(1):74. https://doi.org/10.1186/s12992-024-01078-0
2. Cowger W, Willis KA, Bullock S, et al. Global producer responsibility for plastic pollution. *Sci Adv.* 2024;10(17):eadj8275. https://doi.org/10.1126/sciadv.adj8275
3. Human Rights Council. The imperative of defossilizing our economies. Available at: https://www.ohchr.org/en/documents/thematic-reports/ahrc5942-imperative-defossilizing-our-economies-report-special. Accessed January 8, 2026.
4. Monclús L, Arp HPH, Groh KJ, et al. Mapping the chemical complexity of plastics. *Nature.* 2025;643(8071):349–355. https://doi.org/10.1038/s41586-025-09184-8
5. Geyer R, Jambeck JR, Law KL. Production, use, and fate of all plastics ever made. *Sci Adv.* 2017;3(7):e1700782. https://doi.org/10.1126/sciadv.1700782
6. Carney-Almroth B, Carmona E, Chukwuone N, Dey T. Addressing the toxic chemicals problem in plastics recycling. Available at: https://www-cambridge-org.libproxy.lib.unc.edu/core/journals/cambridge-prisms-plastics/article/addressing-the-toxic-chemicals-problem-in-plastics-recycling/552E550968DC2E0119DB937925505DC6. Accessed January 8, 2026.
7. County of Los Angeles. LA County sues Pepsi and Coca-Cola over plastic beverage pollution and deceiving public on plastic recycling. Available at: https://lacounty.gov/2024/10/30/la-county-sues-pepsi-and-coca-cola-over-plastic-beverage-pollution-and-deceiving-public-on-plastic-recycling. Accessed January 8, 2026.
8. Anastasiou K, Baker P, Hadjikakou M, Hendrie GA, Lawrence M. A conceptual framework for understanding the environmental impacts of ultra-processed foods and implications for sustainable food systems. *J Clean Prod.* 2022;368:133155. https://doi.org/10.1016/j.jclepro.2022.133155
9. Mirzabaev A, Stringer L, Benjaminsen T, Gonzalez P. Desertification. Available at: https://www.ipcc.ch/srccl/chapter/chapter-3. Accessed January 8, 2026.
10. Food and Agriculture Organization of the United Nations. Agricultural trade in the Global South. Available at: https://www.fao.org/family-farming/detail/en/c/1648805. Accessed January 8, 2026.
11. Goyal M, Hickel J, Jha P. Increasing inequality in agri-food value chains: global trends from 1995–2020. *Glob Food Secur.* 2025;46:100883. https://doi.org/10.1016/j.gfs.2025.100883
12. Ataman D. The packaging advantage: how recyclability drives consumer loyalty. Available at: https://www.foodnavigator-usa.com/Article/2025/12/03/why-recyclable-packaging-drives-consumer-loyalty. Accessed January 8, 2026.
13. Lacy-Nichols J, Williams O. "Part of the solution": food corporation strategies for regulatory capture and legitimacy. *Int J Health Policy Manag.* 2021;10(12):845–856. https://doi.org/10.34172/ijhpm.2021.111

The Politics of Ultraprocessed Foods: Dietary Guidelines for Americans

Marion Nestle, PhD, MPH

ABOUT THE AUTHOR

Marion Nestle is with the Department of Nutrition and Food Studies, New York University, New York, NY.

See also Ultraprocessed Food, pp. 898–1029.

AJPH July 2026, Vol. 116, No. 7

On January 7, 2026, the Trump administration's Departments of Health and Human Services (HHS) and Agriculture (USDA) jointly released the 2025–2030 Dietary Guidelines for Americans (https://cdn.realfood.gov/DGA.pdf). For the first time since they were established in 1980, these called for "a dramatic reduction in highly processed foods laden with refined carbohydrates, added sugars, excess sodium, unhealthy fats, and chemical additives." The actual guideline, one of eight, says "Limit highly processed foods, added sugars, & refined carbohydrates."

Although these statements do not use the term "ultraprocessed," that is clearly what they mean. The guidelines are based on a commissioned scientific foundation report that refers repeatedly to ultraprocessed foods and cites major studies of their health effects.[1] Those studies, largely observational, used the Nova classification system to divide foods into four categories based on their degree of processing: unprocessed or minimally processed (Nova 1), processed culinary ingredients (Nova 2), processed (Nova 3), and ultraprocessed (Nova 4).[2] The scientific foundation report notes three reasons for avoiding the Nova 4 term: no consensus definition of "ultraprocessed" exists, defining refined starches and sugars as Nova 2 underestimates dietary intake of Nova 4 foods, and the Nova system classifies some nutrient-dense foods as ultraprocessed. On this basis, the guidelines use "highly processed" as a euphemism.

Even so, the very mention of processing in the US dietary guidelines must be considered an important forward step. In advising limits on highly processed foods, HHS and USDA reversed the decision made by the Biden administration's Dietary Guidelines Advisory Committee (DGAC). That committee judged the category of ultraprocessed to be too ambiguously defined, and the observational evidence for its harm to health too subject to error, to warrant an "eat less" recommendation.[3] I view this decision as overly cautious. Yes, observational studies can only demonstrate association, not causation, but of more than 100 studies of ultraprocessed diets and health, nearly all found such diets to increase risks for chronic disease and overall mortality.[2]

Furthermore, the DGAC excluded consideration of the one exceptionally well-controlled randomized clinical trial available at the time. The participants in that study were housed in a metabolic ward—they could not lie or cheat about what they were eating—and given a diet of either minimally processed or nutritionally comparable ultraprocessed foods. The study results were unexpected and dramatic; the participants consumed an average of 500 calories a day more on the ultraprocessed diet, without realizing it.[4] The DGAC eliminated this trial from consideration because it had set criteria for inclusion that required studies to last longer and involve more participants.[5] I thought the DGAC should have made an exception for this trial; metabolic ward studies are enormously expensive and few human volunteers are willing to be locked in one for more than a few weeks.

At issue is the preponderance of research; scientists can interpret it differently. The Trump administration's commissioned research review found "robust and consistent adverse associations between HPF [highly processed food] consumption and a broad range of chronic health outcomes, often in a dose–response fashion," and concluded that "the current evidence base provides a strong rationale for immediate action at the individual, population, institutional, and policy levels."[6] Many researchers and nutrition professionals, including me, agree with this assessment.[7]

This guideline is new, but most of the other 2025 dietary guidelines are consistent with long-standing scientific consensus on the benefits of eating more vegetables, fruits, and whole grains, and limiting intake of added sugars, sodium, and alcohol, although they call for greater restriction of sugars and less precise (vague) restriction of alcohol. The guidelines sharply diverge from consensus in recommending a doubling of protein—a euphemism for meat—and in not emphasizing plant foods more strongly. They promote greater intake of meat along with full-fat dairy, butter, and beef tallow, but inconsistently limit saturated fat to 10% of calories.

The agencies' fact sheet makes the politics explicit; it uses the word "evangelizing." Its major point: previous governments have lied to you about dietary risks, and you need to take personal responsibility for what you eat. In doing so, the guidelines reject concerns about health equity—and, therefore, policies that might address social determinants of health—as deserving of consideration.[8] Despite promises that the guidelines would be free of conflicts of interest, four of the nine writers of the research reviews report financial ties to meat and dairy industry groups, and three more disclose ties to other food industries.[3] The conflicted interests and emphasis on animal-based foods make these guidelines appear to have been captured by the meat and dairy industries.[9]

I cannot determine whether these guidelines were influenced more by corporate capture or by the personal ideologies of the agency secretaries; they, after all, selected the individuals who wrote the research reviews and are responsible for what the guidelines say. I also do not know how even "highly processed" made it into the guidelines in the face of what surely must have been intense food industry opposition. The food industry, joined by some nutrition scientists, much prefers guidelines based on nutrient content: sugar, salt, fat. Doing so permits the few frequently cited nutrient-dense Nova 4 products—some whole wheat breads, yogurts, and power bars, and plant-based meats—to be considered processed, not ultraprocessed.

Critics of the ultraprocessed concept endlessly invoke the same arguments: there is no scientific consensus on the meaning of the term, and the concept risks undermining "established, evidence-based nutrition strategies," thereby shifting "the focus away from the most important thing about food which is the nutrition aspect."[10] But thoughtful rebuttals to these arguments note that food misclassifications do not appear to change study conclusions; well-controlled clinical trials have now been repeated with similar, biologically plausible results; the mechanisms of action of ultraprocessed foods are under study; and even "healthy" ultraprocessed foods induce greater calorie consumption.[1]

Behind food industry arguments is the enormous profitability of ultraprocessed products. Indeed, the very purpose of ultraprocessing is profit maximization—using low-cost ingredients to create irresistible and long-lasting products—so much so that this goal is built into its Nova definition.[1,8] The food industry's objection to the inclusion of processing as a consideration in dietary guidelines comes down to this: eating less is bad for business.

The call for limits on ultraprocessed foods may be groundbreaking in US dietary guidelines, but in 2015, Brazil issued guidelines that included advice to "Make natural or minimally processed foods the basis of your diet."[11] Unlike US guidelines. these were based on the idea that healthy diets should derive from socially and environmentally sustainable food systems. This is a major conceptual difference from the US approach, which emphasizes personal responsibility above everything else.

When individuals are deemed entirely responsible for their own dietary intake, government policies need focus only on education. If objections to the guidelines from the food industry have been mild so far, it is surely because its leaders know that education is not enough to change dietary behavior. They much prefer education to policies aimed at regulating product contents and marketing. But to really help people reduce intake of ultraprocessed foods, we need a wide range of policy options—taxes, subsidies, marketing, procurement, product placement[12]—aimed at making healthier foods more available, accessible, and affordable. AJPH

CORRESPONDENCE

Correspondence should be sent to Marion Nestle, Department of Nutrition and Food Studies, New York University, New York NY 10003 (e-mail: marion.nestle@nyu.edu). Reprints can be ordered at https://www.ajph.org by clicking the "Reprints" link.

PUBLICATION INFORMATION

Full Citation: Nestle M. The politics of ultraprocessed foods: dietary guidelines for Americans. *Am J Public Health*. 2026;116(7):912–914.

Acceptance Date: March 8, 2026

DOI: https://doi.org/10.2105/AJPH.2026.308530

ORCID iD:

Marion Nestle https://orcid.org/0000-0001-8700-6963

CONFLICTS OF INTEREST

Marion Nestle earns honoraria from lectures and royalties from books about the politics of food.

REFERENCES

1. US Dept of Health and Human Services and US Dept of Agriculture. The scientific foundation for the dietary guidelines for Americans, 2025–2030. Available at: https://cdn.realfood.gov/Scientific%20Report.pdf. Accessed March 4, 2026.
2. Monteiro CA, Louzada ML, Steele-Martinez E, et al. Ultra-processed foods and human health: the main thesis and the evidence. *Lancet.* 2025; 406(10520):2667–2684. https://doi.org/10.1016/S0140-6736(25)01565-X
3. US Dept of Health and Human Services and US Dept of Agriculture. Scientific Report of the 2025 Dietary Guidelines Advisory Committee. December

2024. Available at: https://www.dietaryguidelines.gov/2025-advisory-committee-report. Accessed April 3, 2026.

4. Hall KD, Ayuketah A, Brychta R, et al. Ultra-processed diets cause excess calorie intake and weight gain: an inpatient randomized controlled trial of ad libitum food intake. *Cell Metab.* 2019; 30(1):67–77.e3. https://doi.org/10.1016/j.cmet.2019.05.008
5. LaMotte S. They're up to 70% of the American diet. But the US has no policy on ultraprocessed foods. *CNN Health.* November 22, 2024. Available at: https://www.cnn.com/2024/11/22/health/ultraprocessed-food-us-dietary-guidelines-wellness. Accessed February 27, 2026.
6. Goran M. The Scientific Foundation for the Dietary Guidelines for Americans: Appendices. Appendix 4.1: highly processed foods & health. US Dept of Health and Human Services and US Dept of Agriculture. January 7, 2026. Available at: https://cdn.realfood.gov/Scientific%20Report%20Appendices.pdf. Accessed April 3, 2026.
7. Baker P, Slater S, White M, et al. Towards unified global action on ultra-processed foods: understanding commercial determinants, countering corporate power, and mobilising a public health response. *Lancet.* 2025;406(10520):2703–2726. https://doi.org/10.1016/S0140-6736(25)01567-3
8. US Dept of Health and Human Services and US Dept of Agriculture. Fact sheet: Trump administration resets US nutrition policy, puts real food back at the center of health. January 7, 2026. Available at: https://www.hhs.gov/press-room/fact-sheet-historic-reset-federal-nutrition-policy.html. Accessed February 27, 2026.
9. Neves FS, Nilson EAF, Mendes LL, et al. The 2025–2030 US Dietary Guidelines: an analysis of scientific integrity and global health governance. *Lancet Reg Health Am.* 2026;56:101402. https://doi.org/10.1016/j.lana.2026.101402
10. Food Navigator—Europe. Industry takes aim at Lancet's deadly UPF report. November 20, 2025. Available at: https://www.foodnavigator.com/Article/2025/11/20/lancet-upf-report-sparks-industry-pushback-over-policy-and-evidence-gaps/#:~:text=Most%20question%20the%20scientific%20basis,clarity%20instead%20of%20damning%20reports. Accessed February 27, 2026.
11. Brazil Ministry of Health. Dietary guidelines for the Brazilian population. 2015. Available at: https://bvsms.saude.gov.br/bvs/publicacoes/dietary_guidelines_brazilian_population.pdf. Accessed February 27, 2026.
12. Scrinis G, Popkin BM, Corvalan C, et al. Policies to halt and reverse the rise in ultra-processed food production, marketing, and consumption. *Lancet.* 2025;406(10520):2685–2702. https://doi.org/10.1016/S0140-6736(25)01566-1

Food Environment Policies to Address the Market Power of Ultraprocessed Food Corporations

Gyorgy Scrinis, PhD

ABOUT THE AUTHOR

The author is with the School of Agriculture, Food and Ecosystem Sciences, Faculty of Science, University of Melbourne, Melbourne, Australia.

See also Ultraprocessed Food, pp. 898–1029.

Ultraprocessed foods (UPFs) are beginning to dominate dietary patterns around the world and to displace minimally processed and freshly prepared foods and meals from many people's diets. A growing body of evidence has implicated diets high in UPFs with a range of poor health outcomes.[1] The central role of the large packaged and fast-food corporations in driving the production, distribution, and consumption of UPFs has also been demonstrated in the public health and food systems literature.[2]

However, the food environment policies introduced for addressing the quality and consumption of processed foods in many countries have not been designed to substantially reduce the production and consumption of UPFs or to address the power of corporations driving their production and consumption.[3] These policies include front-of-pack labeling, food and beverage taxes, restrictions on marketing to children, and the availability of these products in schools. Here I highlight two important limitations of many of these policies.

First, despite the growing consensus around the concept of UPFs, these policies define and identify the products requiring regulation primarily in terms of their nutrient composition and mainly target foods high in fats, sugars, and salt (i.e., HFSS foods). This nutrient focus enables food companies to nutritionally reformulate these products by substituting single ingredients, yet the reformulated products typically remain extensively processed.[4] Large corporations are well equipped to respond to and benefit from—and have in fact invented and driven—this reformulation agenda.[5]

Second, these food environment policies are designed to regulate discrete HFSS foods one product at a time rather than addressing these products as part of a group, class, brand, or portfolio of products. In targeting discrete products and marketing practices, these policies are agnostic as to who produces, retails, and markets the products. These policies thereby treat all producers and retailers of HFSS foods and UPFs alike and ignore the structural role that corporations play in driving their consumption. Such one-product-at-a-time policies are therefore unlikely to facilitate more substantial changes and improvements in population dietary patterns.

Many of these food environment policies also continue to ultimately place the responsibility on consumers to make the appropriate "healthy choices." There are, however, ways in which these same policies can be redesigned and extended so as not only to directly target UPFs—as many experts are now proposing—but to also directly target the product portfolios, brands, strategies, and power of UPF corporations.[3]

UPF corporations are defined here as large national and transnational companies in the packaged, fast-food, and retail sectors for which the majority of their food and beverage portfolios consist of UPF/HFSS products and brands or that control a significant market share of subcategories of UPF/HFSS products. I refer to the UPF products manufactured and sold by these corporations as "corporate-UPF" products. The corporate-UPF category is a means of socializing the otherwise technical operational definition of UPFs and of integrating the technological and political–economic dimensions of UPF products and systems.[6]

Rather than approaching UPF corporations as if they were simply very large commercial enterprises, the distinct character and forms of power embedded in these corporations need to be understood and addressed. Since the early 20th century, these corporations have pioneered and shaped the development of UPF products; developed sophisticated distribution, packaging, and marketing strategies; and transformed food environments and national and global food systems to

AJPH July 2026, Vol. 116, No. 7

enable the production and distribution of these products.[2,5]

The rise of UPF production and consumption, as well as the very poor nutritional composition of most UPF products, is a direct result of the market power of these corporations and of the power imbalances between the corporations and other food producers and consumers. This argument is partially supported by a European study showing that higher levels of corporate market share of food and beverage markets correlate with higher levels of HFSS and UPF consumption in those markets.[7] Any attempt to arrest the growth of UPF consumption should target these primary structural drivers, not just the intermediate food environment drivers of consumption. The market concentration of these corporations has also strengthened their political power and influence over many governments' food policies, which has thereby restricted and shaped the kinds of policies that have been introduced to date.[2,8,9]

Food environment policies can be designed to directly and differentially address the power, products, and practices of UPF corporations within food environments, with the aim of reducing their power and influence. Two such policy approaches are proposed here.

One approach is to differentially or exclusively target and regulate the corporate-UPF products and practices of large UPF corporations. This may entail applying regulations only to these large corporations or applying stronger regulatory measures to these corporations in comparison with those applied to other producers and retailers of HFSS or UPF products. For example, front-of-pack labeling, marketing restrictions, and taxes can be applied only to the HFSS or UPF products and marketing practices of large corporations, or, alternatively, stronger regulations (e.g., higher sugar taxes) can be applied to the foods and beverages produced by these corporations than to the more or less identical products manufactured or sold by smaller companies. The aim of these differential policies would be to directly challenge some of the power imbalances between corporations and other food producers rather than targeting only the end products of these power imbalances.

There are few existing policies that aim to differentially target and penalize large food corporations. However, the UK government has recently announced its intention to monitor the nutritional quality of total food sales and set mandatory targets for all large food companies and supermarkets.[10]

A second and complementary policy approach would be to regulate the entire portfolios and marketing practices of UPF corporations.[3] A key market strategy of these corporations is to design, manufacture, distribute, and market their portfolios of brands and products systematically and as a single unit. Their corporate portfolios account for a large proportion of the UPFs consumed and therefore a substantial proportion of the dietary patterns of high-UPF consumers. These corporations also tend to focus their retail and marketing strategies at the level of brands and not just on specific products.[11]

For these reasons, policy responses should shift to the entire portfolios of products of corporations and brands, such that the portfolio or brand becomes the unit of regulation, rather than regulating one product at a time. These brands and portfolios can be monitored for their overall quality, such as in terms of nutrient profile or proportion of UPFs relative to total sales.[12] Those portfolios found to be of poor overall quality could then be collectively subject to regulatory penalties and restrictions, including their better-quality products. For example, food and beverage tax or marketing restrictions could be levied directly on the entire portfolio of a corporation or a brand rather than on only specific HFSS or UPF products.

Given that UPF corporations have already transformed food environments and food systems in ways that support their interests, there is ultimately a need to redesign food systems so that they empower other food producers, retailers, and consumers to produce, distribute, and consume better-quality and freshly prepared processed foods and meals.[3] AJPH

CORRESPONDENCE

Correspondence should be sent to Gyorgy Scrinis, PhD, School of Agriculture, Food and Ecosystem Sciences, Faculty of Science, University of Melbourne, Melbourne, Australia (e-mail: gyorgys@unimelb.edu.au). Reprints can be ordered at https://www.ajph.org by clicking the "Reprints" link.

PUBLICATION INFORMATION

Full Citation: Scrinis G. Food environment policies to address the market power of ultraprocessed food corporations. *Am J Public Health*. 2026; 116(7):915–917.

Acceptance Date: March 30, 2026

DOI: https://doi.org/10.2105/AJPH.2026.308570

ORCID iD:

Gyorgy Scrinis https://orcid.org/0000-0003-3897-4778

CONFLICTS OF INTEREST

The author has no conflicts of interest to declare.

REFERENCES

1. Monteiro CA, Louzada ML, Steele-Martinez E, et al. Ultra-processed foods and human health: the main thesis and the evidence. *Lancet.* 2025; 406(10520):2667–2684. https://doi.org/10.1016/S0140-6736(25)01565-X
2. Baker P, Slater S, White M, et al. Towards unified global action on ultra-processed foods: understanding commercial determinants, countering corporate power, and mobilising a public health

response. *Lancet.* 2025;406(10520):2703–2726. https://doi.org/10.1016/S0140-6736(25)01567-3

3. Scrinis G, Popkin BM, Corvalan C, et al. Policies to halt and reverse the rise in ultra-processed food production, marketing, and consumption. *Lancet.* 2025;406(10520):2685–2702. https://doi.org/10.1016/S0140-6736(25)01566-1
4. Scrinis G, Monteiro CA. Ultra-processed foods and the limits of product reformulation. *Public Health Nutr.* 2018;21(1):247–252. https://doi.org/10.1017/S1368980017001392
5. Scrinis G. Reformulation, fortification and functionalization: big food corporations' nutritional engineering and marketing strategies. *J Peasant Stud.* 2016;43(1):17–37. https://doi.org/10.1080/03066150.2015.1101455
6. Scrinis G, Monteiro C. From ultra-processed foods to ultra-processed dietary patterns. *Nat Food.* 2022;3(9):671–673. https://doi.org/10.1038/s43016-022-00599-4
7. Van Dam I, Allais O, Vandevijvere S. Market concentration and the healthiness of packaged food and non-alcoholic beverage sales across the European single market. *Public Health Nutr.* 2022;25(11):3131–3136. https://doi.org/10.1017/s1368980022001926
8. Clapp J, Vriezen R, Laila A, et al. Corporate concentration and power matter for agency in food systems. *Food Policy.* 2025/07/01/ 2025;134: 102897. https://doi.org/10.1016/j.foodpol.2025.102897
9. Mialon M, da Silva Gomes F. Public health and the ultra-processed food and drink products industry: corporate political activity of major transnationals in Latin America and the Caribbean. *Public Health Nutr.* 2019;22(10):1898–1908. https://doi.org/10.1017/s1368980019000417
10. UK government. Fit for the Future: 10 year health plan for England. 2025. Available at: https://www.gov.uk/government/publications/10-year-health-plan-for-england-fit-for-the-future
11. Boyland E, Davies N, Wilton M, et al. Impact of food, beverage, and alcohol brand marketing on consumptive behaviors and health in children and adults: a systematic review and meta-analysis. *Obes Rev.* 2025;26(9):e13932. https://doi.org/10.1111/obr.13932
12. Bandy L, Jewell J, Luick M, et al. The development of a method for the global health community to assess the proportion of food and beverage companies' sales that are derived from unhealthy foods. *Global Health.* 2023;19(1):94. https://doi.org/10.1186/s12992-023-00992-z

Practical and Equity Considerations for Ultraprocessed Foods Policies

Julia A. Wolfson, PhD, MPP

ABOUT THE AUTHOR

Julia A. Wolfson is with the Department of International Health and the Department of Health Policy and Management, Johns Hopkins Bloomberg School of Public Health, Baltimore, MD.

See also Ultraprocessed Food, pp. 898–1029.

AJPH July 2026, Vol. 116, No. 7

Ultraprocessed foods (UPFs), industrially processed food and beverage products that contain ingredients and additives with little to no culinary use,[1] have become the subject of widespread public health concern. UPFs dominate the food supply[2] and make up the majority of food intake among children, adolescents, and adults in the United States.[3,4] A robust and growing body of evidence shows adverse associations between UPF intake and numerous health outcomes, including obesity, diabetes, cardiovascular disease, and cancer.[5] Although the precise mechanisms through which UPFs affect health are not yet fully understood, given current evidence, policies to reduce UPF intake are warranted. However, to be successful, policies must consider and address societal and behavioral determinants of UPF consumption, including the time and cognitive burden related to procuring and preparing minimally processed foods.

In many respects, the food industry has followed the tobacco industry's playbook by designing UPFs that intentionally promote overconsumption, are heavily marketed, and are widely available. A strong public health response to confront food industry power is required to address UPFs and their role in the food system. However, UPFs are different from tobacco in that we can't "just say no." Unlike smoking, we must eat. Avoiding UPFs in today's food system takes substantial effort, mental energy, money, and time. This work falls primarily on women and is more burdensome for lower-income households for whom alternatives to UPFs are much less accessible. Therefore, to be effective, public health policies must grapple with the practical realities surrounding daily food preparation and the equity implications of policies to limit UPFs.

Although many UPFs are "discretionary" or "junk" foods such as sweet and savory snacks, candy, sweetened beverages, or desserts, UPFs are not limited to these "foods to avoid."[1] UPFs also include products used to prepare meals in home kitchens and in institutional food settings (e.g., schools, hospitals, work cafeterias), including many packaged breads, frozen meals, ready-to-heat products, shelf-stable packaged foods such as boxed macaroni and cheese, many breakfast cereals, processed meats, meat and dairy alternative products such as soy milk or tofu, and condiments, sauces, and other products that are used in everyday meal preparation.[1] Such products enable quick meal preparation, and thus are now widely incorporated into home cooking practice. Although cooking at home is indeed associated with better diet quality (among adults and, to a lesser extent, children) and lower UPF intake (among both adults and children),[4,6,7] even among those in households in which dinner is cooked seven days per week, UPFs make up more than 50% of energy intake among adults and more than 60% among children.[4,6] Additionally, the proportion of energy intake from UPFs has increased in food consumed at home over the last two decades, indicating that UPFs play a large and growing role in meals cooked at home.[8]

There are many good reasons for this—first and foremost, the additional time and cognitive load required to plan, procure, and prepare minimally processed meals. This responsibility falls mostly on women,[9,10] a fact that is often a footnote in discussions about the need to reduce UPF intake and cook more healthy home-cooked meals. Although men spend more time cooking than in the past,[10] the gender distribution of home-cooking time is vastly unequal, and women shoulder more of the "invisible labor" related to domestic chores and parenting while also balancing work and other responsibilities. Preparing minimally processed meals (and snacks) also requires cooking skills, self-efficacy, and confidence. Investing in building those skills (e.g., via hands-on food and cooking skills education throughout public schooling and in community-based programs) should be a priority if we expect to reduce UPF intake. Shifting societal norms and expectations around the gender balance of household labor should also be central.

Affordability and availability are additional key considerations for recommendations to consume fewer UPFs. Both household food insecurity and Supplemental Nutrition Assistance Program (SNAP) participation are associated with higher intake of UPFs.[11] UPFs are more shelf stable and offer an affordable and less effortful way to feed a family on a limited budget, making them a logical strategy for families struggling to put food on the table. Food insecurity itself is stressful, which could make UPFs more attractive both because they are designed to be rewarding and because they are less labor intensive and stressful to procure, manage, and prepare. SNAP benefits are inadequate to afford a healthy diet composed primarily of minimally processed foods,[12] and are likely to become more inadequate given recent policy changes. Alternatives to UPFs are also less readily available and affordable in low-income areas that lack grocery stores. Therefore, public health UPF policies are unlikely to succeed if the upstream issues of availability and affordability of realistic alternatives to UPFs that fit into people's daily lives are not addressed. Policies to both increase purchasing power (e.g., higher minimum wage laws, higher SNAP benefits) and reduce the cost of unprocessed and minimally processed foods (e.g., shifting agricultural subsidies and trade policies) are needed. Without doing so, income-related disparities in healthy food access, diet quality, and diet-related health will only widen.

In institutional settings such as schools, policies to eliminate UPFs face many of the same practical challenges. When many UPFs are no longer allowed, who will cook the minimally processed alternatives? Do viable minimally processed alternatives exist at the price and scale needed? Many school districts do not have the staff, or budgets, to accommodate the longer shifts and additional work needed to do more minimally processed food preparation. Many schools also do not have the kitchen equipment necessary to store and prepare more perishable foods. Any policies to reduce UPFs in schools should be accompanied by the financial investments needed for schools to make these changes. These are key implementation challenges that must be addressed for schools to be able to comply with regulations to reduce or remove UPFs from schools.

It is possible that in the face of regulation, the food industry will reformulate products to remove banned ingredients or otherwise comply with regulations, thereby making "less processed" but still convenient ready-to-heat or ready-to-eat products available to consumers and institutions without necessitating major burdens or behavior change by individuals. However, these supply-side changes will depend on whether the food industry views reformulation as a profitable exercise. Furthermore, reformulated products that have removed certain banned ingredients may be more expensive, which again raises equity concerns.

There are many logical reasons for why we all use UPFs in our daily lives, even when we may know better. These practical realities create barriers to choosing less-processed UPF alternatives that are likely to limit the effectiveness of any UPF public health policy (e.g., labeling, tax, placement, ingredient or product ban). Structural and societal changes are needed to shift gender norms around cooking responsibilities. Policies are needed to invest in culinary skills education for all, reduce the relative unavailability and unaffordability of healthier foods compared with UPFs, and raise incomes and SNAP benefits such that everyone can afford a healthy, minimally processed diet, no matter how much time they have to cook. It is critical that we proceed quickly, but also carefully and thoughtfully, to implement policies to reduce UPF intake in ways that do not adversely and inequitably burden individuals, often women, trying their best to feed their families. AJPH

CORRESPONDENCE

Correspondence should be sent to Julia A. Wolfson, PhD, MPP, Associate Professor, Department of International Health, Johns Hopkins Bloomberg School of Public Health, 615 North Wolfe St, Baltimore, MD 21205 (e-mail: jwolfso7@jhu.edu).

PUBLICATION INFORMATION

Full Citation: Wolfson JA. Practical and equity considerations for ultraprocessed foods policies. *Am J Public Health*. 2026;116(7):918–920.

Acceptance Date: March 13, 2026

DOI: https://doi.org/10.2105/AJPH.2026.308540

ORCID iD:
Julia A. Wolfson https://orcid.org/0000-0001-9155-2609

CONFLICTS OF INTEREST

The author has no conflicts of interest to report.

REFERENCES

1. Monteiro CA, Cannon G, Levy RB, et al. Ultra-processed foods: what they are and how to identify them. *Public Health Nutr.* 2019;22(5):936–941. https://doi.org/10.1017/S1368980018003762
2. Ravandi B, Ispirova G, Sebek M, Mehler P, Barabási A-L, Menichetti G. Prevalence of processed foods in major US grocery stores. *Nat Food.* 2025;6(3):296–308. https://doi.org/10.1038/s43016-024-01095-7
3. Juul F, Parekh N, Martinez-Steele E, Monteiro CA, Chang VW. Ultra-processed food consumption among US adults from 2001 to 2018. *Am J Clin Nutr.* 2022;115(1):211–221. https://doi.org/10.1093/ajcn/nqab305
4. Tucker AC, Martinez-Steele E, Leung CW, Wolfson JA. Associations between household frequency of

cooking dinner and ultraprocessed food consumption and dietary quality among US children and adolescents. *Child Obes.* 2024;20(1):11–22. https://doi.org/10.1089/chi.2022.0200

5. Lane MM, Gamage E, Du S, et al. Ultra-processed food exposure and adverse health outcomes: umbrella review of epidemiological meta-analyses. *BMJ.* 2024;384:e077310. https://doi.org/10.1136/bmj-2023-077310
6. Wolfson JA, Martinez-Steele E, Tucker AC, Leung CW. Greater frequency of cooking dinner at home and more time spent cooking are inversely associated with ultra-processed food consumption among US adults. *J Acad Nutr Diet.* 2024;124(12):1590–1605.e1. https://doi.org/10.1016/j.jand.2024.03.005
7. Wolfson JA, Leung CW, Richardson CR. More frequent cooking at home is associated with higher Healthy Eating Index-2015 score. *Public Health Nutr.* 2020;23(13):2384–2394. https://doi.org/10.1017/S1368980019003549
8. Wolfson JA, Tucker AC, Leung CW, Rebholz CM, Garcia-Larsen V, Martinez-Steele E. Trends in adults' intake of un-processed/minimally processed, and ultra-processed foods at home and away from home in the United States from 2003–2018. *J Nutr.* 2025;155(1):280–292. https://doi.org/10.1016/j.tjnut.2024.10.048
9. Carducci B, Fanzo J, Wolfson JA. Household cooking and eating practices across food system typologies in 135 countries from 2018 to 2022. *Health Promot Int.* 2025;40(2):daaf029. https://doi.org/10.1093/heapro/daaf029
10. Taillie LS. Who's cooking? Trends in US home food preparation by gender, education, and race/ethnicity from 2003 to 2016. *Nutr J.* 2018;17(1):41. https://doi.org/10.1186/s12937-018-0347-9
11. Leung CW, Fulay AP, Parnarouskis L, Martinez-Steele E, Gearhardt AN, Wolfson JA. Food insecurity and ultra-processed food consumption: the modifying role of participation in the Supplemental Nutrition Assistance Program (SNAP). *Am J Clin Nutr.* 2022;116(1):197–205. https://doi.org/10.1093/ajcn/nqac049
12. Zhang FF, Liu J, Rehm CD, Wilde P, Mande JR, Mozaffarian D. Trends and disparities in diet quality among US adults by Supplemental Nutrition Assistance Program participation status. *JAMA Netw Open.* 2018;1(2):e180237. https://doi.org/10.1001/jamanetworkopen.2018.0237

Ultraprocessed Foods in the Global Food System: The Role of US Tobacco Companies

Tera L. Fazzino, PhD, Sydney Kong, Gayeon Lee, MA, and Madison Stewart

See also Ultraprocessed Food, pp. 898–1029.

We sought to characterize the involvement of US tobacco companies in the global food industry, where they disseminated ultraprocessed and hyper-palatable foods, and the methods they used to expand globally. We reviewed and extracted data from 113 primary source industry documents.

US tobacco companies developed billion-dollar food businesses that were prominent internationally between the 1980s and mid-2000s. Tobacco companies developed their international food businesses with the same strategies they used to establish their international tobacco businesses.

Our findings suggest that US tobacco companies used their extensive experiences from their tobacco businesses to maximize the successes of their international food businesses in disseminating ultraprocessed foods globally. Regulation of the multiple addictive products that tobacco companies have disseminated to markets globally may be needed to protect public health. (*Am J Public Health*. 2026;116(7):921–931. https://doi.org/10.2105/AJPH.2026.308501)

AJPH July 2026, Vol. 116, No. 7

Many foods in the global food environment can harm public health.[1,2] Ultraprocessed foods undergo extensive industrial processing, contain few or no whole foods, and are designed for appeal and convenience.[3,4] Ultraprocessed foods are often designed with hyper-palatable nutrient combinations (e.g., high fat and sodium, fat and sugar)[5,6] and may have addictive qualities[7] that promote overconsumption.[1] Excess consumption of ultraprocessed foods can yield substantial health consequences, from obesity and metabolic disease to cardiovascular disease[2] and mental health conditions (e.g., food addiction).[8] The risks of ultraprocessed foods to the population are similar in magnitude to other prominent contributors to premature mortality, including tobacco use.[2] Ultraprocessed foods, particularly those that are hyper-palatable, are prominent in the United States and many countries in Europe,[5,9] and their availability has increased markedly in countries in South America, Asia, and Africa.[10]

US tobacco companies, which specialize in creating addictive cigarettes, owned US food companies between the 1980s through mid-2000s and were influential in spreading ultraprocessed foods into the US food system.[11] Leading US tobacco companies Philip Morris (PM) and RJ Reynolds (RJR) made a major entrance into the food industry in the 1980s,[11] at a time when the companies had strong cash flows yet experienced growing scrutiny regarding their tobacco products.[12] Thus, the tobacco companies invested heavily in food and beverage companies, which facilitated their asset diversification, reduced financial risk, and helped boost their corporate image.[12]

Buying into the food industry also facilitated the tobacco companies in applying the knowledge, skills, and strategies developed from their tobacco businesses to another business domain in ultraprocessed foods and beverages.[13] For example, PM applied its aggressive marketing tactics developed from its tobacco businesses to market ultraprocessed foods to the US public.[14,15] Furthermore, US tobacco companies and their food companies were systematically involved with developing hyper-palatable foods, which have elevated addictive properties.[11] Thus, US tobacco companies played a major role in spreading ultraprocessed and hyper-palatable foods into the US food system.

The tobacco companies also expanded their food businesses internationally during the 1980s through mid-2000s.[16,17]

However, little is known about the ways in which US tobacco companies developed their international food businesses or the degree to which their foods were prominent in global markets. Thus, the purpose of our study was to review primary source industry documents to characterize the degree of involvement of US tobacco companies in food markets globally and the methods used to expand their food businesses globally.

METHODS

A multistep snowball search process was used in identifying industry documents to review and analyze for the study. The search was conducted in the University of California, San Francisco's Industry Documents Library, a publicly available industry document repository that includes documents from industries that harm public health.[18] The goal of the search was to identify documents containing information on the international food business activities of major tobacco companies PM and RJR. The search was conducted in the full library collection, which included tobacco and food industry document collections. Inclusion criteria were as follows: (1) documents reporting activities of PM or RJR and documents referencing international activities. The search was broad to capture relevant documents that could detail international activities related to food. There were no exclusion criteria. The search process consisted of 5 iterations and is detailed in Table A (available as a supplement to the online version of this article at http://www.ajph.org). The search was conducted between March and October 2025.

A total of 113 documents were extracted, met the inclusion criteria, and were included in the study. The documents consisted of summary reports of company activities that were used internally (e.g., annual reports), summary documents sent to outside entities such as shareholders and the US federal government (e.g., 10-K reports), company plans (e.g., 5-year plans), and draft business presentations.

The industry documents were reviewed by 2 independent reviewers who used line-by-line coding to search for relevant content. Reviewers used a standardized process to collect data on strategies used by tobacco companies to develop their international food businesses, including (1) the metrics of food market involvement (e.g., market share, market segment coverage, sales); (2) strategies used to develop international food businesses, with attention to whether practices were informed by the parent tobacco business activities; and (3) strategies used to develop food products and promote sales internationally, with attention to potential tobacco business-informed approaches.

After document review and data extraction, data were organized into descriptive statistical categories to summarize international food market coverage for both companies, reported by geographic region (and country when available). Common strategies for business development activities and product development approaches were identified and discussed, with discrepancies or disagreements resolved by revisiting the source document text and identifying a resolution. In addition to the search described, the reviewers extracted all food and beverage products and brands that were reportedly sold internationally (outside of the domestic United States) and owned by a parent tobacco company. The data were organized by global region and by country (when available) and consolidated into product lists by global region and country (when available).

RESULTS

PM and RJR developed multibillion-dollar international food businesses during the 1980s through mid-2000s.[16,17] Both companies used strategies from developing their international tobacco businesses to inform the development of their international food businesses. Specifically, to establish and expand their tobacco businesses in international markets, the companies acquired local tobacco companies or established joint ventures with local companies to build their market presence in target regions and developed strong distribution and sales systems to support business growth.[19,20] These efforts were complemented sociopolitically with the establishment of local political connections to support business development.[19] Through these processes, RJR built a successful international tobacco business in Europe and parts of Asia[19] and PM established its international tobacco businesses primarily in Europe and South America.[21]

Beginning in the 1980s, RJR and PM used these strategies to grow their international food businesses.[22] In addition, the tobacco companies established points of synergy across their tobacco and food operations to maximize efficiency and sales in international markets.[13] Alongside these business development approaches, the companies expanded food sales by promoting greater use of their food products among international populations using strategies that originated from their tobacco businesses. Note that in parallel with business and product development activities, the tobacco companies established strong connections sociopolitically in international regions, which served to facilitate business-friendly policies and preempt restrictions and legislation.[12,19,23] Although their substantive activities in this domain require a separate investigation, we note them here as part of the context of the tobacco companies' broader activities designed to promote their food business expansion internationally.

A narrative description of strategies PM and RJR used to develop their international food businesses is provided in the sections to follow. We initially describe food business development efforts, followed by synergistic company activities across tobacco and food and, finally, strategies employed to promote food product use adapted from the tobacco businesses. Table 1 shows the countries (76 in total) in which the tobacco companies conducted their international food businesses. Table 2 presents information on acquisitions of international food companies. Lists of products sold by region and country are provided in Tables B through H (available as supplements to the online version of this article at http://www.ajph.org). Note that RJR divested from the food industry in 2000, selling its food business to PM. Thus, overlap in the tables regarding products and companies owned is due to this ownership change during the period in question.

Philip Morris International Food Business Summary

PM's conceptualization of its food business was as a consumer packaged goods business, considered alongside the company's other businesses in tobacco and alcohol.[24] To illustrate their perspective, PM leaders summarized the company's major activities in 1994 as "acquiring strategic consumer packaged goods operations . . . around the world," including "businesses in tobacco in four Central and Eastern European countries . . . food businesses on five continents . . . as well as a 20% stake in Molson [an alcoholic beverage company] of Canada."[24] Accordingly, PM pursued similar international business development approaches across food, tobacco, and alcohol businesses and coordinated efforts across business domains for maximal efficiency.[24] (PM owned alcohol companies, and we include information in this area as a context for PM's broader consumer packaged goods activities. However, a separate study of PM activities is needed to comprehensively detail the company's activities in the alcohol industry.)

Regarding its international food business, PM's primary activities were in Europe and Canada, with smaller sales contributions from the Asia Pacific region and South America (Table 1).[17,25] PM's core food business focus internationally began with coffee, processed cheese, confectionary items, and sugary beverages and later expanded to grocery products, snacks, and convenience meals.[25] PM's food business was among the largest in international markets[25]; PM sold food products in 76 countries (Table 1) and sold 829 food and beverage products (nonalcoholic) internationally (details are provided in the appendix, available as a supplement to the online version of this article at http://www.ajph.org).

To promote business growth, PM aggressively acquired smaller food companies in Europe and Asia,[26] and its acquisitions were extensive (52 companies overall; Table 2). One example of a key acquisition in Europe was the Swiss chocolate company Jacobs Suchard, which provided PM with business infrastructure and scaling in the region alongside leading market shares in confectionary.[26] As a result of its efforts, PM established leading market positions in Europe, with more than 70% of total international food sales becoming leading products by the 1990s.[17] Similarly, PM established successful joint ventures with food companies in Asia including Dong Suh Foods in South Korea and Ultra Jaya in Indonesia (Table 2), which facilitated cheese production in the regions. By the late 1990s, PM had strong market positions in cheese, sauces and dressings, coffee, and sugary drinks (e.g., Tang) in many Asian countries and had growing shares of snacks and confectionary products.[22]

Philip Morris Synergistic Activities

PM had a business presence in both the tobacco and food markets in Europe and engaged in synergistic activities designed to benefit both businesses in the region.[24] By the early 1990s, PM was aware that public perception of PM as a tobacco company was low in Europe; however, its food-based brands such as Jacobs Suchard were viewed favorably.[27] Thus, PM developed a strategy to jointly communicate about its tobacco and food businesses in public-facing interactions (e.g., media, press releases), as their market research indicated that public perception of PM improved with knowledge of its food business involvement.[27]

In the early 1990s, PM also coordinated activities regarding sourcing of supplies and ingredients, product sales, and distribution across its tobacco and food businesses. For example, PM sought to "fully exploit our purchasing power with suppliers by coordinating with other PM organizations" such as Kraft International to purchase supplies and ingredients needed for both

TABLE 1— Countries in Which US Tobacco-Owned Food Companies Sold Food and Beverage Products

Region	Country	Philip Morris	RJ Reynolds
North America	Canada	X	X
	Mexico	X	X
Central and South America	Argentina	X	X
	Brazil	X	X
	Chile	X	
	Colombia	X	X
	Costa Rica	X	
	Ecuador	X	X
	El Salvador	X	
	Guatemala	X	
	Honduras	X	
	Nicaragua	X	X
	Panama	X	
	Peru	X	X
	Uruguay	X	X
	Venezuela	X	X
Caribbean Islands	Antilles[a]	X	
	Bahamas	X	
	Bermuda	X	
	British Virgin Islands	X	
	Cayman Islands	X	
	Dominican Republic	X	
	Jamaica	X	X
	Puerto Rico[b]	X	X
	Trinidad	X	
Europe	Austria	X	
	Belgium	X	
	Bulgaria	X	
	Czech Republic	X	
	Denmark	X	
	Estonia	X	
	Finland	X	X
	France	X	X
	Germany	X	X
	Greece	X	
	Hungary	X	
	Ireland	X	
	Italy	X	X
	Lithuania	X	
	Netherlands	X	
	Norway	X	
	Poland	X	
	Portugal	X	X
	Romania	X	
	Slovakia	X	

Continued

TABLE 1— Continued

Region	Country	Philip Morris	RJ Reynolds
	Spain	X	X
	Sweden	X	
	Switzerland	X	
	Turkey	X	
	Ukraine	X	
	United Kingdom	X	X
Asia	Bahrain	X	
	China	X	X
	India	X	X
	Indonesia	X	
	Japan	X	X
	Malaysia	X	X
	Pakistan	X	
	Philippines	X	
	Russia	X	
	Singapore	X	X
	South Korea	X	X
	Taiwan	X	X
	Thailand	X	X
	Vietnam	X	
Pacific	Australia	X	
	New Zealand	X	X
Middle East and Africa	Egypt	X	
	Iran	X	
	Israel	X	
	Kuwait	X	
	Morocco	X	
	Nigeria	X	
	Tunisia	X	X
	Saudi Arabia	X	
	South Africa	X	X

[a]Islands consisting of Aruba, Bonaire, Curacao, Saba, Sint Eustatius, and Sint Maarten.
[b]US territory not previously covered in mainland US report.

cigarettes and food in Europe.[28] In addition, PM established joint product distribution activities across tobacco and food businesses in the southern Mediterranean and Eastern European regions.[26] Finally, in 1992 PM established cross-border sourcing of its food products in Europe, a practice it adopted on the basis of the 20-year success of its cross-border tobacco sourcing in the European region.[28]

PM also established joint tobacco and food distribution and marketing systems in regions targeted for business expansion in the 1990s. For example, in South America, PM integrated the management of its established tobacco business with its growing food business, which it considered "a step forward in achieving the scale we need to succeed" in the region.[12] Furthermore, PM tested joint sales and distribution approaches in key areas, such as Brazil, that informed broader synergy activities in the region and internationally. For example, PM tested a pilot joint sales and delivery system for 2 large cities in Brazil and sought to coordinate the distribution and sales of tobacco and food products through its common retail channels in city areas.[29] Alongside the retail channels, PM identified microdistributors to generate

TABLE 2— International Food Companies Acquired by US Tobacco Companies

Country	Name of Company Acquired	Type of Food Company	Acquiring Company	Year of Acquisition
North America				
Canada	Aylmer	Canned fruits and vegetables	RJR	1987[a]
Canada	Canada Dry	Carbonated soft drink	RJR	1984
Canada	Group Café	Coffee	PM	1990
Canada	Nabob	Coffee	PM	1994
Mexico	Lance	Cookie	RJR	1992
Central and South America				
Argentina	Alimentos Especiales	Coffee	PM	1992
Argentina	Establecimiento Modelo Terrabusi S.A.	Biscuit	RJR	1994
Argentina	Monthelado	Ice cream	PM	1993
Argentina	Productos Capri S.A.C.I.I	Biscuit	RJR	1996
Argentina	Productos Mayco S.A.I C.I.E	Biscuit	RJR	1996
Argentina	Tita	Biscuit	RJR	1994
Brazil	Avare	Milk products	RJR	1995
Brazil	Companhia Produtos Pilar	Biscuit	RJR	1996
Brazil	Gumz	Milk products	RJR	1995
Brazil	Industrias Alimenticias Maguary	Fruit juice	RJR	1992
Brazil	Iracema Industrias de Caju SA	Cashew producer	RJR	1987
Brazil	Kibon	Ice cream	PM	1985
Brazil	Q-Refres-Ko	Powdered drink/confectionary	PM	1993
Panama	Gallito Products	Chocolate	PM	1993
Venezuela	La Favorita	Cracker	RJR	1992
Caribbean Islands				
Jamaica	Butterkist Ltd.	Biscuit	RJR	1998
Europe				
Bulgaria	Republika	Confectionary	PM	1993
Czech Republic	Dadak	Coffee and spice	PM	1993
Denmark	Scandinavisk Kaffekompagni	Coffee	PM	1989
France	Cote d'Or	Chocolate	PM	
France	Grand M'ere	Coffee	PM	1992
France	ULC Bahlsen	Frozen dessert	RJR	1987
Germany	Jacobs Kronung	Coffee	PM	1991[a]
Germany/Switzerland	Milka	Chocolate	PM	1990[a]
Greece	Fiesta	Coffee	PM	1992
Greece	Pavildes	Confectionary	PM	1992
Hungary	Csemerge	Confectionary	PM	1992
Italy	Caramba	Coffee	PM	1990
Italy	Fini SpA	Meat and pasta	PM[b]	1989
Italy	Negroni	Processed meat	PM	1990
Italy	Simmenthal	Canned meat	PM	1989
Italy	Splendid	Coffee	PM	1991
Lithuania	Kaunaa	Chocolate	PM	1993
Norway	Disena	Cheese	PM[b]	
Norway	Freia Marabou	Confectionary and snacks	PM	1993
Norway	Maarud	Fresh cheese	PM	1992

Continued

TABLE 2— Continued

Country	Name of Company Acquired	Type of Food Company	Acquiring Company	Year of Acquisition
Poland	Chorzele	Cheese	PM[b]	1994
Poland	Oltza	Confectionary	PM	1993
Romania	Poiana	Chocolate	PM	1994
Russia	Petroconf		PM[b]	
Slovak Republic	Figaro	Confectionary	PM	1992
Spain	El Almendro	Confectionary	PM	1992
Spain	El Caserio	Processed cheese	PM	1992
Spain	Galletas Fontaneda, S.A.	Biscuit	RJR	1996
Spain	Industrial Quesera Menorquina	Cheese	PM	1991
Spain	Royal Brands	Food and biscuit	RJR	1993
Spain	Saimaza	Coffee	PM	1989
Spain	Tabacalera, S.A.[c]	Spanish government's food and tobacco company	RJR	1987
Sweden	KF Co-op	Coffee	PM	1994
Switzerland	Jacobs Suchard	Chocolate	PM	1990
Switzerland	Toblerone	Chocolate	PM	1991[a]
Turkey	Kar Gida	Salted snacks	PM	2003
Turkey	Marsa J.V.	Dairy	PM	1993
Ukraine	Ukrania	Confectionary	PM	1995
United Kingdom	Bird's	Desserts	RJR	1980[a]
United Kingdom	Kenco	Coffee	PM	1987
United Kingdom	Lyons Tetley	Coffee	PM	1994
United Kingdom	Terry's of York	Confectionary	PM	1993
United Kingdom	Walkers and Smith	Crisp and snack	RJR[d]	
Asia				
China	Shunde	Chewing gum	PM[e]	
India	Britannia Industries[c]	Biscuit	RJR	1987
India/Pakistan	Associated Biscuits International	Biscuit	PM[d]	
Indonesia	Ultra Jaya[c]	Cheese company	PM	1994
South Korea	Dong Suh Foods[c]	Cheese and grocery	PM	1985
Taiwan	Luck Enterprises Corporation Ltd.[c]	Biscuit	RJR	1996
Taiwan	Premier Foods	Coffee	PM	1992
Pacific				
Australia	ETA Peanut Butter	Peanut butter	PM	1992
Australia	Twin Valley	Dairy	PM	1992
New Zealand	Abels Industries, Inc.[c]	Biscuit	RJR	1987[a]
New Zealand	Butlands	Cheese/grocery	PM	1989
Middle East and Africa				
Egypt	Family Nutrition	Biscuit	RJR	2003
South Africa	Royal Beech-Nut Ltd.[c]		RJR	1995
Tunisia	Royal Food Products		RJR	1994

Note. PM = Philip Morris; RJR = RJ Reynolds.
[a]Date is approximate, derived from source document publication date.
[b]Year of divestiture: 1998.
[c]Joint venture or partial ownership of company.
[d]Year of divestiture: 1990.
[e]Year of divestiture: 1999.

sales in lower volume city areas, and these companies contracted to sell PM's tobacco and food products for sales commissions (6% for cigarettes and 15% for foods).[29]

PM also used parallel business development practices across international tobacco and food operations in Asia. For example, in China, PM pursued simultaneous business expansions in tobacco and food as a result of concurrent opportunities.[30] PM established cooperative agreements and joint ventures with Chinese tobacco and food companies in the 1970s through 1980s, and by the 1990s it had success in selling both tobacco products (e.g., Marlboro cigarettes) and food products (e.g., Tang, cheese) in the country.[30]

Philip Morris Strategies to Promote Use

In the early 1990s, PM recognized that continued business growth would require "greater penetration in existing markets,"[31] a premise that informed its food and tobacco product development strategies internationally. In service of this goal for food, PM sought to increase food product use among international populations, the same strategy used to promote cigarette use internationally at the time. Regarding food, PM identified a plan to invest in growing snacks as a way to promote greater product use and sales in all global food sectors.[22]

To address this opportunity in Europe, PM manipulated the size of products to promote more frequent use of desserts as snacks (e.g., snack size)[22] and sold larger-sized versions of popular cream cheese products "to increase consumption among current users."[22] (Additional examples are provided in the appendix.) Notably, the manipulation of product size (for smaller and larger intakes) was consistent with the company's approach to promoting use of its cigarettes internationally at the time, which included selling "slim" cigarettes that purportedly had lower nicotine or tar and selling "king size" cigarettes for greater use occasions.[20,21]

PM also created food product line extensions that addressed health concerns of customers, similar to its approach with cigarette line extensions at the time. For example, PM pursued the development of "fat replacement technology," which was used to create highly flavored yet low-fat or fat-free products between 1989 and 2003, with the explicit goal of retaining users[32] who might otherwise stop using high-fat products because of health concerns. These strategies paralleled PM's strategies in selling low-tar and low-nicotine cigarettes in international markets during the same period.[33] Such products were intended to be perceived as "safer" by consumers[33] yet still had full flavor profiles, which was a product development strategy designed to retain smoking customers who were concerned about health consequences and might otherwise quit smoking.[34]

RJ Reynolds International Food Business Summary

RJR had a dual focus on its "consumer product businesses" in tobacco and food, and by the late 1980s the 2 business areas had "the size, the product mix, the successful experience, and the distribution and merchandising networks to remain a world-class competitor."[23] Also by the late 1980s, RJR had "very strong positive cash flows" and made "major investments in market, research and development, and new manufacturing technology" to serve the company's focus in the areas of both tobacco and food.[23]

Regarding its international food business operations, RJR's major business activities were in Mexico, Central America, and South America, followed by smaller businesses in Europe, Canada, and the Asia Pacific region.[35] RJR's core food business areas were in biscuits, powdered and dry mix desserts and baking products, sugary drinks (e.g., Tang), snacks, confectionary products, and canned fruits and vegetables.[36] RJR was among the largest international packaged food companies,[35] sold food products in 30 countries (Table 1), and sold 195 food and beverage products internationally (see the appendix).

In the early 1990s, RJR established its primary food business activities in 17 countries in Central and South America (Table 1), with its largest markets in Brazil, Venezuela, and Mexico.[35] For scaling in the region, RJR acquired a number of local cookie and snack companies with leading market positions (Table 2).[35] Along with building infrastructure, the acquisitions provided RJR leading market shares in a country while simultaneously eliminating competition from the national market leader. By the mid-1990s, RJR was among the largest packaged food businesses in the region and was the market leader in biscuits and powdered and dry mix desserts in many countries.[35]

RJR replicated its acquisitions strategy in Europe and Asia (Table 2), which solidified its leading market position in biscuits in many countries[35] (see the appendix for more details). In the broader regions across Europe and Asia, RJR sought opportunities to leverage both tobacco and food business development. In 1994, RJR acquired a tobacco processing plant in Russia and a confectionary company in Kazakhstan; RJR

AJPH July 2026, Vol. 116, No. 7

planned to jointly manufacture a variety of food products and high-quality tobacco products for local sale and export.[37] Similarly, RJR assigned the Planters Lifesavers Company to be managed by the international tobacco division with the goal of aligning common sales and distribution procedures for international markets.[36]

RJ Reynolds Strategies to Increase Use

RJR pursued international growth by disseminating its most popular food products to new markets, an approach that originated from its international tobacco business.[19] Specifically, a key strategy that RJR used in the 1970s to enter new international tobacco markets was to introduce highly competitive products (e.g., Winston brand cigarettes) to new markets in Europe (e.g., France, Italy) and Asia (e.g., the Philippines, Malaysia).[19] This approach was highly successful and almost doubled RJR's total international cigarette sales volume between 1974 and 1984.[19]

In the mid-1980s through 1990s, RJR used this same approach to enter new international food markets. RJR introduced its core cookie brands Oreo and Chips Ahoy! in Mexico and introduced Planters snack products to Germany and France, both of which were well received by consumers and served to further expand RJR's market reach.[37] In the late 1990s, RJR launched an "aggressive expansion of the worldwide biscuit business" with a focus on Oreo, Ritz, Chips Ahoy!, and Air Crisps[38]; the initiative was highly successful and more than doubled the number of international markets in which the company's foods were sold between 1993 and 1998.[35]

RJR also developed high-flavor food products that could be marketed as light and perceived as healthier (lower harm), consistent with its practices of selling high-flavor, low-tar cigarettes at the time internationally.[20] For example, in the 1990s, RJR Nabisco's research division was focused on developing low-fat products that had strong flavor and could serve as alternatives for health-conscious customers.[38] The company developed its own proprietary fat replacement technology, Salatrim, and subsequently developed a number of high-flavor, low-fat products (e.g., Air Crisps, fat-free Fig Newtons) that it disseminated widely to international markets.[38]

DISCUSSION

In this article, through an analysis of primary source industry documents, we have reported on the development and global expansion of US multinational food companies owned by US tobacco companies between the 1980s and the mid-2000s.[11] Our findings contextualize the proliferation of ultraprocessed and hyper-palatable foods in the global food system[9,10] and reveal the framework that tobacco companies used to expand their global food businesses. Overall, our results reveal that PM and RJR established their international food businesses with the same strategies they used to establish their international tobacco businesses. Furthermore, the tobacco companies leveraged business synergies in sales, distribution, and marketing across tobacco and food products to maximize business success in both domains.

In addition, the tobacco companies used product development strategies originally designed for cigarettes (e.g., high-flavor, low-tar cigarettes) to develop new food products (e.g., high-flavor, low-fat foods) with the goal of retaining customers and promoting use among populations globally. Our findings suggest that US tobacco companies used their extensive resources and experiences from their tobacco businesses to develop and maximize the successes of their international food businesses in disseminating ultraprocessed foods globally. Although the tobacco companies divested from the food system in 2000 to 2007, their impact in the US food system has been long-standing,[11] and their effects are likely similarly enduring in the global food system.

Our findings suggest that the tobacco companies were able to pursue international food company growth at a scale that likely dwarfed those of other food companies because of the combination of their financial resources, breadth of products, and scale of business infrastructure. Furthermore, given that the tobacco companies established formal synergy activities across their businesses,[13] the development of their international food businesses was likely accelerated by the regular exchange of cross-business knowledge, skills, and technological advances. In this regard, a review of leading global competitors across tobacco, food, and mixed packaged goods companies in 1989 identified PM and RJR as having the most well-balanced product portfolios across tobacco and food and the most opportunity to transfer knowledge, skills, and technology across their tobacco and food businesses.[13] Thus, the tobacco companies appeared to have a major advantage over their competitors with respect to maximizing the success of their international food businesses and disseminating ultraprocessed foods globally.

One notable outcome of the tobacco companies' synergistic tobacco and food business activities was the use of product development strategies across both tobacco and food. Product development strategies consisted of those designed to increase use (via product size manipulation) as well as those intended to encourage use of alternative low/light products over cessation. Although tactics to increase food product use have existed for decades in the international food industry, our findings suggest that these approaches may have been informed by or originated from tobacco company strategies with cigarettes.[21] This premise is consistent with a recent review that robustly detailed the commonalities between the development of cigarettes and ultraprocessed foods to maximize their appeal and addictiveness.[7]

Our study further contributes to the literature by providing specific instances in which a tobacco company used the same product development strategies for tobacco and food at the same time in international markets (PM during the 1990s) as well as instances in which a tobacco company's use of a cigarette product development strategy was later applied to its food products (RJR). Our results are also aligned with a previous study reporting that PM applied tailored marketing strategies for selling cigarettes to Black Americans to selling ultraprocessed foods to Black and Hispanic communities in the United States.[15] Thus, our findings highlight a major consequence of cross-industry activities: well-established strategies to promote the use of cigarettes may have been applied to food product portfolios that were disseminated to populations globally.

Our study involved several limitations. For example, the documents reviewed were derived from a single archive, which may have limited the representativeness of the documents included. Also, although the archive contains a large collection of documents, the documents were not comprehensive, as most were obtained through litigation efforts. However, given the summary-style nature of many of the reports reviewed, we believe that the documents likely contained sufficient detail to provide a representative summary of company activities in international food markets during the study period. In addition, the tobacco document collection was substantially larger than the food document collection. However, most tobacco documents also reported on food business activities given the summary-style nature of many of the documents reviewed. Another limitation is that the documents contained limited detail at the country level for some regions (e.g., Western vs Central and Eastern Europe, South and Southwest Asia vs Southeast Asia).

CONCLUSIONS AND PUBLIC HEALTH IMPLICATIONS

Our findings suggest that US tobacco companies developed their food companies into multibillion-dollar international food businesses between the 1980s and mid-2000s using strategies informed by tobacco business development. Our results can be leveraged to inform food system surveillance efforts and policy initiatives globally. Regarding surveillance, countries might consider establishing a baseline of ultraprocessed or hyper-palatable food availability in their food environments to monitor food system health; such efforts could be informed by our lists of affected market segments and brands in each region and country (as reported in the appendix). Regarding policy approaches, a global precedent has been set for how to address addictive products introduced by tobacco companies; governments globally have regulated aspects of tobacco products to protect public health.[39] Thus, countries can learn from these efforts and apply similar restriction and regulation activities to ultraprocessed foods.

However, the tobacco companies are currently invested in a number of additional health-harming products including alcohol, vaping products, and cannabis[40] and have since divested from the food industry. Thus, there may be a global need to consider regulation of multiple addictive products disseminated by tobacco companies at any point in time given our finding that the application of company knowledge to new addictive products may be accelerated within such companies, potentially presenting quick and enduring risks to global public health. AJPH

ABOUT THE AUTHORS

Tera L. Fazzino is with the Department of Psychology and Cofrin Logan Center for Addiction Research and Treatment, University of Kansas, Lawrence. Gayeon Lee and Sydney Kong are graduate students in the Department of Psychology and Cofrin Logan Center for Addiction Research and Treatment, University of Kansas. Madison Stewart is an undergraduate student in the Department of Psychology and Cofrin Logan Center for Addiction Research and Treatment, University of Kansas.

CORRESPONDENCE

Correspondence should be sent to Tera L. Fazzino, PhD, University of Kansas, 1415 Jayhawk Blvd, 4th Floor, Lawrence, KS 66046 (e-mail: tfazzino@ku.edu). Reprints can be ordered at https://www.ajph.org by clicking the "Reprints" link.

PUBLICATION INFORMATION

Full Citation: Fazzino TL, Kong S, Lee G, Stewart M. Ultraprocessed foods in the global food system: the role of US tobacco companies. *Am J Public Health*. 2026;116(7):921–931.

Acceptance Date: February 13, 2026.

DOI: https://doi.org/10.2105/AJPH.2026.308501

ORCID iDs:

Tera L. Fazzino https://orcid.org/0000-0002-2896-9791

Sydney Kong https://orcid.org/0009-0003-1877-061X

Gayeon Lee https://orcid.org/0000-0001-5577-1361

AJPH July 2026, Vol. 116, No. 7

CONTRIBUTORS

T. L. Fazzino conceptualized and designed the study and developed the methodology. S. Kong, G. Lee, and M. Stewart conducted data curation and investigation activities under the supervision of T. L. Fazzino. T. L. Fazzino led the formal analysis with participation from S. Kong, G. Lee, and M. Stewart. G. Lee conducted validation activities related to data curation and analysis. T. L. Fazzino wrote the original draft, and S. Kong, G. Lee, and M. Stewart reviewed and edited the article.

ACKNOWLEDGMENTS

Tera L. Fazzino's time during the study was partially supported by the National Institute of General Medical Sciences and the Office of the Director of the National Institutes of Health under award P20GM152280.

CONFLICTS OF INTEREST

The authors declare no conflicts of interest.

HUMAN PARTICIPANT PROTECTION

No protocol approval was needed for this study because no human participants were involved.

REFERENCES

1. Juul F, Martinez-Steele E, Parekh N, Monteiro CA. The role of ultra-processed food in obesity. *Nat Rev Endocrinol.* 2025;21(11):672–685. https://doi.org/10.1038/s41574-025-01143-7
2. Lane MM, Gamage E, Du S, et al. Ultra-processed food exposure and adverse health outcomes: umbrella review of epidemiological meta-analyses. *BMJ.* 2024;384:e077310. https://doi.org/10.1136/bmj-2023-077310
3. Monteiro CA, Levy RB, Claro RM, de Castro IRR, Cannon G. A new classification of foods based on the extent and purpose of their processing. *Cad Saude Publica.* 2010;26(11):2039–2049. https://doi.org/10.1590/S0102-311X2010001100005
4. Monteiro CA, Cannon G, Moubarac JC, Levy RB, Louzada MLC, Jaime PC. The UN Decade of Nutrition, the NOVA food classification and the trouble with ultra-processing. *Public Health Nutr.* 2018;21(1):5–17. https://doi.org/10.1017/S1368980017000234
5. Sutton CA, Stratton M, L'Insalata AM, Fazzino TL. Ultraprocessed, hyper-palatable, and high energy density foods: prevalence and distinction across 30 years in the United States. *Obesity (Silver Spring).* 2024;32(1):166–175. https://doi.org/10.1002/oby.23897
6. Fazzino T, Rohde K, Sullivan D. Hyper-palatable foods: development of a quantitative definition and application to the United States food system database. *Obesity (Silver Spring).* 2019;27(11):1761–1768. https://doi.org/10.1002/oby.22639
7. Gearhardt AN, Brownell KD, Brandt AM. From tobacco to ultraprocessed food: how industry engineering fuels the epidemic of preventable disease. *Milbank Q.* Published online 2026;104(1):76–115. https://doi.org/10.1111/1468-0009.70066
8. Pereira T, Mocellin MC, Curioni C. Association between ultraprocessed foods consumption, eating disorders, food addiction and body image: a systematic review. *BMJ Open.* 2024;14(12):e091223. https://doi.org/10.1136/bmjopen-2024-091223
9. Jun D, Knowles K, Fazzino T. Examination of hyper-palatable foods and their nutrient characteristics using globally crowdsourced data. *PLoS One.* 2025;20(6):e0325479. https://doi.org/10.1371/journal.pone.0325479
10. Baker P, Machado P, Santos T, et al. Ultra-processed foods and the nutrition transition: global, regional and national trends, food systems transformations and political economy drivers. *Obes Rev.* 2020;21(12):e13126. https://doi.org/10.1111/obr.13126
11. Fazzino TL, Jun D, Chollet-Hinton L, Bjorlie K. US tobacco companies selectively disseminated hyper-palatable foods into the US food system: empirical evidence and current implications. *Addiction.* 2024;119(1):62–71. https://doi.org/10.1111/add.16332
12. Philip Morris Companies. Philip Morris Latin America Inc. strategic plan. Available at: https://www.industrydocuments.ucsf.edu/docs/nzwp0169. Accessed September 10, 2025.
13. Philip Morris Companies Inc. Report on the PM Companies Technical Synergy Committee. Available at: https://www.industrydocuments.ucsf.edu/docs/gpdd0084. Accessed October 20, 2025.
14. Nguyen KH, Glantz SA, Palmer CN, Schmidt LA. Tobacco industry involvement in children's sugary drinks market. *BMJ.* 2019;364:l736. https://doi.org/10.1136/bmj.l736
15. Nguyen KH, Glantz SA, Palmer CN, Schmidt LA. Transferring racial/ethnic marketing strategies from tobacco to food corporations: Philip Morris and Kraft General Foods. *Am J Public Health.* 2020;110(3):329–336. https://doi.org/10.2105/AJPH.2019.305482
16. Bernstein Research. RJR Nabisco, Inc. strategic analysis financial forecast 1986. Available at: https://www.industrydocuments.ucsf.edu/docs/yrmx0118. Accessed September 29, 2025.
17. Goldman Sacks. Philip Morris Companies: an in-depth analysis of Kraft. Available at: https://www.industrydocuments.ucsf.edu/docs/nnfh0131. Accessed September 10, 2025.
18. University of California, San Francisco. Industry Documents Library. Available at: https://www.industrydocuments.ucsf.edu/home. Accessed September 10, 2025.
19. RJ Reynolds. RJ Reynolds strategic assessment. Available at: https://www.industrydocuments.ucsf.edu/docs/xxkv0139. Accessed October 21, 2025.
20. RJ Reynolds Inc. R.J. Reynolds Industries, Inc. 1977 annual report. Available at: https://www.industrydocuments.ucsf.edu/docs/ghxh0099. Accessed October 21, 2025.
21. Philip Morris Companies. Philip Morris EEC region operations three-year plan 1988–1990. Available at: https://www.industrydocuments.ucsf.edu/docs/zxnj0113. Accessed October 21, 2025.
22. Philip Morris Companies. Kraft Foods International strategic plan summary. Available at: https://www.industrydocuments.ucsf.edu/docs/zgkg0155. Accessed September 10, 2025.
23. Carbonell R. Remarks by Dr. Robert J. Carbonell, senior executive vice president and chief administrative officer, RJR Nabisco Inc. Available at: https://www.industrydocuments.ucsf.edu/docs/fhvw0003. Accessed October 21, 2025.
24. Philip Morris. Remarks by senior executives: Philip Morris Companies Inc. Available at: https://www.industrydocuments.ucsf.edu/docs/phyg0077. Accessed October 20, 2025.
25. Philip Morris Companies. Kraft strategic plan and general foods strategic plan summary 1989. Available at: https://www.industrydocuments.ucsf.edu/docs/qtlm0111. Accessed September 10, 2025.
26. Philip Morris Inc. Kraft general foods international five-year plan summary. Available at: https://www.industrydocuments.ucsf.edu/docs/pkcf0116. Accessed September 10, 2025.
27. Philip Morris Companies. The Reputation of Philip Morris KGF in Europe. Available at: https://www.industrydocuments.ucsf.edu/docs/mrxv0111. Accessed September 10, 2025.
28. Philip Morris Companies Inc. Philip Morris EEC region operations three-year plan. Available at: https://www.industrydocuments.ucsf.edu/docs/sffb0120. Accessed October 21, 2025.
29. Philip Morris Companies. Philip Morris marketing and Kraft Suchard Brazil joint sales and distribution project questions and answers. Available at: https://www.industrydocuments.ucsf.edu/docs/xskx0085. Accessed October 21, 2025.
30. Philip Morris Companies. Philip Morris Asia Inc. and Philip Morris China Inc. Available at: https://www.industrydocuments.ucsf.edu/docs/hhpg0093. Accessed October 21, 2025.
31. Philip Morris Companies. PM presentation on an American approach to the new Europe. Available at: https://www.industrydocuments.ucsf.edu/docs/jjbb0077. Accessed September 10, 2025.
32. Philip Morris Companies. *Ymbl0000 Philip Morris Companies, Inc Five Year Plan 1989-1993.* UCSF Industry Documents Library, Philip Morris Records, Master Settlement Agreement; 1989. Available at: https://www.industrydocuments.ucsf.edu/docs/ymbl0000/
33. Philip Morris Companies. Philp Morris USA R&D strategic plan 1991–1995. Available at: https://www.industrydocuments.ucsf.edu/docs/nypf0189. Accessed October 21, 2025.
34. Philip Morris Companies. Philip Morris EEC region three-year plan 1994–1996. Available at: https://www.industrydocuments.ucsf.edu/docs/nznd0116. Accessed October 21, 2025.
35. RJR Nabisco. RJR Nabisco 1998 annual report. Available at: https://www.industrydocuments.ucsf.edu/docs/pfvf0097. Accessed October 13, 2025.
36. RJR Nabisco. RJR Nabisco Securities and Exchange Commission form 10-K. Available at: https://www.industrydocuments.ucsf.edu/docs/rscv0082. Accessed October 21, 2025.
37. RJR Nabisco. Annual report: 1994 was the year when a "new" RJR Nabisco began to emerge. Available at: https://www.industrydocuments.ucsf.edu/docs/txll0081. Accessed October 21, 2025.
38. RJR Nabisco. Strategic plan 1998–2000. Available at: https://www.industrydocuments.ucsf.edu/docs/kgkb0019. Accessed September 29, 2025.
39. WHO Study Group on Tobacco Product Regulation. Report on the scientific basis of tobacco product regulation: ninth report of a WHO study group. Available at: https://iris.who.int/server/api/core/bitstreams/62dd3c46-9bf4-4ebe-a0f6-7bded964c84b/content. Accessed October 23, 2025.
40. Dewhirst T. "Beyond nicotine" marketing strategies: Big Tobacco diversification into the vaping and cannabis product sectors. *Tob Control.* 2023;32(3):402–404. https://doi.org/10.1136/tobaccocontrol-2021-056798

What Do Nova and the Ultraprocessed Food Concept Offer to Policymakers? From Updating Dietary Guidance to Regulatory Action and Advancing Sustainable Food System Transitions

Carlos A. Monteiro, MD, PhD, Phillip Baker, PhD, Camila Corvalan, MD, MPH, PhD, and Barry M. Popkin, PhD

See also Ultraprocessed Food, pp. 898–1029.

This article outlines applications of the Nova food classification system in policies aimed at reducing the share of ultraprocessed food (UPF) in population diets. Such policies are lagging far behind the growing scientific and public attention to UPFs and the mounting evidence of their harms, reflecting industry opposition and institutional inertia but also valid scientific critiques and policy concerns.

We examine how Nova and the UPF concept can inform and improve dietary guidance, dietary monitoring and target-setting, food regulation, and sustainable food system transitions.

We position UPF-based policies as complementary to, rather than in competition with, existing policies aimed at addressing dietary nutrient imbalances, offering a constructive way forward to enhance the promotion of healthy diets and facilitate the transition to healthier and sustainable food systems. (*Am J Public Health*. 2026;116(7):932–939. https://doi.org/10.2105/AJPH.2026.308509)

AJPH July 2026, Vol. 116, No. 7

As defined by the Nova food classification system, ultraprocessed foods (UPFs) are ready-to-consume industrial formulations of food substances and additives designed and marketed to displace unprocessed and minimally processed foods, as well as the preparation of dishes and meals based on them.[1,2] UPFs now dominate population diets in many high-income countries, and are rapidly expanding in the diets of populations in low- and middle-income countries.[3,4] A growing body of evidence links the ultraprocessed dietary pattern to multiple chronic disease outcomes.[3] In total, more than 3000 articles listed on PubMed use the UPF descriptor, jumping from just 1 in 2009 to 890 in 2025, indicating a rapid growth in research.

Yet government policy responses are lagging far behind this growing scientific attention and evidence of harm, with few governments having translated this accumulating knowledge into comprehensive policies.[5] This partly reflects the political influence of the UPF industry's leading corporations and front groups, which have sought to block, delay, and dilute policy responses, including by sharing disinformation about Nova, its UPF concept, and the supporting evidence base.[6] Policy responses are likely also delayed by institutional constraints, including the long review cycles associated with dietary guideline revisions and related food policies. Finally, this delay also reflects legitimate debate about what the Nova system and the UPF concept can offer to policymakers, and how these can be operationalized into policy applications. Critics often question the clarity of UPFs' operational definition, the legal feasibility of applying it in policy contexts, and whether it provides added value beyond existing methods for identifying unhealthy foods based on nutrient imbalances.

In this essay, we take several steps. First, we describe the Nova system and the contrasting dietary patterns that it reveals. Second, we set out how Nova has been used in research, along with a summary of the body of evidence that supports urgent government policy interventions, to halt and reverse the global rise in the ultraprocessed dietary pattern. Third, we outline how the Nova system has been—and can be further—used in policymaking aimed at promoting healthy diets, protecting public health, and supporting the transition to sustainable food systems. We argue that UPF-based policies complement, rather than compete with, existing policies based on addressing dietary nutrient imbalances. By bridging science and policy, and integrating with rather than replacing existing policy approaches, we hope to propose a constructive way forward for addressing an urgent global health challenge.

THE NOVA SYSTEM AND ITS DEFINITION OF DIETARY PATTERNS

Initially proposed in 2009 and updated in subsequent years, the Nova classification system categorizes foods and food products—including individual ingredients used in culinary preparations—into 4 groups based on the extent and purpose of their industrial processing (Box 1).[1,2,7]

Collectively, the dietary share of Nova Groups 1 to 3 reflects adherence to long-established, whole-food and meal-based dietary patterns, which are consistently associated with health benefits across diverse global contexts. Well-studied traditional Mediterranean, Nordic, Meso-American, and other territorial diets constitute a diverse range of Nova Group 1 foods, along with moderate amounts of Groups 2 and 3 used in the preparation of dishes and meals. Together, these 3 groups form the foundation of culturally relevant cuisines, biodiverse food systems, and food economies that have long supported the livelihoods of billions of farmers and vendors worldwide.[5]

In contrast, the growing dietary share of UPFs reflects the displacement of long-established dietary patterns by the ultraprocessed dietary pattern—based on products manufactured largely by transnational corporations, derived from a limited number of high-yield crops, and produced using ingredients and processing techniques that represent, in the context of human evolution, entirely novel exposures in the human diet.[6] Although UPFs are also produced by small and medium-sized firms, it is transnational corporations who spread UPFs globally, spend large sums on marketing, and block government regulation through their political influence, and are therefore the primary drivers of this dietary displacement.[6]

APPLYING NOVA IN RESEARCH

To study the health impacts of the ultraprocessed dietary pattern and track how it is replacing long-established dietary patterns, researchers have used Nova's simple operational definition of UPFs: food and drink formulations that contain

BOX 1— The Nova Food Classification System

Group 1, *unprocessed or minimally processed foods*, includes vegetables, fruits, roots, tubers, grains, legumes, nuts, meat, milk, and eggs in their natural state or modified through methods such as chilling, freezing, pasteurization, fermentation, drying, and grinding. These techniques, often replicable in home or restaurant kitchens, largely preserve the structural integrity of the original foods; do not involve the addition of salt, sugar, or fat; and primarily serve to extend shelf life and facilitate or diversify their use in freshly prepared dishes and meals. This group also includes human breast milk, the food produced and delivered through breastfeeding, or when modified by chilling, freezing, or pasteurization.

Group 2, *processed culinary ingredients*, consists of substances extracted from Group 1 foods (or obtained directly from nature) that are used to prepare a wide variety of freshly made dishes and meals based on Group 1 foods. These ingredients are not intended to be consumed on their own. Examples include cooking oils, butter, lard, sugar, honey, and salt.

Group 3, *processed foods*, refers to Group 1 foods modified by the industry using methods similar to those applied to minimally processed foods, but with the addition of salt, sugar, oils, or fats to enhance preservation or sensory qualities. Processed foods—consumed by human societies for centuries or even millennia—are often incorporated into freshly prepared dishes and meals. Examples include vegetables in brine, fruits in syrup, tinned fish, breads, and cheeses.

Group 4, *ultraprocessed foods*, are industrial formulations made from inexpensive ingredients, engineered and marketed to displace the other 3 Nova groups and the preparation of dishes and meals based on them while maximizing industry profits. These products result from multiple processing steps applied to a few high-yield crops or their isolated components, such as extracted carbohydrates, proteins, fats, and fibers. The techniques used often have no equivalents in domestic kitchens and include processes such as hydrolysis, hydrogenation, extrusion, the incorporation of cosmetic additives, and packaging with synthetic materials.

The manufacture of UPFs typically involves a wide array of ingredients. These include salt, sugar, and fats, as well as substances used exclusively in industrial settings, such as protein isolates, hydrogenated or interesterified oils, modified starches, and added fibers. A long list of additives—particularly those with cosmetic functions, such as colorings, flavorings, emulsifiers, thickeners, and nonnutritive sweeteners, is also common. Whole foods are generally absent or make up only a minimal proportion of the total ingredients.

The processes and ingredients used to manufacture UPFs make them both highly profitable—because of their low-cost components—and likely to displace the other 3 Nova groups. This is largely attributable to their convenience (e.g., long shelf life and ready-to-eat, -heat, or -drink formats) and their hyper-palatability, or even addictive properties, which result from specific combinations of sugars and fats, carbohydrates and sugars, or carbohydrates and salt, along with the extensive use of cosmetic additives.

Examples include sodas; flavored "fruit" or "chocolate" drinks; flavored sweetened dairy drinks; extruded, flavored, sweetened breakfast cereals; potato chips, cereal bars, and other sweet or savory snacks; mass-produced packaged breads and buns; sausages, nuggets, hamburgers, and other reconstituted meat products; industrial sauces and spreads; instant noodles and other shelf-stable or frozen ready meals; and ice cream and many other industrial desserts.

either a food substance used exclusively or predominantly in industrial settings or an additive with a cosmetic function.[1,2,7]

Importantly, these food substances and additives are considered by Nova as markers of ultraprocessing because they are essential components of the UPF manufacturing process and business model. They serve 4 main purposes: to replace whole-food components with cheaper and long-duration alternatives, thereby reducing costs and extending shelf-life (e.g., protein isolates, added fibers, and hydrogenated oils); to stabilize processed mixtures and make them palatable (e.g., emulsifiers and thickeners); to enhance palatability and promote overconsumption by making reconstituted food components look and taste irresistible (e.g., flavors, flavor enhancers, colors, emulsifiers, emulsifying salts, sweeteners, thickeners, and antifoaming, bulking, carbonating, foaming, gelling, and glazing agents); and to help manufacturers sidestep existing regulations (e.g., modified starches replacing fats, nonsugar sweeteners replacing sugar, or flavor enhancers reducing sodium content). While salt, sugar, fats, and noncosmetic additives are also common in UPFs—often in large amounts—these components may also occur in processed foods (Nova Group 3) and therefore do not serve as specific markers of ultraprocessing.[1]

More than 100 large, mostly high-quality cohort studies using Nova's operational definition of UPFs have shown that a higher dietary share of these foods—or greater exposure to the ultraprocessed dietary pattern—is linked to increased risks of many adverse health outcomes. These include obesity, type 2 diabetes, dyslipidemias, hypertension, and cardio- and cerebrovascular diseases, and respiratory, gastrointestinal, hepatic, renal, and mental health disorders, as well as all-cause premature mortality.[3] Four crossover, randomized controlled trials and 1 community trial, also using Nova's operational definition of UPFs, have further corroborated part of these associations, linking ultraprocessed diets to increased energy intake and the accumulation of body and fat mass, relative to diets based on minimally processed foods.[3]

Mechanistic studies using the same definition have identified several factors likely responsible for the wide range of harmful effects linked to ultraprocessed diets. Besides major nutrient imbalances (e.g., excessive sugar and saturated fat, along with insufficient intake of protein, fiber, and micronutrients), these factors include features that encourage overeating (e.g., high energy density, hyper-palatability, soft texture, reduced chewing, and fast consumption); loss of beneficial bioactive compounds (e.g., flavonoids and phytoestrogens), and elevated levels of harmful xenobiotics, such as processing-related contaminants (e.g., acrylamide), chemicals leached from packaging (e.g., bisphenol), and various additives and mixtures of additives.[3,8]

The evidence outlined here meets all relevant Bradford Hill criteria, widely used in epidemiology for establishing causality.[3]

Studies of trends from the 1980s to the 2010s in 8 out of 9 middle- and high-income countries with 3 or more repeated national surveys using Nova and the operational definition of UPFs have shown an increase in the dietary share of UPFs. In 1 country, the United Kingdom, where UPFs represent more than half of total energy intake, this share remained stable.[3] Analysis of more recent data on per-capita annual sales of UPFs in 93 countries (2007–2022) has shown increasing sales in low- and middle-income countries and in most world regions, with stable sales in high-income countries and regions, where sales reached 200 kilograms per person or more by 2007.[3]

APPLYING NOVA IN POLICYMAKING

When taken together, the evidence on UPF harms and trends provides a strong rationale for policy intervention, which we consider across diverse applications of Nova, in the following sections.

Dietary Guidance

National dietary guidelines are essential to orient food education activities aimed at promoting healthy and sustainable diets and function as reference points for wider food policies and regulation. Policymakers can directly integrate Nova into dietary guidelines by recommending a variety of unprocessed and minimally processed foods (Nova Group 1), mostly plant-sourced, as the basis of diets; using small amounts of culinary ingredients like oils, fats, salt, and sugar (Nova Group 2) when seasoning food or cooking; and using, also in small amounts, processed foods (Nova Group 3)—preferably those low in added sugars, sodium, and saturated fats—to add variety to freshly prepared meals. UPFs (Nova Group 4), identified using Nova's operational definition, as in research, should be limited or avoided when possible.[9]

Brazil, in 2014, was the first country to use Nova in framing its national dietary guidelines, which included the recommendation to not replace unprocessed or minimally processed foods and their culinary preparations with UPFs.[10] The guidelines acknowledge the importance of eating context, recommending eating with others when possible, and that, when eating outside of the home, to preference vendors serving freshly made meals based primarily on minimally processed foods. Since then, 14 countries have also integrated Nova into national dietary guidelines, recommending avoiding or limiting UPFs: Belgium, Chile, Colombia, Ecuador, France, India, Israel, Malaysia, Maldives, Mexico, Peru, Sri Lanka, Uruguay, and Zambia.[11,12] Nova-based recommendations have been tailored to promote culturally appropriate dishes, meals, and cuisines, constituting Nova Groups 1 to 3, and are intended to complement—rather than replace—other recommendations to encourage healthy and sustainable diets, including limiting sugar, sodium, and red and processed meat.[13,14]

Nova's operational definition of UPFs has also been adopted by consumer food education apps, including OpenFoodFacts, a barcode-scanning app that provides Nova classifications and NutriScore ratings,[15] and Perfact, a web-based platform that helps users identify non-UPFs in online food purchases.[16] The operational definition of UPFs has been used in thousands of media articles published by global news outlets,[6] often with the simple guidance to avoid products containing ingredients not commonly used in home kitchens.

By emphasizing food processing, Nova can also help to communicate how food is made, what food is made from, and who makes it. School lesson plans can use Nova to build food literacy, helping students to understand how industrial processing affects diet quality, health, and the environment; how to distinguish between Nova groups; the importance of food processing in human evolution, economies, and food culture; and how to identify misleading marketing practices. School kitchen gardens and cooking classes can reinforce ecological connections to food and emphasize preparing meals from Nova Groups 1 to 3. Behavior change communication, including mass-media campaigns, can use clear, actionable dietary messages—for example, to choose foods made from real ingredients or to avoid or limit ultraprocessed products.

Dietary Monitoring and Target Setting

Monitoring population dietary patterns is essential for assessing the progress of policies aimed at promoting healthy and sustainable diets. Adherence to the ultraprocessed dietary pattern can be monitored by using 2 metrics, which are suitable for integration into existing dietary monitoring systems.

A first metric is the share of UPFs in population diets, measured as the average percentage of total food energy (kilocalories) or weight (grams), assessed using Nova's operational definition of UPFs, as applied in research and dietary guidelines. Many studies have used this metric to document country-level transitions from long-established dietary patterns based on Nova Groups 1 to 3 to those increasingly dominated by UPFs.[3] For example, a Brazilian study showed a deceleration in the increase of the dietary share of UPFs in the overall population and a reduction in this share among more-educated and higher-income individuals, following the implementation of the 2014 Nova-based dietary guidelines.[17]

A second metric is the Nova UPF-score, which counts the number of commonly consumed UPF subgroups reported by the population on the previous day using brief, country-adapted screening tools lasting 2 to 3 minutes.[18,19] This metric has been validated against Nova's operational definition of UPFs in 5 countries[18–21] and is acknowledged jointly by the World Health Organization (WHO), Food and Agricultural Organization of the United Nations (FAO), and United Nations Children's Fund (UNICEF) as 1 of the 4 key metrics for the global monitoring of diet quality.[22] These metrics can be considered for integration into, for example, the WHO's Global Nutrition Monitoring Framework; the WHO, UNICEF and World Bank's Joint Child Malnutrition Estimates; and FAO's food balance sheets.

Both of these metrics can inform international and national target setting for policies aiming to reduce the share of UPFs in diets[23]—for example, achieving a population-level dietary share from UPFs of less than a certain percentage range (e.g., less than 10%), complementing existing nutrient-based targets like the WHO recommendation of consuming less than 5% to 10% of calories from free sugars. The establishment of feasible targets will be context dependent, based, first of all, on a given country's stage in the transition to the ultraprocessed dietary pattern.[9]

Regulation

The Nova classification system is grounded in evidence that the displacement of traditional dietary patterns by an ultraprocessed dietary pattern is adversely impacting population health. Existing food regulatory systems are poorly designed to respond to this challenge.[24] Codex and national food regulators permit many additives commonly used in ultraprocessing and, hence, support the proliferation—rather than curtailment—of UPFs in diets. Reform proposals have called for changing the mandates, governance, and risk assessment frameworks used by food regulators, including by expanding the concept of food safety to incorporate cumulative long-term additive exposures and chronic disease endpoints associated with ultraprocessed diets.[9,24,25] In the United States, this includes calls to substantially reform or abolish the Generally Recognized as Safe pathway for additive approval.[26] These are important considerations for food regulatory reform over coming years.

More immediately, the UPF concept can be operationalized to identify food products for regulation, including taxation, labeling, marketing controls, and public procurement, among other key interventions to reduce the share of UPFs in diets.[27,28] Achieving this requires careful consideration of both public health objectives and the complexities of practical implementation. One such challenge is that food substances used exclusively or predominantly in industrial settings, and additives with cosmetic functions number in the thousands and continue to grow each year. Moreover, these markers of food ultraprocessing are not always consistently disclosed on ingredient lists, and some cosmetic additives may also serve other functional roles in processing, which manufacturers are not required to declare.

While these limitations may not affect most UPF categories (e.g., carbonated soft drinks, confections, packaged snacks, sweetened breakfast cereals, reconstituted meat products, and so on), because such products typically contain multiple markers of ultraprocessing, they may lead to misclassification in some cases. These inaccuracies are manageable in research (e.g., through sensitivity analyses) and in monitoring or consumer education (where minor misclassifications have limited impact), but they may pose legal challenges when applied in regulatory contexts. Feasibility could be strengthened by requiring food manufacturers to report, in a standardized way, all additives and substances that are markers of ultraprocessing.[1] It is also essential to recognize that food regulatory criteria must be tailored to national contexts, depending on the proportion of UPFs in the food supply, local legislative frameworks, the autonomy of regulatory bodies, and anticipated industry responses. Here we propose 2 pathways forward to identifying UPFs for regulatory purposes.

Pathway 1—Regulation based on Nova's operational definition of ultraprocessed foods. The first approach is to regulate all food and drink products that meet Nova's operational definition of UPFs—formulations containing either a food-derived substance used exclusively or predominantly in industrial settings or an additive with a cosmetic function.[29] This would involve developing classification algorithms similar to those used in the aforementioned consumer applications like OpenFoodFacts and Perfact.

Importantly, regulation of UPFs using this approach should be viewed as complementing—not competing with—existing regulations targeting products with high levels of added sugar, sodium, and saturated unbalanced nutrient profiles. For example, a proposal to combine UPF warnings with NutriScore rankings on front-of-pack labels has been shown to be both well-understood and accepted by consumers.[30] Nor should this approach be viewed as replacing single nutrient–based regulations—for example, sodium reduction or transfat elimination—or those restricting the use of food additives with evidence of harm.

This approach has several strengths: it directly translates scientific evidence into policy, it applies a UPF definition already familiar to many consumers and health professionals, and it can build on existing consumer information tools. Its main advantage is scientific fidelity—targeting what has been empirically shown to be harmful by studies using the Nova UPF definition. However, a drawback is the potential for legal challenges attributable to ambiguities in ingredient labeling and inconsistent classification of certain additives across jurisdictions.

Pathway 2—Expanded nutrient-based regulation incorporating ultraprocessed food markers. The second option seeks to capture most UPFs while addressing the legal complexities outlined previously. It involves regulating unhealthy foods more broadly without strictly distinguishing between ultraprocessed products, those with poor nutrient profiles, and those that fall into both categories.

This approach is supported by studies from Brazil,[31] the United States,[32] and the United Kingdom,[33] demonstrating substantial but not complete overlap between Nova-defined UPFs and foods with high levels of added sugar, sodium, or saturated fat. These findings suggest that expanding current nutrient-based criteria to include a limited set of easily identifiable UPF markers—such as nonnutritive sweeteners, colorings, and flavorings—would allow regulators to cover most unhealthy products, including all with unbalanced nutrient profiles and nearly all UPFs. Under this model, regulations would apply to food items that (1) exceed thresholds for critical nutrients (e.g., saturated fat, added and total sugars, and sodium); (2) contain selected, easily identifiable markers of ultraprocessing (e.g., nonnutritive sweeteners, colorants, and flavorings); or (3) meet both conditions.

This approach is more legally defendable, aligns well with existing regulatory frameworks including nutrient profiling models, and would maintain high coverage of both foods with unbalanced nutrient profiles and UPFs, thereby enhancing regulatory effectiveness. Another important benefit is that it would prevent UPF manufacturers from gaming existing nutrient profiling models to avoid regulation. Its main limitation is that it does not align perfectly with the research evidence base, which has primarily relied on Nova's full operational definition of UPFs.

In contexts where nutrient profile–based regulations are already in place, this second approach would require only the integration of selected markers of ultraprocessing into existing criteria. Nonsugar sweeteners (including artificial, natural noncaloric, and caloric sweeteners) have already been integrated in nutrient-based regulatory framework in countries adopting the Pan-American Health Organization (PAHO) nutrient profile model,[34] such as Mexico, Argentina, and Colombia. In other contexts, criteria for identifying unhealthy foods should be developed to encompass both unbalanced nutrient profiles—such as those recommended by PAHO or other WHO regional offices—and selected UPF markers. Market-specific analyses of product composition[26,27] can inform the selection of nutrient thresholds and UPF markers.

This second pathway should not be interpreted as simply collapsing the UPF concept into a nutrient-profiling framework. Integration should prioritize regulatory approaches that clearly signal products to be avoided or limited, rather than positioning UPFs along a spectrum of perceived healthfulness. For example, threshold-based warning labels are more effective than graded schemes like the Health Star Rating system.[9]

Sustainable Food Systems Transition

Nova can also help in guiding policymakers seeking to strengthen local and territorial markets, and the transition to sustainable food systems provisioning nutritious, locally produced, culturally appropriate, and underutilized traditional foods.[6]

By recognizing profit maximization as the core purpose of ultraprocessing, the Nova classification foregrounds the business practices and financial incentives that drive UPF expansion.[6,35] The much higher average profitability of UPF manufacturers relative to firms producing Nova Groups 1 to 3 foods is essential to understand and for policy to respond to.[6,36] This is because higher profit margins both attract investment and incentivize ultraprocessing as a business model, while generating surplus resources that corporations can reinvest into marketing, product engineering, supply chain expansion, and political influence to further generate UPF market growth.[6,37] This results in the structural displacement of Nova Group 1 to 3 food producers and thereby undermines local agri-food systems supporting the food security and livelihoods of billions. This displacement coincides with a growing share of food-related income flowing from food producers in low- and middle-income countries to UPF corporations headquartered largely in high-income countries.[6,38,39]

Food policies informed by Nova would seek to counter this wealth and income extraction and rebalance power within food systems by limiting the structural dominance and profitability of UPF producers while fostering the conditions for alternative food economies, territorial markets, and traditional industries to grow and thrive.[6,9,27] The objective is to protect and stop the displacement of local agri-food systems and strengthen them to produce diverse Nova Group 1 to 3 foods that form the basis of long-established healthy dietary patterns. This could involve restricting foreign investment by UPF manufacturers and limiting their entry into national markets; dietary guidelines recommending to preference local producers, vendors, and culturally appropriate foods; repurposing public subsidies away from commodity crops that serve as inputs for UPF production toward diversified agroecological systems and producers; investing in infrastructure, research, and workforce development that supports short supply chains, local food vendors, and culturally appropriate diets; using state procurement (e.g., school feeding programs) to create demand for locally sourced foods; and imposing much stricter controls on UPF marketing.[6,9,37,40]

CONCLUSION

The evidence linking the ultraprocessed dietary pattern to diseases affecting nearly all body organ systems, along with documentation of the displacement of long-established, whole-food, and meal-based healthy dietary patterns by

UPFs, underscores the urgent need for policy action. By integrating Nova and the UPF concept into dietary guidance, monitoring systems, regulatory frameworks, and wider food policies, policymakers can complement existing nutrient-based policies and strengthen efforts to promote healthy diets and facilitate sustainable food system transitions. AJPH

ABOUT THE AUTHORS

Carlos A. Monteiro is with the Center for Epidemiological Studies in Health and Nutrition, School of Public Health, University of São Paulo, Brazil. Phillip Baker is with the School of Public Health, University of Sydney, Australia. Camila Corvalan is with the Institute of Nutrition and Food Technology, University of Chile, Santiago, Chile. Barry Popkin is with the Gillings School of Global Public Health, University of North Carolina at Chapel Hill.

CORRESPONDENCE

Correspondence should be sent to Carlos A. Monteiro, Ave Dr Arnaldo 715, Sao Paulo 01416-001, Brazil (e-mail: carlosam@usp.br). Reprints can be ordered at https://www.ajph.org by clicking the "Reprints" link.

PUBLICATION INFORMATION

Full Citation: Monteiro CA, Baker P, Corvalan C, Popkin BM. What do Nova and the ultraprocessed food concept offer to policymakers? From updating dietary guidance to regulatory action and advancing sustainable food system transitions. *Am J Public Health*. 2026;116(7):932–939.

Acceptance Date: February 17, 2026.

DOI: https://doi.org/10.2105/AJPH.2026.308509

ORCID iDs:

Carlos A. Monteiro https://orcid.org/0000-0002-3777-1533

Barry M. Popkin https://orcid.org/0000-0001-9495-9324

CONTRIBUTORS

All authors contributed equally to the work.

CONFLICTS OF INTEREST

The authors report no conflicts of interest.

HUMAN PARTICIPANT PROTECTION

This essay is based on previously published studies and does not involve any new studies with human participants performed by the authors.

REFERENCES

1. Monteiro CA, Cannon G, Levy RB, et al. Ultra-processed foods: what they are and how to identify them. *Public Health Nutr*. 2019;22(5):936–941. https://doi.org/10.1017/S1368980018003762
2. Monteiro CA, Cannon G, Moubarac J-C, Levy RB, Louzada MLC, Jaime PC. The UN Decade of Nutrition, the Nova food classification and the trouble with ultraprocessing. *Public Health Nutr*. 2018;21(1):5–17. https://doi.org/10.1017/S1368980017000234
3. Monteiro CA, Louzada ML, Steele-Martinez E, et al. Ultra-processed foods and human health: the main thesis and the evidence. *Lancet*. 2025;406(10520):2667–2684. https://doi.org/10.1016/S0140-6736(25)01565-X
4. Baker P, Machado P, Santos T, et al. Ultra-processed foods and the nutrition transition: global, regional and national trends, food systems transformations and political economy drivers. *Obes Rev*. 2020;21(12):e13126. https://doi.org/10.1111/obr.13126
5. Northcott T, Lawrence M, Parker C, Reeve B, Baker P. Regulatory responses to ultraprocessed foods are skewed towards behaviour change and not food system transformation. *Nat Food*. 2025;6(3):273–282. https://doi.org/10.1038/s43016-024-01101-y
6. Baker P, Slater S, White M, et al. Towards unified global action on ultraprocessed foods: understanding commercial determinants, countering corporate power, and mobilizing a public health response. *Lancet*. 2025;406(10520):2703–2726. https://doi.org/10.1016/S0140-6736(25)01567-3
7. Martinez-Steele E, Khandpur N, Batis C, et al. Best practices for applying the Nova food classification system. *Nat Food*. 2023;4(6):445–448. https://doi.org/10.1038/s43016-023-00779-w
8. Juul F, Martinez-Steele E, Parekh N, Monteiro CA. The role of ultraprocessed food in obesity. *Nat Rev Endocrinol*. 2025;21(11):672–685. https://doi.org/10.1038/s41574-025-01143-7
9. Scrinis G, Popkin B, Corvalan C, et al. Policies to halt and reverse the rise in ultraprocessed food production, marketing, and consumption. *Lancet*. 2025;406(10520):2685–2702. https://doi.org/10.1016/S0140-6736(25)01566-1
10. Monteiro CA, Cannon G, Moubarac J-C, et al. Dietary guidelines to nourish humanity and the planet in the twenty-first century. A blueprint from Brazil. *Public Health Nutr*. 2015;18(13):2311–2322. https://doi.org/10.1017/S1368980015002165
11. Anastasiou K, De Melo PR, Slater S, et al. From harmful nutrients to ultraprocessed foods: exploring shifts in 'foods to limit' terminology used in national food-based dietary guidelines. *Public Health Nutr*. 2023;26(11):2539–2550. https://doi.org/10.1017/S1368980022002580
12. Koios D, Machado P, Lacy-Nichols J. Representations of ultraprocessed foods: a global analysis of how dietary guidelines refer to levels of food processing. *Int J Health Policy Manag*. 2022;11(11):2588–2599. https://doi.org/10.34172/ijhpm.2022.6443
13. What Are Healthy Diets? Joint Statement by the Food and Agriculture Organization of the United Nations and the World Health Organization. Geneva, Switzerland: World Health Organization, Food and Agriculture Organization of the United Nations; 2024.
14. Sustainable Healthy Diets: Guiding Principles. Rome, Italy: Food and Agriculture Organization of the United Nations, World Health Organization; 2019.
15. OpenFoodFacts. Available at: https://world.openfoodfacts.org. Accessed February 16, 2025.
16. Perfact. Available at: http://perfact.co. Accessed February 16, 2025.
17. Louzada M, Cruz G, Silva KAAN, et al. Consumption of ultraprocessed foods in Brazil: distribution and temporal evolution 2008–2018. *Rev Saude Publica*. 2023;57:12. https://doi.org/10.11606/s1518-8787.2023057004744
18. Correa-Madrid MC, Correa Guzmán N, Bergeron G, Restrepo-Mesa SL, Cediel G. Validation of the Nova score for the consumption of ultraprocessed foods by young women of Medellín, Colombia. *Ann N Y Acad Sci*. 2023;1528(1):69–76. https://doi.org/10.1111/nyas.15054
19. Costa C, Faria F, Gabe KT, et al. Nova score for the consumption of ultraprocessed foods: description and performance evaluation in Brazil. *Rev Saude Publica*. 2021;55:13. https://doi.org/10.11606/s1518-8787.2021055003588
20. Kébé SD, Diouf A, Sylla PMDD, et al. Assessment of ultra processed foods consumption in Senegal: validation of the Nova-UPF screener. *Arch Public Health*. 2024;82(1):4. https://doi.org/10.1186/s13690-024-01239-y
21. Freire WB, Tello B, Guerrón PB. Validation of Nova 27 Ultra-Processed Food Screener: adaptation and performance in Ecuador. *Public Health Nutr*. 2025:28(1):e105. https://doi.org/10.1017/S1368980025100475
22. Guidance for Monitoring Healthy Diets Globally. Geneva, Switzerland: World Health Organization, Food and Agriculture Organization of the United Nations, United Nations Children's Fund; 2024.
23. Lawrence M. Ultra-processed foods: a fit-for-purpose concept for nutrition policy activities to tackle unhealthy and unsustainable diets. *Public Health Nutr*. 2023;26(7):1384–1388. https://doi.org/10.1017/S1368980022002117
24. Lawrence M, Parker C, Johnson H, et al. An ecological reorientation of the Codex Alimentarius Commission could help transform food systems. *Nat Food*. 2024;5(7):557–562. https://doi.org/10.1038/s43016-024-01009-7
25. Zokaityte A. EU food law and ultraprocessed food markets: safety from what and for whom? *J Consum Policy*. 2025;48(1):51–74. https://doi.org/10.1007/s10603-025-09582-5
26. Pomeranz JL, Broad Leib EM, Mozaffarian D. Regulation of added substances in the food supply by the Food and Drug Administration Human Foods Program. *Am J Public Health*. 2024;114(10):1061–1070. https://doi.org/10.2105/AJPH.2024.307755
27. Northcott T, Lawrence M, Parker C, Baker P. Ecological regulation for healthy and sustainable food systems: responding to the global rise of ultraprocessed foods. *Agric Hum Values*. 2023;40(3):1333–1358. https://doi.org/10.1007/s10460-022-10412-4
28. Popkin BM, Barquera S, Corvalan C, et al. Towards unified and impactful policies to reduce ultraprocessed food consumption and promote healthier eating. *Lancet Diabetes Endocrinol*. 2021;9(7):462–470. https://doi.org/10.1016/S2213-8587(21)00078-4
29. Mozaffarian D. Regulatory policy to address ultra-processed foods. *N Engl J Med*. 2025;392(24):2393–2396. https://doi.org/10.1056/NEJMp2503241

30. Srour B, Hercberg S, Galan P, et al. Effect of a new graphically modified Nutri-Score on the objective understanding of foods' nutrient profile and ultraprocessing: a randomised controlled trial. *BMJ Nutr Prev Health.* 2023;6(1):108–118. https://doi.org/10.1136/bmjnph-2022-000599
31. Canella DS, Pereira Montera V, Oliveira N, Mais LA, Andrade GC, Martins APB. Food additives and PAHO's nutrient profile model as contributors' elements to the identification of ultraprocessed food products. *Sci Rep.* 2023;13(1):13698. https://doi.org/10.1038/s41598-023-40650-3
32. Popkin BM, Miles DR, Taillie LS, Dunford EK. A policy approach to identifying food and beverage products that are ultraprocessed and high in added salt, sugar and saturated fat in the United States: a cross-sectional analysis of packaged foods. *Lancet Reg Health Am.* 2024;32:100713. https://doi.org/10.1016/j.lana.2024.100713
33. Kesaite V, Chavez-Ugalde Y, White M, Adams J. Overlap between ultraprocessed food and food that is high in fat, salt or sugar: analysis of 11 annual waves of the UK National Diet and Nutrition Survey 2008/2009–2018/2019. *BMJ Nutr Prev Health.* 2025;8(1):e001035. https://doi.org/10.1136/bmjnph-2024-001035
34. Pan American Health Organization Nutrient Profile Model. Washington, DC: Pan American Health Organization; 2016.
35. Monteiro CA, Cannon G. The impact of transnational "Big Food" companies on the South: a view from Brazil. *PLoS Med.* 2012;9(7):e1001252. https://doi.org/10.1371/journal.pmed.1001252
36. Wood B, Robinson E, Baker P, et al. What is the purpose of ultraprocessed food? An exploratory analysis of the financialisation of ultraprocessed food corporations and implications for public health. *Global Health.* 2023;19(1):85. https://doi.org/10.1186/s12992-023-00990-1
37. Wood B, Garton K, Milsom P, et al. Using a systems thinking approach to map the global rise of ultraprocessed foods in population diets. *Obes Rev.* 2025;26(4):e13877. https://doi.org/10.1111/obr.13877
38. Goyal M, Hickel J, Jha P. Increasing inequality in agri-food value chains: global trends from 1995–2020. *Glob Food Sec.* 2025;46:100883. https://doi.org/10.1016/j.gfs.2025.100883
39. Wood B, McCoy D, Baker P, Williams O, Sacks G. The double burden of maldistribution: a descriptive analysis of corporate wealth and income distribution in four unhealthy commodity industries. *Crit Public Health.* 2023;33(2):135–147. https://doi.org/10.1080/09581596.2021.2019681
40. Fuel to Fork: What will it take to get fossil fuels out of our food systems? Brussels, Belgium: International Panel of Experts on Sustainable Food Systems; 2025.

Tobacco Industry Contributions to the Development of Ultraprocessed Food in the United States, 1985–2007: A Case Study of Lunchables

Laura A. Schmidt, PhD

See also Ultraprocessed Food, pp. 898–1029.

We need to know how ultraprocessed foods (UPFs) are designed and formulated to better understand why these products cause overeating and weight gain, and how to apply appropriate guardrails. This information, however, is typically kept hidden by UPF companies as proprietary trade secrets. Using previously undisclosed internal company documents, this study traced product development for Lunchables, a prepackaged meal brand developed at Kraft General Foods while it was owned by the tobacco giant Philip Morris Companies.

Findings show that a key reason Philip Morris purchased food companies was to increase revenues by sharing proprietary research and development assets across tobacco and food product lines. Philip Morris applied its product development approach for making cigarettes to Lunchables in 2 important ways: First, it applied its "consumer-driven product development" strategy that optimized products for consumer pleasure and appeal. Second, Phillip Morris applied its "better-for-you" reformulation strategy, first used to create filtered Marlboro cigarettes, to develop Low-Fat Lunchables in efforts to keep consumers worried about childhood obesity loyal to the brand.

These findings speak to the need for public health research and policies that extend existing models for regulating tobacco to UPFs. (*Am J Public Health*. 2026;116(7):940–949. https://doi.org/10.2105/AJPH.2026.308491)

AJPH July 2026, Vol. 116, No. 7

In 2023, 2 new formulations of Kraft–Heinz's grab-and-go prepackaged meal brand, Lunchables, qualified for the US National School Lunch Program (NSLP) serving 30 million low-income children. With Lunchables "built for schools," Kraft-Heinz told investors that the NSLP was a "$25 billion growth opportunity."[1] A year later, the company abruptly withdrew Lunchables from the NSLP, citing poor market performance. This came on the heels of a *Consumer Reports* study that found high concentrations of sodium and heavy metals in Lunchables[2] and reports that school districts were hesitant to dispense them because of nutritional concerns.[1] Citing a decline in consumer trust because of "negative publicity," the Kraft–Heinz CEO said, "This is a brand that is focused on families and kids. So rebuilding that trust just takes some time."[3]

Among other health challenges, nearly 20% of US children have obesity—a rate nearly quadruple what it was in the 1970s, before ultraprocessed foods (UPFs), like Lunchables, became widespread in the US food supply.[4] UPFs—industrially produced foods that use multiple physical processing steps and chemical additives not used in home cooking—contribute 62% of daily calories to the diet of US children today.[5] Linked to poor diet quality and health outcomes, UPFs are rapidly displacing traditional diets in most parts of the world.[6] In clinical trials of adults, they are causally linked to overeating and weight gain.[7] Epidemiological studies associate UPF dietary share with population-level obesity rates, along with diabetes, cardiovascular disease, and premature death.[6,8] Lunchables is a quintessential child-focused UPF brand made with processed meats and cheeses, refined carbohydrates, and sugar-sweetened beverages (SSBs) that largely fails to meet child nutrition standards.[9] Even reformulated "better-for-you" Lunchables for the NSLP contain highly processed ingredients and cosmetic additives, including emulsifiers, enzymes, preservatives, and artificial flavorants (Appendix A, available as a supplement to the online version of this article at https://ajph.org).

Between 1963 and 2008, the largest US food companies were owned by the largest tobacco firms, RJ Reynolds (Del Monte, Nabisco) and Philip Morris (Kraft, General Foods). Two previous studies found that, during this 45-year period, tobacco companies applied cigarette marketing strategies to promote their UPF product lines.[10,11] This study adds to the picture by examining tobacco companies' technical contributions to the design and formulation of UPF products. Research of this kind is important because clinical trials find that "hyper-palatable" UPF formulations cause more overeating[12] and that tobacco-owned UPF brands were disproportionately hyper-palatable.[13] Scientists, policymakers, and parents need information on how UPFs are designed and formulated to better understand why these foods are overeaten and produce weight gain, and to apply appropriate guardrails.[14] However, this information is often kept secret by UPF companies as proprietary intellectual property.

Lunchables were in premarket development at General Foods in 1985 when Philip Morris Companies (PMC) acquired the company and subsequently brought Lunchables to market, developing the brand over 23 years. It is possible to pierce the secrecy surrounding the design and formulation of some UPF products, including Lunchables, because this process is described in internal company documents (e.g., executive correspondence, research and development [R&D] records) in the UCSF Industry Documents Library—an archive launched following class action litigation of the tobacco industry (Appendix B, available as a supplement to the online version of this article at https://ajph.org).[15] This information, triangulated with public-facing documents (e.g., corporate websites, journalism) reveals that a key reason why PMC diversified into the food industry was to boost growth and revenues by sharing proprietary R&D across tobacco and food product lines. PMC applied its technical knowledge for making cigarettes to Lunchables in 2 important ways: first, by applying its "consumer-driven product development" process that optimized products for pleasure, and second, by applying its approach to formulating "better-for-you" products for health-conscious consumers.

BOOSTING PROFITS BY SHARING TOBACCO AND FOOD R&D

PMC ("Altria Group" since 2003) acquired the Lunchables brand during a period of significant corporate growth through acquisitions and mergers. As Figure 1 shows, by 1985, when PMC bought General Foods, it already owned an alcohol subsidiary (Miller Brewing Company, acquired 1970) and an SSB company (7-UP, 1978). These acquisitions were designed to competitively position PMC against its largest US competitor, RJ Reynolds, which was also acquiring food (Del Monte, 1979; Nabisco, 1985), alcohol (Heublein, 1985), and SSB (Pacific Hawaiian Products, 1963) companies.

In 1987, PMC bought Kraft and merged it with General Foods to create the second-largest food corporation in the world, Kraft General Foods (KGF). By 1989, PMC had installed tobacco executives in KGF's leadership[16] and restructured the firm into 7 different operating units with a combined sales of $22.5 billion.[17] In 1990, the long-standing tobacco executive Geoff Bible became CEO of KGF[18] in a move that PMC's chairman, Hamish Maxwell, said would promote "significant cross-fertilization between our businesses."[19(p8)] Emphasizing the similarities between tobacco products and food, Maxwell told investors that PMC had become the largest consumer packaged goods firm in the world:

> We are the largest publicly held cigarette company, the second-largest food company and second-largest beer company in the world today. In aggregate, we are the world's largest consumer packaged goods company—marketing products to millions of people daily. All of our major businesses share common characteristics. They market low-priced consumer packaged goods with huge retail markets. Most of our products are sold around the world; using common marketing approaches and similar retail outlets. Most products are agriculturally based and are resistant to economic change.[20(p36)]

PMC's diversification strategy was designed to exploit "technical synergies" across its tobacco, alcohol, SSB, and food product lines. In 1988, PMC launched a Technical Synergies Committee comprising product development leads from its tobacco, alcohol, and food subsidiaries. Viewed as "a large component of the battle to dominate the world's consumer product business,"[21(p33)] the Committee's mission was "to increase effectiveness and

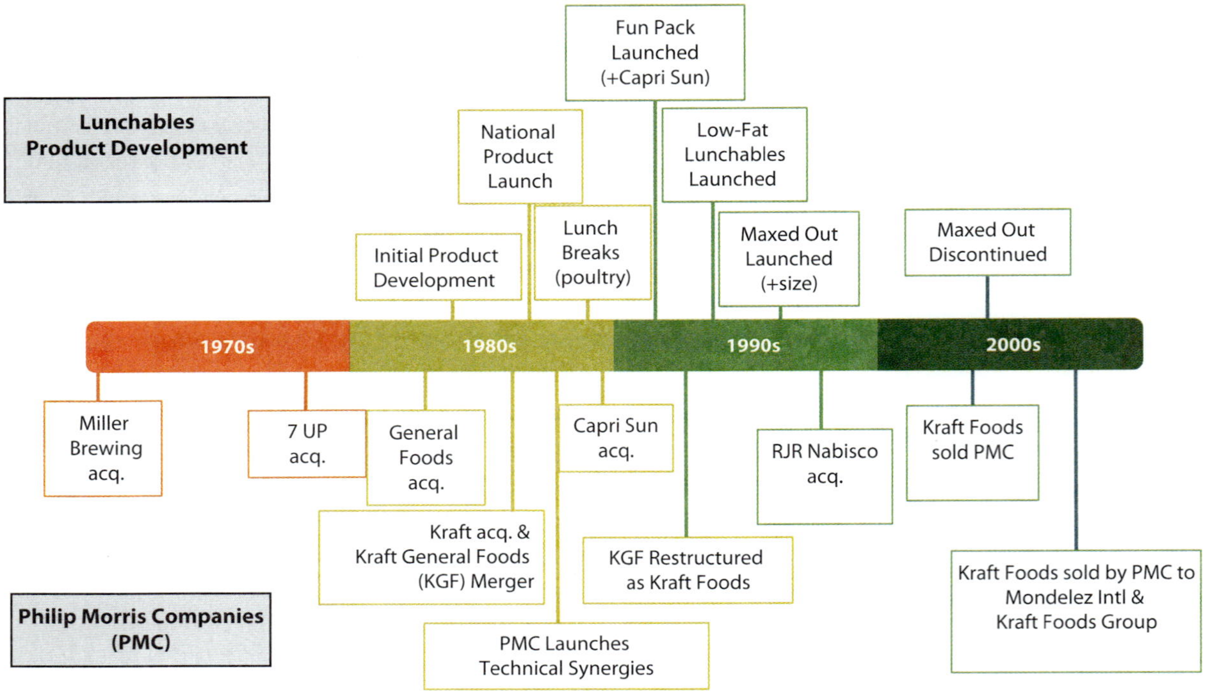

FIGURE 1— Milestones for Lunchables Product Development and Philip Morris Companies

Note. acq. = acquired.
Source. Moodys Investor Service.[23]

reduce costs of R&D throughout PM Companies wherever possible through well-designed interactions among all of the technical centers."[22(p10)] The Synergies Committee began with a companywide assessment of "PM's technology portfolio," including skills, people, research capabilities, equipment, facilities, "emerging technologies," and "coordinated/joint research" to facilitate the "transfer of technologies or skills"[21(p3–4)] across tobacco, food, and alcohol R&D departments. At the time, PMC had a vast global R&D enterprise comprising 2840 engineers and scientists. One third was devoted to tobacco, and the remainder to food and beverage R&D.[21]

In 1989, Bob McVicker, vice president of technology at KGF, took leadership of the Technical Synergies Committee to serve as "an active participant in the synergy effort so that we could all rapidly benefit from Kraft's complementary technologies, and they from ours."[21(p38)] The companywide assessment found numerous opportunities for collaboration. As its 1989 report described, the Committee found that "there were some technologies that were being pursued by more than one operating company at that time; if these efforts could be coordinated, we could avoid duplication and benefit from the differences in perspective."[21(p3–4)]

Throughout the 1990s, the Technical Synergies Committee coordinated and streamlined R&D sharing across PMC's 6 tobacco, food, and alcohol subsidiaries (Figure 2).[23] Shared R&D assets included chemical additives, processing and packaging technologies, research, research partnerships, and supply chains.[20] Specific synergies projects utilized "biotechnology in developing innovative natural food flavors" and flavor encapsulation technology (chemically coating flavor compounds for timed release and extended shelf life) for use in cigarettes and food. An "antifreeze protein project" applied genetically engineered yeast developed by Miller Brewing to solve KGF's problems with inhibiting ice crystal formation to improve frozen food texture.[21](p5–6) Collaborative studies focused on chemical flavorants for cigarettes and food, and the development of a companywide "crop protection agent" (e.g., pesticide) database.[22(p11)]

Lunchables, launched nationally in 1988, embodied PMC's approach to leveraging technical synergies. By design, Lunchables allowed product developers to combine numerous PMC ingredients and products in a single snack tray (Figure 3, panel a). As PMC's

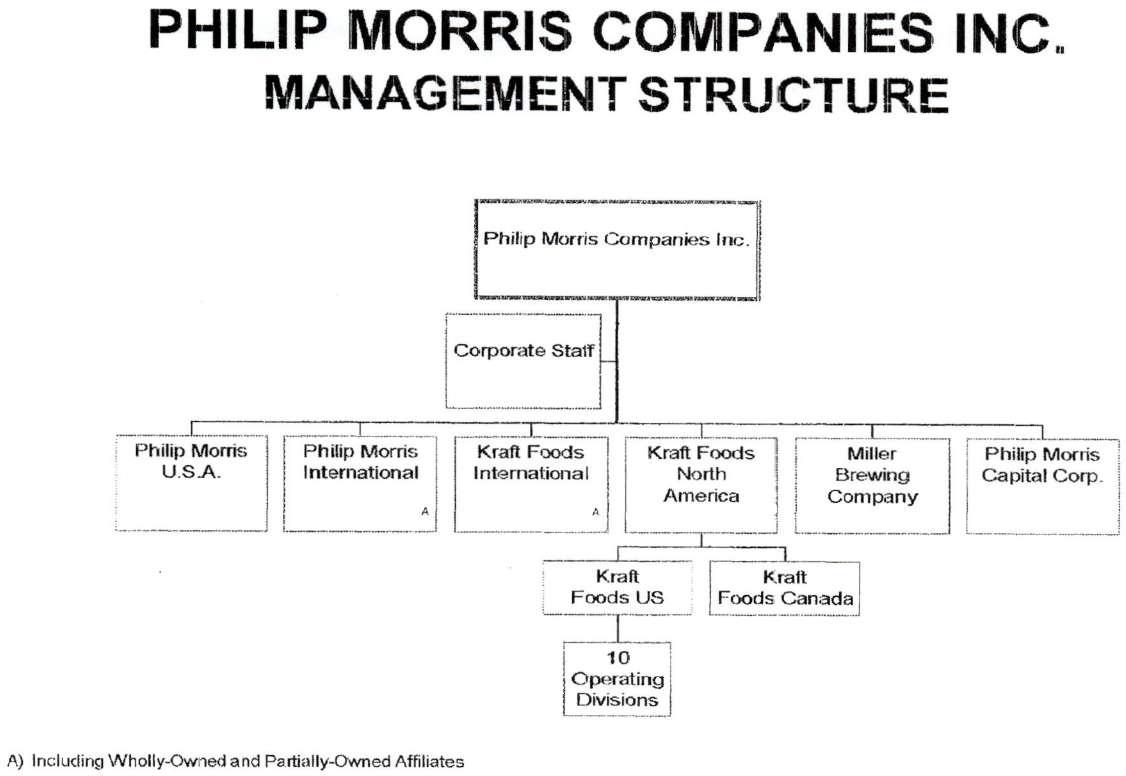

FIGURE 2— Philip Morris Companies Management Structure, 1995

Source. Moodys Investor Service.[23]

vice chairman pointed out, the "new Lunchables line has benefitted from Kraft's technical and production of knowledge in cheese. . . . One way of sharing expertise is through cross-unit working groups."[20(p27)] Lunchables was lauded by the Synergies Committee as a model of the "benefits we can expect from the corporation's technical synergies."[21(p41)] When, in 1991, PMC spent $115 million to acquire the SSB company Capri Sun, the new aseptic "juice" pouches were added to make the "Lunchables Fun Pack." When PMC bought Del Monte's pudding division in 1995, the Jell-O brand made "Lunchables with Pudding."[24] By then, Lunchables had become a $200 million food category, in part, through "simplifying the organization" via synergies. PMC's leadership credited synergies for making Lunchables KGF's "fastest growing business."[24(p23)]

CIGARETTE PRODUCT DESIGN APPROACH APPLIED TO LUNCHABLES

Key to optimizing technical synergies was sharing expertise in "consumer-driven product development" between PMC's tobacco and food product developers. PMC's approach was to embed market researchers in "cross-functional teams," working alongside product engineers. This allowed consumer testing to drive decision-making at each step of the product development cycle, from prototyping to design, formulation, and packaging. As KGF's CEO Bible explained at a 1990 companywide R&D symposium, PMC's goal was to optimize products in ways that fulfilled the consumer's deepest "needs and preferences" using synergies:

> Cigarettes may not have much to do with cheese or beer or mayo. But test methodologies excavating one hierarchy of needs might well apply to the other. . . . As far as I'm concerned, understanding the customer is the heart and soul of Philip Morris companies—at KGF, Miller, or anywhere else in the corporation. If the customer doesn't care about a new product—what else matters? . . . Remember, our mission is to plumb the sometimes murky recesses of the customer's attitudes, behavior and hierarchy of needs and excavating any needs that may remain unarticulated, locked away in a corner somewhere. That supreme thought should guide our behavior throughout

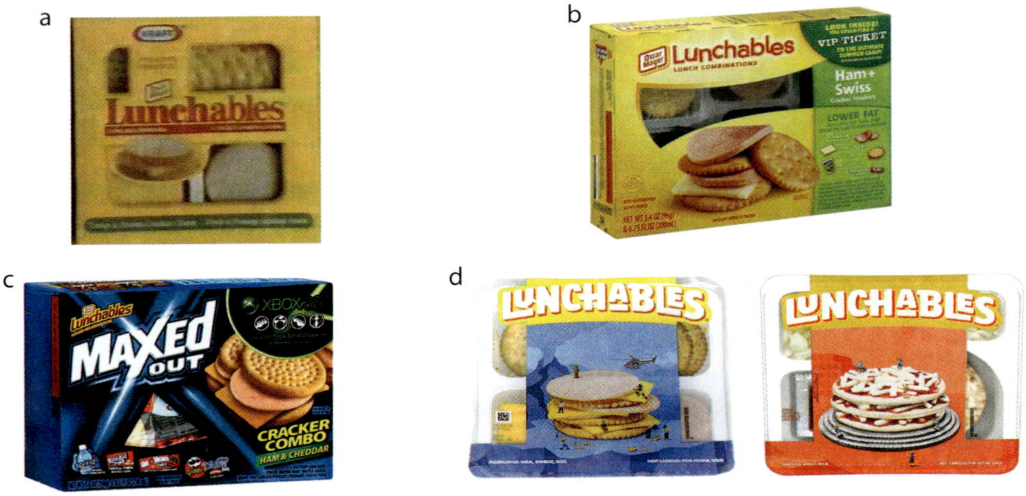

FIGURE 3— **Lunchables Product Evolution Showing (a) Original (1988), (b) Low Fat (1995), (c) Maxed Out (1999), and (d) US National School Lunch Program (2023)**

Sources. (a) https://www.youtube.com/watch?v=eYvlFTxSWmk; (b) https://www.historyoasis.com/post/discontinued-lunchables; (c) https://duckduckgo.com/?t=ftsa&q=maxed+out+lunchables&ia=images&iax=images&iai=https%3A%2F%2Fimages.freshop.com%2F00044700360675%2F1d2ca4ce78bd24330 14f773654fb5f30_large.png; (d) https://vegnews.com/lunchables-toxic-chemicals.

> the new-product development process. . . . We don't create demand. We excavate it. We prospect for it. We dig until we find it.[25(p109–110)]

Later in this R&D symposium, product developers for Lunchables explained how a consumer-driven approach had "optimized" their product concept. The Lunchables cross-functional team had started the design process by asking, "What do consumers want?" Focus groups with children led developers to believe the product could fulfill the child's deepest desires for play and autonomy: "Kids loved them" because the children wanted "control over their lunch," and also wanted "permission to play with their food."[25(p265)] Early prototypes for Lunchables used a "Food Playground" paradigm, where the cross-functional design team built 17 prototypes through interactive play in a "room full of food" with "plastic and scissors."[25(p260)] As a KGF executive later reflected on Lunchables with Pizza, "We're letting kids know that they can have their favorite food, pizza—anytime and anywhere."[24(p31)]

Consumer testing also focused on the market segment, "Busy mothers/working women 25–49." In focus groups for early design prototypes, mothers called Lunchables "cute" and suggested a desire for convenience. Central location testing found that mothers weighed convenience against child health concerns: "easy to pack, easy to clean up, last-minute lunch," and "better than junk food."[25(p267)] Consumer testing by the firm, BehaviorScan, found that mothers liked Lunchables' tray format, but needed the reassurance of familiar contents,[26] such as PMC's Oscar Mayer processed meat and Kraft cheese, made visible through plastic windows in the cardboard packaging (Figure 3, panel a). With a bright yellow band around the box, suggestive of a gift, Lunchables' packaging was designed to alleviate mothers' guilt about opting for a prepackaged meal. Lunchables' lead designer later explained, "The box was there as a gift, something precious to elevate its specialness."[26(p205)]

PMC continued to build the Lunchables brand until 2007, when it sold Kraft. Product development during this period focused on the prolific release of new product line extensions—novel flavor, size, and packaging variations used to penetrate new market segments and revitalize flagging sales (Figures 1 and 3). Although the cumulative total is unknown, as of July 2025, the Kraft–Heinz website listed 52 Lunchables line extensions.[27] Even before the 1988 national launch, KGF had been testing line extensions for vending machines and "man-size" portions.[28,29] In 1991, it released 4 new line extensions of Lunchables with Dessert "to maximize total customer appeal and synergy with the Jell-O brand" and as "an important defensive tool" against the Sara Lee Corporation, which was marketing "knock-off

Lunchables."[30] After "sparking huge growth," PMC executives described the 1994 "Lunchables Fun Pack" as the "perfect example of how we grow through innovation."[31(p1)]

Throughout the 1990s, the Technical Synergies Committee supported continuous innovation in Lunchables line extensions by sharing processing and packaging technologies across PMC's tobacco and food subsidiaries. Synergies promoted high-speed aseptic packaging,[21] innovations in "taste enhancers and modifiers," the "control of flavor delivery" and "flavor release," as well as the continued "transfer of people across tobacco, food and beer."[32(p10,30)] Consumer-driven product development fostered new line extensions optimized for consumer pleasure. The 1991 invention of "Lunchables with Pizza" brought major growth to the brand. Although mothers in focus groups were revolted by the cold sauce and unmelted cheese, test children embraced the idea of building their own pizza.[33] As a PMC executive told shareholders, "we expect our growth to continue as we answer some of America's insatiable appetite for pizza—with new Pizza Lunchables. No one else could put together such a great combination with Kraft cheese and Oscar Mayer luncheon meats. That's what synergy is all about!"[31(p29)]

MARLBORO'S "BETTER-FOR-YOU" STRATEGY AND LOW-FAT LUNCHABLES

As public concern about childhood obesity grew in the 1990s, the brand image of Lunchables faced challenges. In 1994, a prominent pediatrician called Lunchables a "nutritional disaster."[33(p2)] In 1997, the American College of Cardiology called them a "blood pressure bomb."[34] Eventually, Kraft was forced to withdraw the profitable line extension, "Lunchables Maxed Out," from the market (Figure 3, panel c). With its exaggerated portion sizes, totaling 9 grams of saturated fat and 54 grams of sugar, Maxed Out brought too much negative publicity, according to the business press.[26,35]

In 1988, PMC's Corporate Products Development Committee announced that "principal R&D priorities under Synergies" were "cholesterol reduction" and calorie limits, while maintaining "fundamentals of taste."[29] Business reporters described a "down-with-cholesterol movement" throughout the food industry, noting the technical challenges inherent in making reduced fat products deliver the taste and "mouth feel" of real fat.[36] Internal PMC memos suggested heightened pressures on R&D as the firm's competitors launched cholesterol-free mayonnaise and simulated fat substitutes, such as Olestra.[21] In product development discussions, PMC managers observed that "the arena of nutritionally controlled foods is very dynamic and growing. It is critical we keep current on technology applications, marketplace initiatives and consumer understandings."[25(p492)]

By 1990, these pressures had led KGF to leverage its Louis Rich line of poultry products to launch a "white meat Lunchables," called "Lunch Breaks," to "preempt" competitors trying to "lure away current Lunchables users through a 'better for you' posturing."[30(p1)] Like its competitors, KGF was struggling with the palatability of fat substitutes: "Reduced fat cheeses were not included in the Lunch Breaks product line because of their poor appearance and taste." Consumer testing found that "lower fat process cheeses do not peel properly, while lower fat natural cheeses form calcium crystals that consumers perceive as mold."[37]

In a 1990 speech to newly hired managers, PMC's CEO, Maxwell, emphasized that the push to design products for health-conscious consumers extended to all of PMCs product lines, from tobacco to food:

> One of the key consumer trends we are most attentive to is increasing public concern about health. . . . We want to respond to the whole range of consumer concerns. We've modified our food products to remove fat or lessen the calories, and we've developed lighter cigarette products.[19(p6)]

Maxwell believed the "better-for-you" market was "the most powerful driving force in the cigarette market since 1954" and that PMC had a first mover advantage because of its early success with a filtered version of Marlboro cigarettes for men.[38(p26)] PMC's market advantage was independently confirmed by a competitor analysis commissioned by British American Tobacco that assessed PMC's better-for-you product portfolio (Figure 4).[39] Their analysis concluded that Marlboro's success with "getting the guilt out of the product" gave PMC an edge in making better-for-you foods and beverages:

> Philip Morris' successes have predominantly involved marketing products which deliver fully on consumer expectations but with the key additional benefit of 'reduced guilt' (greater permissibility). Marlboro cigarettes is the best example. . . . Its success came through not only delivering full flavour with a less negative health positioning but also in appealing to male smokers. . . . The successful formula developed with Marlboro was repeated with Miller

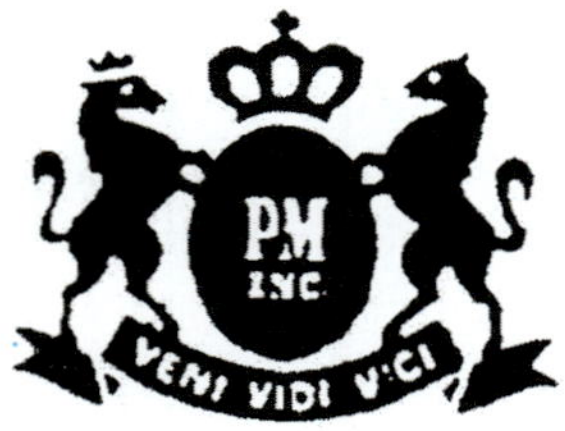

PHILIP MORRIS

A COMPETITOR REVIEW

Getting The Guilt Out Of The Product

Philip Morris' successes have predominantly involved marketing products which deliver fully on consumer expectations but with the key additional benefit of "reduced guilt" (greater permissibility). Marlboro cigarettes is the best example. This brand was amongst the first to use a filter although it was not the first. Its success came through not only delivering full flavour with a less negative health positioning but also in appealing to male smokers (see advertisement below). Thus Marlboro became the number one cigarette brand worldwide from a starting position of having less than one percent of the US market and a mostly female consumer base.

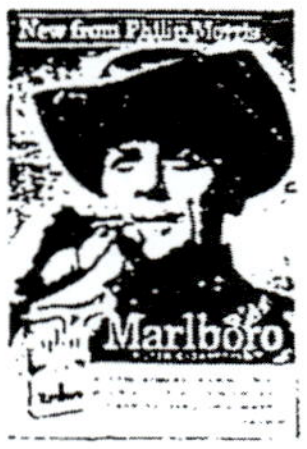

The Original Marlboro Man Ad.

Caption Reads:

"This new, easy-drawing filter cigarette
that delivers the most on flavour.
Long size. Regular filter price.
Light up a Marlboro and be glad you changed
to a filter cigarette."

The successful formula developed with Marlboro was repeated with Miller Lite beer. Low calorie beers did not appeal to male drinkers until Philip Morris improved their image by using football players in the marketing. The success of this brand, thus generated, has been a key factor in taking Miller from seventh place to second in the US beer market.

Seven-Up's promotion under the banner "Caffeine: Never Had It, Never Will" was similar although in this case the non-presence of a perceived negative was stressed rather than any positive elements of the brand. The launch of the first 99% caffeine-free cola "Like" reinforced this campaign and the Seven-Up company achieved a strong growth rate over this period. More recently Philip Morris have launched Sharp alcohol-free beer and very low nicotine cigarettes.

Technologies behind further potential products of this type had been separately developed by both Kraft and General Foods and they have been quickly assimilated into the relevant portfolios resulting in the launch of a range of fat-free products (Figure 4). Further products of this nature are expected, especially if Kraft's Olestra-type fat replacer "Trailblazer" receives FDA approval.

FIGURE 4— Competitor Review of Philip Morris Companies' Better-For-You Product Portfolio, 1990

Source. British American Tobacco.[39]

> Lite Beer. . . . Seven Up's promotion under the banner "Caffeine: Never Had It, Never Will!" was similar.[39(p15)]

PMC's 1990 strategic plan expanded investments for R&D to "develop products which address the consumers' desire to reduce their health concerns," led by the Technical Synergies Committee.[40(p3)] This included the development of a low-nicotine cigarette, designed to address rising consumer concerns about tobacco addiction while "maintaining our smoking population."[41(p363)] To achieve this, the Synergies Committee coordinated a companywide application of carbon dioxide supercritical fluid extraction technology (CO_2 SFE), a new processing technology for extracting compounds from plant and animal tissue matrices using CO_2 under high pressure. KGF had been using CO_2 SFE to decaffeinate coffee beans for Maxwell House Coffee. Under Synergies, the technology was successfully applied to remove nicotine from tobacco for a new cigarette: "Without the knowledge, experience and facilities of General Foods, Philip Morris USA could not have placed our new product in test market until late 1991."[21(p4)] To compensate for flavor loss resulting from de-nicotinizing tobacco, PCM's scientists used neuroperception research (e.g., electroencephalogram-based olfactometer studies) to identify chemical flavor additives that produced "commercially acceptable cigarette products" with 95% of the nicotine extracted.[42(p899)]

Under Synergies, PMC's scientists and engineers applied the same combination of technologies—CO_2 SFE and neuroperception research on chemical flavor additives—to create more palatable "fat replacement ingredients." The Technical Synergies Committee reported in 1989 that "We are aggressively pursuing the transfer of supercritical fluid extraction technology from coffee to tobacco to fats and other substances. 95% of all SCE capacity in the world belongs to PM."[21(p30–31)] KGF was under market pressure to move beyond "traditional technologies believed at their limits" that substituted starches, gums, and water for fat.[25(p277)] In testing, consumers found the "texture okay" in existing fat-free formulations, but the "flavor not up to standards."[25(p301)] Marketing recommended that KGF roll out a new fat-free formulation as a "preemptive" move in the "Better For Me" market. While consumers had significant "concerns about ingredient safety" with fat-free mayonnaise and processed meat, marketing researchers found that adding a simple "All Natural" label provided adequate "ingredient reassurance."[25(p303)]

In 1991, the Technical Synergies Committee reported "promising results" from its "cross-laboratory projects . . . investigating the feasibility of extracting fat with supercritical carbon dioxide extraction from peanuts, chocolate and coconut."[22(p10)] The push for new, more palatable "fat mimetics" brought one of PMC's top neuroperception scientists, Frank Gullotta, into collaboration with KGF's laboratory. KGF product developers believed that Gullotta's research using electroencephalogram-based olfactometers, plus their "Neuro Scan system" and a "new Brain Wave computer system, . . . could be extended . . . to tastants that would be of mutual benefit to PM and KGF."[43(p1)] Gullotta had been conducting research on nicotine addiction and flavor perception in a secret laboratory in Germany, where PMC hoped his research would evade the scrutiny of attorneys and tobacco regulators in the United States.[44] KGF's fat mimetics developers viewed Gullotta "as our one bonafide 'internal expert'" and as "an absolutely key resource for us in this task."[45(p1)] A year later, research techniques developed in Gullotta's lab, including "Electronic Nose/Biosensors," were in use at KGF "to assist with their fat-free research program, . . . toward a better understanding of the processes by which fat affects taste perception."[46(p1)]

In 1995, the Technical Synergies Committee reported some success with its Strategic Research Initiative on "fat mimetics," noting "improved flavor systems for next generation fat free products." Related work on "Fats, Oils and Replacement" was seeking "breakthrough fat mimetics for next generation cheeses, viscous, pourables, desserts, whipped toppings."[47(p8)] That year, Low-Fat Lunchables went to market, the first line extension to apply the new fat extraction technology in processed meat and cheese (Figure 3, panel b). A Kraft vice president noted that fat-free processed meats are "some of the food industry's hottest new products. . . . We've fueled the growth in the most successful segment of the industry in decades . . . the Lunchables category, when we introduced Fun Pack, low fat and pizza lunchables."[24(p2)] In his 1995 annual speech to stockholders, CEO Bible celebrated, "We consistently come up with ways to satisfy consumers, like our 700-million-dollar fat-free food business here in North America . . . like Oscar Mayer Lunchables, one of the best new product success stories in the industry."[48(p4)]

FROM CIGARETTES TO ULTRAPROCESSED FOOD

As the CEO of Philip Morris, Maxwell, observed in 1989, cigarettes and food are very similar businesses. Both are "low-priced consumer packaged goods with huge retail markets."[20(p36)] Manufacturing cigarettes and UPFs, like Lunchables, relied on the same supply chains for refined agricultural ingredients and chemical additives. Both used the same processing and packaging technologies, such as chemically encapsulated flavors and high-speed aseptic packaging. And both benefitted from the same product development approach, one that optimized products for consumer pleasure by using consumer research—from focus groups to neuroscience—to guide each step of the product engineering cycle.

This case study of Lunchables illustrates the pivotal role that tobacco companies played in the food industry during the 1980s and 1990s, when UPFs were scaled up in the US food supply. Because making cigarettes and UPFs were such similar businesses, PMC could profit off their "technical synergies," allowing food and tobacco product lines to coevolve. Processing innovations, such as CO_2 supercritical fluid extraction, could just as easily extract fats from processed meats as nicotine from cigarettes. Consumer-driven product development allowed engineers to design Lunchables to appeal to the child's deepest desires for play and autonomy, just as low-nicotine cigarettes appealed to the adult's desire to "get the guilt out of the product." PMC's "better-for-you" reformulation strategy, used to develop filtered and low-nicotine cigarettes, was equally effective for developing Low-Fat Lunchables, to keep consumers worried about childhood obesity loyal to the brand. Neuroperception research and chemical flavorants helped compensate for flavor loss in low-nicotine cigarettes. And they could do the same for low-fat food, resulting in Low-Fat Lunchables—the first of many "better-for-you" line extensions leading up to the most recent, Lunchables for the US NSLP.

Public health practitioners and policymakers tend to treat tobacco, UPF, and alcohol as separate and distinct commercial determinants of health. Research on their health harms is largely conducted in separate scientific silos that produce separate policy recommendations for preventing chronic disease. While the largest firms in today's consumer packaged goods industry may be less diversified than they were in the 1990s, one can still find numerous examples of child-focused brands that blur the boundaries between industries, such as "alcopops," candy-flavored e-cigarettes, and even cannabis-infused snack foods.[49] Public health research has begun to uncover the common "corporate playbook" used by health-harming industries,[50] and addiction research has identified common mechanisms in tobacco and food addiction.[51] Evaluation studies show that many tobacco control policies are effective for regulating UPF, including taxation, warning labels, and restrictions on child-focused marketing.[52] There are growing international calls to implement these policies to halt the rise in UPF production worldwide, as well as calls within the United States to remove UPFs from school meals, and for civil litigation to recover the health care costs of UPFs to the public.[6,53,54]

In light of Maxwell's observation that cigarettes, beer, and bologna are very similar businesses, we would be wise to accelerate efforts to understand the "synergies" between tobacco and UPFs in public health research and practice. And governments would be wise to find ways to extend existing consumer protection laws and public health regulations protecting children from tobacco products to include UPF. In the 1990s, legal actions against tobacco companies by US state attorneys general opened the door to significant policy advances in tobacco control, in part because internal industry documents showed that tobacco companies were intentionally formulating products to boost consumption.[15] Results from this study show that the same corporate logic was applied to manufacturing UPF products, suggesting the need to explore similar legal remedies. AJPH

ABOUT THE AUTHOR

Laura A. Schmidt is with the Institute for Health Policy Studies and Department of Humanities and Social Sciences, School of Medicine, University of California at San Francisco.

CORRESPONDENCE

Correspondence should be sent to Laura A. Schmidt, 490 Illinois St, Floor 7, San Francisco, CA 94158 (e-mail: laura.schmidt@ucsf.edu). Reprints can be ordered at https://www.ajph.org by clicking the "Reprints" link.

PUBLICATION INFORMATION

Full Citation: Schmidt LA. Tobacco industry contributions to the development of ultraprocessed food in the United States, 1985–2007: a case study of Lunchables. *Am J Public Health*. 2026; 116(7):940–949.

Acceptance Date: February 10, 2026.

DOI: https://doi.org/10.2105/AJPH.2026.308491

ORCID iD:
Laura A. Schmidt https://orcid.org/0000-0003-4346-7260

ACKNOWLEDGMENTS

The author's research is funded by the US National Institutes of Health, National Science Foundation, Department of Agriculture, and private philanthropies.

The author is grateful to James Roake for assistance with archival searches and Leslie Gerstenfeld for assistance with article formatting and graphic design.

CONFLICTS OF INTEREST

The author consults as an expert witness for plaintiffs in litigation involving necrotizing enterocolitis and infant formula marketing.

HUMAN PARTICIPANT PROTECTION

No human participants were involved in this research.

REFERENCES

1. Bernstein L, Weber L, Keating D. How Lunchables ended up on school lunch trays. *Washington Post.* October 17, 2023. Available at: https://www.washingtonpost.com/health/interactive/2023/lunchables-school-lunch-ultraprocessed-foods. Accessed July 22, 2025.
2. Loria K. Should you pack Lunchables for your kid's school lunch? *Consumer Reports.* November 12, 2024. Available at: https://www.consumerreports.org/health/lunch-and-snack-packs/should-you-pack-lunchables-for-your-kids-school-lunch-a1165583878. Accessed July 22, 2025.
3. Meyersohn N. Lunchables were a smashing success. Now they're in crisis. *CNN Business.* November 25, 2024. Available at: https://www.cnn.com/2024/11/25/business/lunchables-in-crisis. Accessed September 25, 2025.
4. Fryar CD, Carroll MD, Afful J. Prevalence of overweight, obesity, and severe obesity among children and adolescents aged 2–19 years: United States, 1963–1965 through 2017–2018. National Center for Health Statistics. February 5, 2021. Available at: https://www.cdc.gov/nchs/data/hestat/obesity-child-17-18/obesity-child.htm. Accessed July 22, 2025.
5. Williams AM, Couch CA, Emmerich SD, Ogburn DF. Ultraprocessed food consumption in youth and adults: United States, August 2021–August 2023. *NCHS Data Brief.* 2025;(536). https://doi.org/10.15620/cdc/174612
6. Scrinis G, Popkin BM, Corvalan C, et al. Policies to halt and reverse the rise in ultraprocessed food production, marketing, and consumption. *Lancet.* 2025;406(10520):2685–2702. https://doi.org/10.1016/S0140-6736(25)01566-1
7. Hall KD, Ayuketah A, Brychta R, et al. Ultraprocessed diets cause excess calorie intake and weight gain: an inpatient randomized controlled trial of ad libitum food intake. *Cell Metab.* 2019; 30(1):67–77.e3. https://doi.org/10.1016/j.cmet.2019.05.008
8. Lane MM, Gamage E, Du S, et al. Ultraprocessed food exposure and adverse health outcomes: umbrella review of epidemiological meta-analyses. *BMJ.* 2024;384:e077310. https://doi.org/10.1136/bmj-2023-077310
9. Harris JL, Kidd B, LoDolce M, Munsell C, Schwartz MB. Rudd Report: Food market facts in focus: Kraft Lunchables. April 2014. Available at: https://uconnruddcenter.media.uconn.edu/wp-content/uploads/sites/2909/2020/09/Rudd Report_Lunchables_4_14.pdf. Accessed May 5, 2026.
10. Nguyen KH, Glantz SA, Palmer CN, Schmidt LA. Transferring racial/ethnic marketing strategies from tobacco to food corporations: Philip Morris and Kraft General Foods. *Am J Public Health.* 2020;110(3):329–336. https://doi.org/10.2105/ajph.2019.305482
11. Nguyen KH, Glantz SA, Palmer CN, Schmidt LA. Tobacco industry involvement in children's sugary drinks market. *BMJ.* 2019;364:l736. https://doi.org/10.1136/bmj.l736
12. Fazzino TL, Courville AB, Guo J, Hall KD. Ad libitum meal energy intake is positively influenced by energy density, eating rate and hyper-palatable food across four dietary patterns. *Nat Food.* 2023;4(2):144–147. https://doi.org/10.1038/s43016-022-00688-4
13. Fazzino TL, Jun D, Chollet-Hinton L, Bjorlie K. US tobacco companies selectively disseminated hyper-palatable foods into the US food system: empirical evidence and current implications. *Addiction.* 2024;119(1):62–71. https://doi.org/10.1111/add.16332
14. Tobias DK, Hall KD. Eliminate or reformulate ultra-processed foods? Biological mechanisms matter. *Cell Metab.* 2021;33(12):2314–2315. https://doi.org/10.1016/j.cmet.2021.10.005
15. Glantz SA, Slade J, Bero L, Hanauer P, Barnes D. *The Cigarette Papers.* Berkeley, CA: University of California Press; 1996. Available at: https://publishing.cdlib.org/ucpressebooks/view?docId=ft8489p25j. Accessed October 6, 2025.
16. Smith P. General Foods - The Year in Review. 1986. Philip Morris. Bates no. 2063252141-2063252168. Available at: https://www.industrydocuments.ucsf.edu/docs/tyjf0021. Accessed July 22, 2025.

17. Endicott RC. Philip Morris ad spending muscles past $2 billion. October 3, 1989. Philip Morris. Bates no. 2063245506-2063245515. Available at: https://www.industrydocuments.ucsf.edu/docs/msfb0016. Accessed September 25, 2025.
18. Cuff DF. Business People; Kraft General Foods gets a new president. *New York Times.* January 19, 1990. Available at: https://www.nytimes.com/1990/01/19/business/business-people-kraft-general-foods-gets-a-new-president.html. Accessed September 25, 2025.
19. Campbell W, Maxwell H. Remarks by Hamish Maxwell and William Campbell, Kraft General Foods Orientation to Management Meeting, July 11–12, 1990. October 17, 1994. Philip Morris. Bates no. 2023439228-2023439237. Available at: https://www.industrydocuments.ucsf.edu/docs/tykb0106. Accessed September 25, 2025.
20. Philip Morris Companies Inc. Presentation to the investment community. May 24, 1989. Tobacco Institute Records. Bates no. TI12330622-TI12330657. Available at: https://www.industrydocuments.ucsf.edu/tobacco/docs/#id=hpmd0026. Accessed July 22, 2025.
21. Houghton K. Report of the Philip Morris Companies Technical Synergy Committee. September 29, 1989. Philip Morris. Bates no. 2063616317-2063616358. Available at: https://www.industrydocuments.ucsf.edu/tobacco/docs/#id=fpvv0123. Accessed July 22, 2025.
22. Unknown. Philip Morris technology assessment. December 1, 2005. Philip Morris. Bates no. 3042356235-3042356246. Available at: https://www.industrydocuments.ucsf.edu/docs/tgpf0151. Accessed September 25, 2025.
23. Moodys Investor Service. Philip Morris Companies Inc. Philip Morris. Bates no. 2048759726-2048759856. Available at: https://www.industrydocuments.ucsf.edu/docs/xqjy0159. Accessed July 17, 2025.
24. Eckert RA, Wauters R. Oscar Mayer Foods Division, PM Corporate Products Committee. October 20, 1995. Philip Morris. Bates no. 2070177703-2070177741. Available at: https://www.industrydocuments.ucsf.edu/docs/mnjw0036. Accessed September 25, 2025.
25. Philip Morris. Philip Morris Product Development Symposium. December 6, 1990. Philip Morris. Bates no. 2023162919-2023163499. Available at: https://www.industrydocuments.ucsf.edu/tobacco/docs/#id=lgkh0143. Accessed July 23, 2025.
26. Moss M. *Salt, Sugar, Fat: How the Food Giants Hooked Us.* 1st ed. New York, NY: Random House; 2013.
27. Kraft-Heinz Inc. Lunchables–products. Available at: https://www.lunchables.com/parents/products. Accessed July 23, 2025.
28. Campbell WI. Minutes Corporate Products Committee Meeting January 23, 1989. February 21, 1989. Philip Morris. Bates no. 2025848982-2025848983. Available at: https://www.industrydocuments.ucsf.edu/tobacco/docs/#id=zmgw0117. Accessed July 22, 2025.
29. Campbell WI. Minutes Corporate Products Committee Meeting September 26, 1988. September 26, 1988. Product Design MSA Collection. Bates no. 2025848988-2025848989. Available at: https://www.industrydocuments.ucsf.edu/tobacco/docs/#id=lynj0037. Accessed July 23, 2025.
30. Murray CL. Philip Morris Corporate Products Committee January 1991. January 1991. Philip Morris. Bates no. 2070041625-2070041627. Available at: https://www.industrydocuments.ucsf.edu/docs/xgjj0033. Accessed September 25, 2025.
31. Storr H, Kilts J. Remarks by Hans Storr and Jim Kilts, Phillip Morris Companies, Inc. October 17, 1995. Philip Morris. Bates no. 2046882264-2046882304. Available at: https://www.industrydocuments.ucsf.edu/docs/tjbw0058. Accessed September 25, 2025.
32. Peters A. PM wide technology synergy re-assessment. August 21, 1996. Philip Morris. Bates no. 2059732784-2059732828. Available at: https://www.industrydocuments.ucsf.edu/docs/xkmd0157. Accessed October 8, 2025.
33. Pinsker J. The 30-year reign of Lunchables. *The Atlantic.* November 17, 2018. Available at: https://www.theatlantic.com/family/archive/2018/11/lunchables-30-years-invented-history/576025. Accessed July 23, 2025.
34. Hinman A. Lunchables may be munchable—but study warns of salt. *CNN Interactive.* March 16, 1997. Available at: https://web.archive.org/web/20210228052447/http://www.cnn.com/HEALTH/9703/16/lunchables. Accessed October 7, 2025.
35. Kleinfield NR. Catching the anti-cholesterol fever. *New York Times.* April 16, 1989. Available at: https://www.nytimes.com/1989/04/16/business/catching-the-anti-cholesterol-fever-catching-the-anti-cholesterol-fever.html. Accessed September 25, 2025.
36. Schultz EJ. How Kraft's Lunchables is evolving in the anti-obesity era. *AdAge.* April 19, 2011. Available at: https://adage.com/article/news/kraft-s-lunchables-evolving-anti-obesity-era/227075. Accessed September 25, 2025.
37. Oscar Mayer Foods, Lord J. Philip Morris Corporate Products Committee 900300 Louis Rich Lunch Breaks. March 1990. Philip Morris. Bates no. 2041053447-2041053451. Available at: https://www.industrydocuments.ucsf.edu/docs/krvm0033/. Accessed May 6, 2026.
38. Tindall JE. Market-Driven Development and Consumer Research Philip Morris Companies Product Development Symposium 901205 - 901206. December 5, 1990. Philip Morris. Bates no. 2504057179-2504057211. Available at: https://www.industrydocuments.ucsf.edu/docs/jsjd0110. Accessed October 8, 2025.
39. Philip Morris. Philip Morris: a competitor review. October 1990. British American Tobacco. Bates no. 201771149-201771192. Available at: https://www.industrydocuments.ucsf.edu/docs/hgvb0192. Accessed September 25, 2025.
40. PM USA R&D strategic plan draft. November 28, 1989. Philip Morris. Bates no. 2021537495-2021537579. Available at: https://www.industrydocuments.ucsf.edu/docs/rrpk0000. Accessed September 25, 2025.
41. Dunsby J, Bero L. A nicotine delivery device without the nicotine? Tobacco industry development of low nicotine cigarettes. *Tob Control.* 2004;13(4):362–369. https://doi.org/10.1136/tc.2004.007914
42. Experientiahf + Phf Reemtsmapm Philip Morris, Philip Morris Board of Directors, Lehman Brothers, et al. The occurrence of n-nitroso compounds in tobacco smoke (and a composite of documents not gone through at time of deposition). December 6, 2002. Philip Morris. Bates no. 3990129842-3990130796. Available at: https://www.industrydocuments.ucsf.edu/docs/xfxv0184. Accessed May 6, 2026.
43. Hayes CS. Philip Morris USA inter-office correspondence subject KGF visit. March 26, 1991. Philip Morris. Bates no. 2028813491-2028813492. Available at: https://www.industrydocuments.ucsf.edu/docs/xzyw0108. Accessed October 6, 2025.
44. US District Court for District of Columbia. Direct testimony of Paul Mele PhD. *United States of America v. Philip Morris USA* Civil Action 99-CV-02496 (GK). Available at: https://www.justice.gov/sites/default/files/civil/legacy/2014/09/11/01_Mele%20Written%20Direct_0.pdf. Accessed May 5, 2026.
45. Leland J. PM Synergy - next steps for chemoperception. February 25, 1998. Philip Morris. Bates no. 2063128469. Available at: https://www.industrydocuments.ucsf.edu/docs/rybw0157. Accessed February 15, 2026.
46. Ellis C. InterOffice correspondence: electronic nose/biosensors. April 1, 1992. Philip Morris. Bates no. 2023114566. Available at: https://www.industrydocuments.ucsf.edu/docs/hpkg0119. Accessed September 25, 2025.
47. Kraft. Philip Morris food & tobacco technical organizations view their roles very similarly. November 14, 1995. Philip Morris. Bates no. 2059733396-2059733406. Available at: https://www.industrydocuments.ucsf.edu/docs/ksld0157. Accessed September 25, 2025.
48. Bible GC. 950000 Annual Meeting of Stockholders Philip Morris Inc. Remarks by Geoffrey C. Bible Chairman and Chief Executive Officer. April 27, 1995. Philip Morris. Bates no. 2046003394-2046003408. Available at: https://www.industrydocuments.ucsf.edu/docs/txng0088. Accessed May 6, 2026.
49. Schmidt LA, Jacobs LM, Matthay EC, et al. Characteristics and trends in child cannabis exposures during legalization in California. *Am J Prev Med.* 2025;69(4):107963. https://doi.org/10.1016/j.amepre.2025.107963
50. Lacy-Nichols J, Marten R, Crosbie E, Moodie R. The public health playbook: ideas for challenging the corporate playbook. *Lancet Glob Health.* 2022;10(7):e1067–e1072. https://doi.org/10.1016/S2214-109X(22)00185-1
51. Gearhardt AN, Bueno NB, DiFeliceantonio AG, Roberto CA, Jiménez-Murcia S, Fernandez-Aranda F. Social, clinical, and policy implications of ultra-processed food addiction. *BMJ.* 2023;383:e075354. https://doi.org/10.1136/bmj-2023-075354
52. Popkin BM, Barquera S, Corvalan C, et al. Toward unified and impactful policies for reducing ultra-processed food consumption and promoting healthier eating globally. *Lancet Diabetes Endocrinol.* 2021;9(7):462–470. https://doi.org/10.1016/S2213-8587(21)00078-4
53. California Governor Newsom signs first-in-the-nation law to ban ultraprocessed foods from school lunches. Governor of California. October 9, 2025. Available at: https://www.gov.ca.gov/2025/10/08/governor-newsom-signs-first-in-the-nation-law-to-ban-ultra-processed-foods-from-school-lunches. Accessed May 5, 2026.
54. ABC News. San Francisco files landmark lawsuit, comparing ultraprocessed food companies to "Big Tobacco." Available at: https://abcnews.go.com/GMA/Food/san-francisco-files-landmark-lawsuit-comparing-ultraprocessed/story?id=128046148. Accessed February 4, 2026.

Nutritional Characteristics of Foods With Addictive Potential: A Machine-Learning Approach

Ashley N. Gearhardt, PhD, Zach Hutelin, Emmanuel Nartey, PhD, Monica L. Ahrens, PhD, Mary Elizabeth Baugh, PhD, RDN, Tera L. Fazzino, PhD, Erica M. LaFata, PhD, Kendrin R. Sonneville, ScD, RD, and Alexandra G. DiFeliceantonio, PhD

See also Ultraprocessed Food, pp. 898–1029.

Objectives. To identify nutritional characteristics associated with the perceived addictive potential of commonly consumed foods in the US food supply, the majority of which are ultraprocessed foods (UPFs).

Methods. In a demographically diverse sample of US adults (n = 1664; 55.2% female), participants rated the perceived addictiveness of 297 commonly consumed foods (74.4% UPFs). Data were collected through Prolific in June 2024. Machine-learning models identified nutritional predictors of addictiveness using both the 15 variables required on US Nutrition Facts labels and an expanded set of 166 nutrient characteristics from the Nutrition Data System for Research.

Results. Models performed comparably and revealed consistent nonlinear associations between nutrient content and perceived addictiveness. Foods higher in carbohydrates, glycemic load, energy density, and fat were rated as more addictive. These nutrient profiles were rare in minimally processed foods but common in UPFs, which frequently exceeded multiple addictive nutrient thresholds simultaneously.

Conclusions. This study identifies a nutritional signature linked to perceived addictive potential. Findings provide a data-driven framework for identifying foods most likely to promote compulsive intake and inform policies aimed at creating a healthier, less addictive food environment. *(Am J Public Health.* 2026;116(7):950–959. https://doi.org/10.2105/AJPH.2026.308500)

AJPH July 2026, Vol. 116, No. 7

Over the past 50 years, diet-related diseases have risen dramatically.[1] Human brains evolved to find energy-dense foods highly rewarding, aiding survival during scarcity,[2,3] but advances in food science and technology have turned these tendencies into liabilities.[3] Although food processing can improve safety, convenience, and nutritional adequacy through fortification and enrichment, some processed foods are low in nutritional value and high in added sugars and fats.[4] These products now dominate the modern food environment and are associated with increased risk of multiple adverse health outcomes, including cancer and metabolic disease.[4]

Advances in food science and technology have enabled the formulation of some processed foods with sensory and nutritional characteristics that enhance reward value, paralleling mechanisms observed in other reinforcing products.[5] This raises the possibility that some foods may promote patterns of intake that resemble addiction-like behavior and contribute to diet-related disease.[5–7] The Yale Food Addiction Scale (YFAS), a validated tool, applies gold-standard substance-use disorder criteria (loss of control, cravings, continued use despite harm, withdrawal, tolerance) to eating behavior.[6,7] Meta-analyses of more than 270 studies estimate that approximately 14% of adults meet the clinical threshold for "food addiction,"[8] comparable to addictions to legal substances, including tobacco (10%)[9] and alcohol (14%).[10] Individuals who meet criteria for YFAS-defined food addiction show poorer health across multiple domains, including an 11- to 19-times higher likelihood of being overweight[11] and a 6.7-fold greater likelihood of type 2 diabetes.[12]

When the YFAS was developed in 2009, the term food addiction was adopted because of limited evidence about which specific foods might be addictive.[13] Subsequent work shows that not all foods equally trigger addictive intake: products high in rapidly absorbed, rewarding components (e.g., refined carbohydrates, added fats, some sweeteners) are most implicated, whereas minimally processed foods (MPFs) rarely are.[14] Individuals meeting criteria for YFAS food addiction consume more nutrient-poor processed foods and fewer minimally processed foods.[15] Thus, foods with certain characteristics rather than all foods are likely to have heightened addictive potential.

Empirical identification of these addictive food characteristics remains limited. Most studies examined fewer than 40 foods and a narrow predictor set (e.g., carbohydrate, fat, glycemic load).[16–18] Yet, the food supply is vast; the 2021–2023 Food and Nutrient Database for Dietary Studies lists over 5000 unique types of foods consumed in the United States.[19] A comprehensive, data-driven approach is needed.

To this end, we surveyed a demographically diverse US sample (n = 1664; 55.2% female) and collected perceived addictiveness ratings for 297 foods. We applied machine learning using (1) the 15 Food and Drug Administration–required Nutrition Facts variables and (2) an expanded set of 166 Nutrition Data System for Research (NDSR; 2024) variables,[20] examining nonlinear relationships, a broad predictor space, and the distribution of a preliminary nutritional signature of addictiveness across Nova processing categories, which were used descriptively rather than as causal explanatory variables.[4]

This work advances an evidence-based understanding of addictive potential by identifying both the foods and nutritional profiles most associated with problematic intake, informing public health messaging, clinical interventions, and regulatory decision-making.

METHODS

We recruited a demographically diverse sample of US adults (n = 1664; 55.2% female) through Prolific in June 2024 (see Appendix Methods, available as a supplement to the online version of this article at http://www.ajph.org). To be eligible, participants had to be aged 18 to 100 years and US residents. Participants provided online informed consent and completed surveys in REDCap.

Procedures

Participants filled out the modified YFAS 2.0, which is a validated self-report instrument designed to assess symptoms of food addiction based on the diagnostic criteria for substance-use disorders (see Appendix Methods).[6] To reduce priming effects, we renamed the measure the "Food Problems Survey" for administration, and the instruction that highlights certain types of food (e.g., sweets, salty snacks) was removed.[6] A full description of task instructions is available in Appendix Methods.

Participants were shown 99 randomly selected food images to rate. We selected the foods from a set of 297 foods representing commonly consumed items in the US food supply, spanning the Nova classification system (for Food Stimulus Development, see Appendix Methods). Prior to completing the rating task, they were prompted to rate "How PROBLEMATIC is this food for you?" with a note to "Remember, by PROBLEMATIC we are referring to problems like losing control, intense cravings or being unable to cut down"; participants used a 100-point visual analog scale with the anchors "not at all" and "very" (Appendix Figure A). This approach reflects established principles from human abuse liability research, which routinely incorporates subjective self-report measures to assess addiction-relevant experiences and has demonstrated reliability, validity, and sensitivity to clinically meaningful differences across addictive substances.[21,22] Participants were not required to identify any foods as problematic. At the 50th photo, we administered an attention check where an image of an empty plate was shown with the words "Rate this 'not at all'" (Appendix Figure A).

Additional Measures

We collected demographic information including race, gender, sex, income, perceived socioeconomic status,[23] education status, height, and weight.

Analytic Plan

Data cleaning. We excluded participants who failed quality checks (e.g., attention check, implausible body mass index [BMI], out-of-range age and height; see Appendix Methods). The final analytic sample included 1664 individuals (mean age = 45.3 years; mean BMI = 27.1 kg/m^2).

Machine-learning models. We aggregated participant ratings of addictive potential to the food level by computing unweighted mean ratings for each food item, which served as the primary outcome variable for the supervised machine-learning models. Models were trained to identify nutritional features associated with higher perceived addictiveness across foods. Additional sensitivity analyses considered weighted food-level mean ratings that accounted for participant sex, income, education level, food security status, and YFAS score (Appendix Methods). Because the analytic unit was the food, we split the data set of 297 foods into training (80%) and test (20%) sets stratified by rating quartiles. Candidate algorithms included LASSO regression, random forest, and extreme gradient boosting, implemented in R version 4.4.0 (R Foundation for Statistical Computing, Vienna Austria). We evaluated model performance with root mean square error (RMSE) and mean absolute error (MAE).

We tested 2 models: (1) a nutrition facts label model, using 15 variables required on US food labels, and (2) an expanded model, using 166 food characteristics from the Nutrition Data System for Research (NDSR[20]; see Appendix Tables A and B for variable list). We selected final models via cross-validation and hyperparameter tuning; additional sensitivity analyses including weighted means were performed (see Appendix Methods).

Feature importance and thresholds. We used permutation-based feature importance to assess the influence of each predictor on model predictions. This approach evaluates the change in model performance when the information from a given predictor is randomly disrupted, with larger performance declines indicating greater influence on perceived food addictiveness. For predictors with a substantial impact (ΔRMSE $\geq$ 0.1), partial dependence plots visualized marginal effects. Distinct nutrient thresholds ("elbows") emerged, suggesting tipping points beyond which perceived addictiveness rises sharply. We identified nutrient elbows (inflection points in partial dependence plots) by multiple raters to estimate thresholds associated with higher addictiveness ratings. Full details on preprocessing, exclusion criteria, and threshold derivation are provided in Appendix Methods.

RESULTS

Participants were on average 45 years old with a median BMI of 27 kilograms per square meters. Most were White (71.4%; n = 1188), and the sample was reasonably balanced by sex (55.2% female; n = 919). About one third held a bachelor's degree (35.4%; n = 589). Most (72.8%; n = 1211) reported high or marginal food security, and 8.6% met the clinical threshold for food addiction based on the modified YFAS 2.0 (Appendix Table C).

Food Characteristics

The final set contained 297 foods (Figure 1, Table 1, Appendix Tables D and E), most of which were ultraprocessed foods (UPFs; 74.4%). Foods had a median energy density of 210 kilocalories (kcal) per 100 grams (g), with 19.5 g of carbohydrates, 8.6 g of fat, and 6.6 g of protein. Median sodium was 311.01 mg of sodium, 3.3 g of total sugars with a median glycemic load of 10.5 (Table 1).

Food Characteristics by Addiction Score Tertile

The foods with the highest addictiveness ratings were pepperoni pizza (fast-food), chocolate chip cookies (store-bought), French fries (fast-food), glazed doughnuts, and plain potato chips (store-bought; Appendix Tables D and E). The foods with the lowest addictiveness ratings were canned split pea and ham soup, canned black bean soup, canned red kidney beans, cooked green peppers, and celery (see Appendix Tables D and E).

On average, foods in the top tertile were rated as somewhat problematic (median = 39.16), with the top 10 foods rated as moderately problematic (median = 50.19). Participants with clinically significant food addiction rated top-tertile foods 21.8 points higher (median = 59.12) than those without food addiction (median = 37.26). For the top 10 foods, ratings were highly problematic among those with food addiction (median = 72.36) versus moderately problematic among those without (median = 48.39). By contrast, bottom-quartile foods were rated as minimally problematic (median = 17.83). Ratings differed by 7.0 points between those with food addiction (mean = 24.04) and those without (mean = 17.04). Results were similar for the bottom 10 foods, with those with food addiction reporting an average score of 15.64, only 5.51 points higher than those without (Appendix Table D).

To examine potential nutritional differences across addictiveness scores, we grouped foods into tertiles according to average addictiveness score and examined the 15 food characteristics found on the nutrition facts label plus glycemic load as it has been previously indicated to be a predictor of food

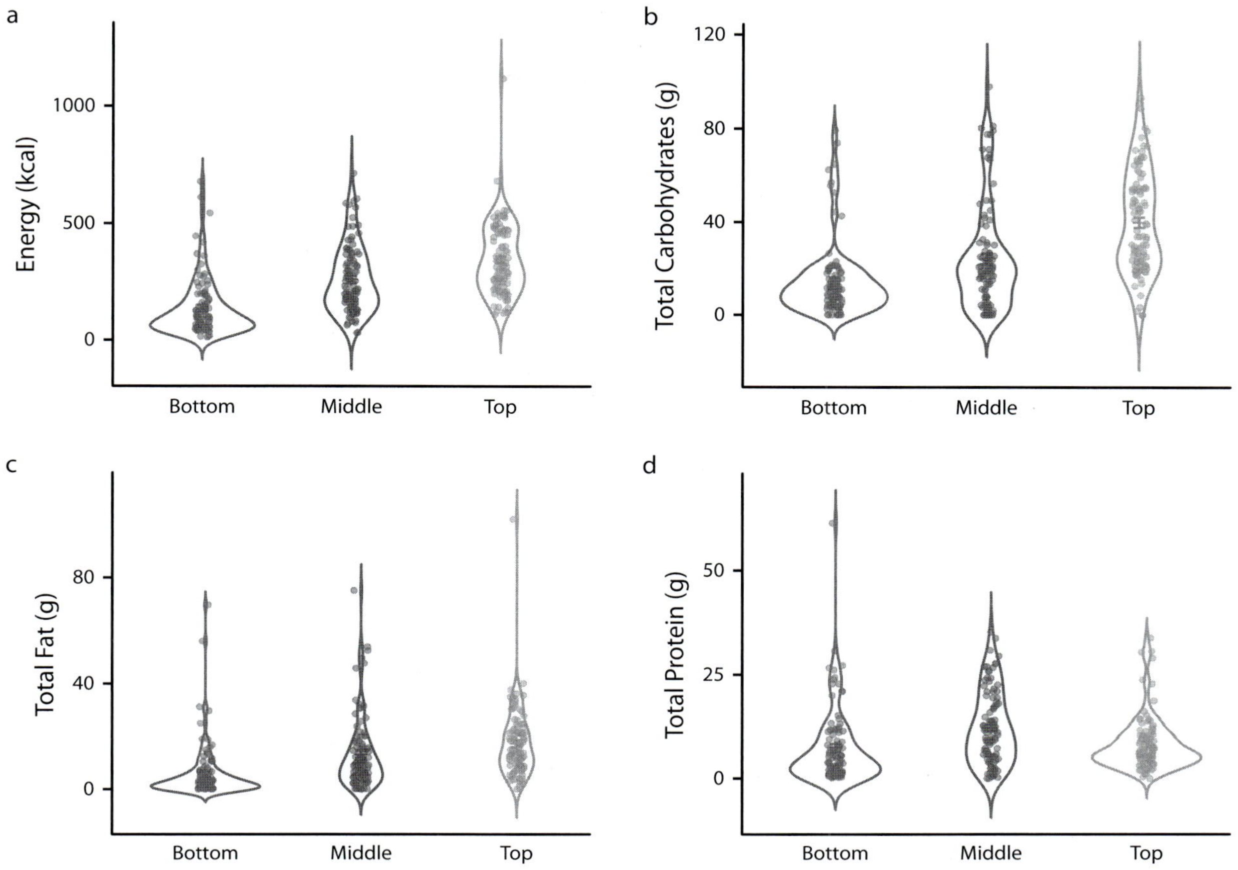

FIGURE 1— Nutrition Information Across Tertiles of Perceived Addictiveness Ratings for (a) Energy, (b) Total Carbohydrates, (c) Total Fat, and (d) Total Protein: United States, 2024

Note. Each point represents a food.

addictiveness[16] (Table 1). We also examined Nova classification. Foods in the top tertile had higher energy (320 kcal), fat (14.0 g), carbohydrate (34.1 g), added sugar (4.8 g), total sugar (5.7 g), and glycemic load (21.5) compared with lower tertiles. In the top tertile of addictiveness score, 91.9% were Nova 4 and 8.1% Nova 3; no Nova 1 foods appeared (Table 1). In the bottom tertile, 23.2% of foods were Nova 1, 23.2% Nova 3, and 53.5% Nova 4 (Table 1).

Nutrition Label Model of Addictive Ratings

Among algorithms evaluated via cross-validation, random forest performed best. This model produced good predictive accuracy on the test data set, with an RMSE of 6.05 and MAE of 4.57, indicating that, on average, the model's predicted addictiveness scores deviated from actual scores by about 4 to 6 points within the empirically observed range of mean ratings (7.9–53.5). Permutation feature importance analysis (Figure 2) revealed that total carbohydrates, energy, total fat, and total trans fats were the most influential predictors of perceived addictiveness ratings. These results were robust to weighted means and train-test resampling (Appendix Methods, Tables F, G, and H). Partial dependence plots (Appendix Figure C) show that higher values of total carbohydrates, energy, and fat were associated with increased predicted addictiveness ratings. By contrast, features such as iron, added sugar, total protein, potassium, and sodium showed more complex or inverse relationships with the predicted outcome.

Expanded Food Characteristics Model

When we used 166 NDSR variables, random forest again outperformed LASSO and XGBoost and achieved strong predictive performance (RMSE = 5.56; MAE = 4.31); sensitivity analyses were also performed on this model and produced similar results

AJPH July 2026, Vol. 116, No. 7

TABLE 1— Characteristics of Foods Rated in the Study, Stratified by Tertile of Addictiveness Rating: United States, 2024

Characteristic	Overall (n = 297), No. (%) or Median (IQR)	Tertile, No. (%) or Median (IQR)			Overall P	Pairwise P		
		Bottom (n = 99)	Middle (n = 99)	Top (n = 99)		Middle vs Bottom Tertile	Top vs Bottom Tertile	Top vs Middle Tertile
Nova					<.001			
Nova 1	28 (9.4)	23 (23.2)	5 (5.1)	0 (0.0)				
Nova 3	48 (16.2)	23 (23.2)	17 (17.2)	8 (8.1)				
Nova 4	221 (74.4)	53 (53.5)	77 (77.8)	91 (91.9)				
Rating	27.1 (19.7, 35.4)	17.8 (14.9, 19.7)	27.1 (24.8, 29.4)	39.2 (35.4, 42.6)	<.001	<.001	<.001	<.001
Energy, kcal	210 (118, 340)	94 (52, 173)	218 (150, 345)	320 (229, 464)	<.001	<.001	<.001	<.001
Total fat, g	8.6 (2.9, 17.6)	2.8 (0.4, 6.6)	9.2 (4.5, 16.6)	14.0 (8.9, 22.6)	<.001	<.001	<.001	<.001
Total saturated fatty acids, g	2.2 (0.9, 5.4)	0.8 (0.1, 2.1)	2.2 (1.2, 4.9)	5.0 (2.3, 9.4)	<.001	<.001	<.001	<.001
Total trans-fatty acids, g	0.07 (0.02, 0.20)	0.02 (0.00, 0.09)	0.06 (0.03, 0.23)	0.13 (0.06, 0.34)	<.001	<.001	<.001	<.001
Cholesterol, mg	11.0 (0.0, 41.1)	3.0 (0.0, 17.2)	16.0 (0.0, 52.8)	14.7 (3.1, 41.4)	<.001	.006	<.001	.85
Sodium, mg	311.0 (165.9, 516.0)	283.0 (58.1, 405.3)	379.0 (213.2, 608.4)	318.4 (172.6, 540.2)	.003	.005	.031	.24
Total carbohydrates, g	19.5 (8.5, 39.7)	10.6 (4.8, 17.9)	18.7 (7.6, 30.2)	34.1 (22.0, 54.9)	<.001	<.001	<.001	<.001
Total dietary fiber, g	1.3 (0.7, 2.4)	1.5 (0.9, 2.8)	1.1 (0.2, 2.5)	1.4 (0.9, 2.3)	.08	.16	.62	.16
Total sugars, g	3.3 (1.4, 11.9)	2.4 (1.2, 6.5)	3.1 (1.2, 8.6)	5.7 (2.0, 30.2)	<.001	.18	<.001	.002
Added sugars (by available carbohydrate), g	0.4 (0.0, 6.9)	0.0 (0.0, 0.8)	0.7 (0.0, 5.8)	4.8 (0.1, 28.6)	<.001	<.001	<.001	<.001
Total protein, g	6.6 (3.3, 12.4)	3.8 (1.2, 10.9)	10.5 (5.3, 18.3)	6.4 (4.3, 10.4)	<.001	<.001	.003	.003
Vitamin D (calciferol), mcg	0.03 (0.00, 0.32)	0.01 (0.00, 0.07)	0.09 (0.00, 0.44)	0.10 (0.00, 0.38)	.002	.006	.006	.76
Calcium, mg	43.9 (16.0, 96.8)	29.0 (13.8, 58.4)	43.0 (15.4, 97.3)	72.3 (24.5, 132.2)	<.001	.054	<.001	.054
Potassium, mg	188.0 (140.3, 256.5)	184.5 (141.8, 259.5)	209.5 (155.0, 292.85)	180.0 (118.8, 245.6)	.06	.41	.41	.054
Iron, mg	1.3 (0.6, 2.1)	0.7 (0.4, 1.5)	1.6 (0.9, 2.5)	1.6 (0.9, 2.1)	<.001	<.001	<.001	.26
Glycemic load (glucose reference)	10.5 (2.8, 22.4)	3.8 (1.5, 7.9)	10.0 (1.8, 17.7)	21.5 (12.9, 35.1)	<.001	<.001	<.001	<.001

Note. IQR = interquartile range. Nova 2 foods (i.e., processed culinary ingredients) are not included as these are not intended to be consumed in isolation. *P* value is based on χ^2 test, Kruskal–Wallis test, or Mann–Whitney *U* test, as appropriate.

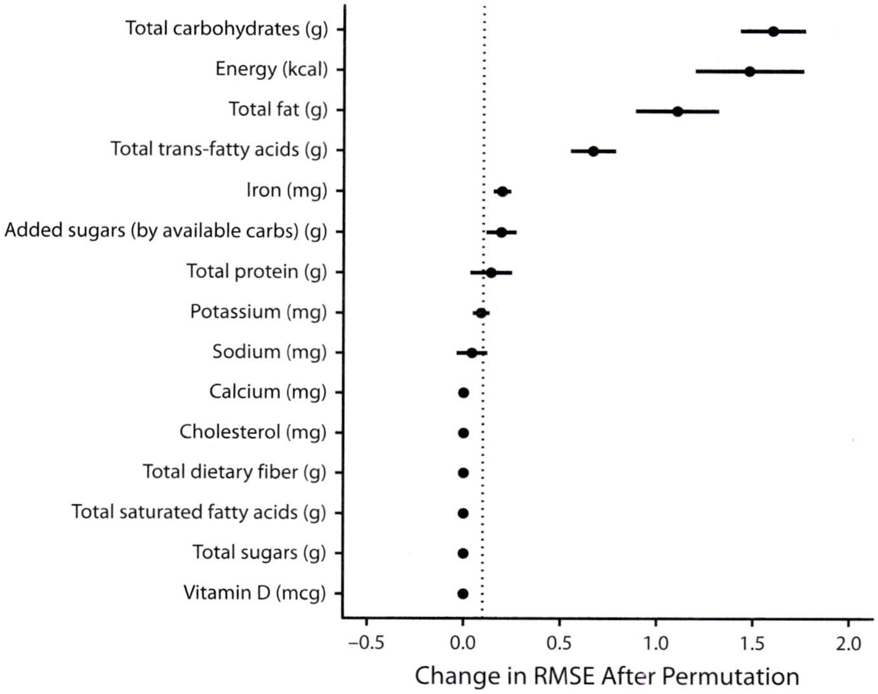

FIGURE 2— Nutrition Facts Label Random Forest Model: United States, 2024

Note. Permutation feature importance plot showing the change in root mean square error (RMSE) after permuting each predictor variable in the nutrition facts label model. Error bars represent 95% confidence intervals. Features with point estimates and error bounds that intersect or lie entirely to the right of the dotted line (ΔRMSE ≥ 0.1) are considered to have a substantial impact on model performance. Based on a 100 g serving, total carbohydrates, energy, and total fat were among the most influential predictors.

(Appendix Tables F, G, and H). Top predictors included glycemic load, available carbohydrate, energy density, and lactose (Figure 3). Partial dependence plots (Appendix Figure D) highlighted nonlinear effects, especially for glycemic load, available carbohydrate, and energy. Total fat, total carbohydrates, palmitic acid, and saturated fats contributed less strongly, whereas water content showed a slight protective association. Overall, multiple carbohydrate-related metrics emerged as key predictors.

Model Thresholds

To identify preliminary nutrient thresholds associated with higher addictiveness, the research team examined elbow points for predictors with dropout RMSE increases of 0.1 or higher. The final elbow thresholds derived from the partial dependence plots highlight distinct nutrient values associated with increased predicted addictiveness.

Across both models, total carbohydrates had elbows of 24.0 g (label model) and 21.4 g (expanded model); energy showed nearly identical thresholds of 201 and 200 kcal, and fat thresholds were 9 g and 7 g. Additional thresholds in the label model included iron (2 mg), protein (6.5 g), potassium (233 mg), trans fat (0.13 g), added sugar (17.5 g), and sodium (238 mg). In the expanded model, additional thresholds were glycemic load (12), available carbohydrate (20 g), lactose (0.12 g), palmitic acid (2 g), water (71 g), and saturated fat (2.9 g).

Despite the expanded model's larger predictor set, both models performed similarly ($P = .21$). Together, carbohydrate quantity and availability, energy density, and fat content consistently emerged as the strongest contributors to perceived addictiveness.

DISCUSSION

In a large, demographically diverse sample of US adults, we identified a distinct nutritional signature associated with perceived food addictiveness across 297 commonly consumed food items. Foods with the highest addictiveness ratings included fast-food pepperoni pizza, store-bought chocolate chip cookies, and glazed doughnuts, whereas the lowest-rated items were canned kidney beans, cooked green peppers, and celery. Foods in the top tertile of perceived addictiveness scored 21.4 points higher on a 100-millimeter

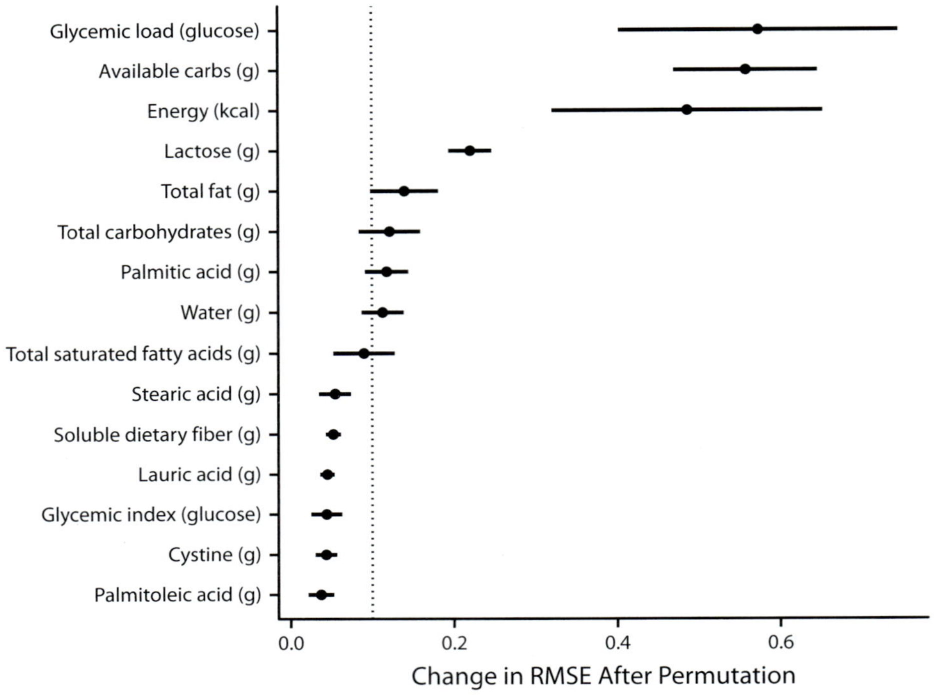

FIGURE 3— Expanded Food Characteristics Random Forest Model: United States, 2024

Note. Permutation feature importance plot showing the change in root mean square error (RMSE) after permuting each predictor variable in the expanded food characteristics model. Error bars represent 95% confidence intervals. Features with point estimates and error bounds that intersect or lie entirely to the right of the dotted line ($\Delta RMSE \geq 0.1$) are considered to have a substantial impact on model performance. Based on a 100 g serving, glycemic load, available carbohydrates, and energy were among the most influential predictors.

AJPH July 2026, Vol. 116, No. 7

visual analog scale than those in the bottom tertile, with the top 10 foods scoring 32.4 points higher. In addiction science, differences of approximately 10 millimeters on such scales are commonly considered clinically meaningful,[21,22] indicating that the observed differences in perceived addictiveness are substantial rather than trivial, although replication using controlled laboratory food administration is needed. Across models using both the 15 Nutrition Facts and 166 NDSR variables, higher total carbohydrates, carbohydrate-related features (glycemic load, lactose, available carbohydrate), energy density, and fat consistently predicted higher addictiveness ratings. This is an initial proof of concept—that a food's perceived addictiveness can be predicted from nutritional features using a scalable machine-learning approach. Importantly, this work represents a first step that requires replication, refinement, and validation in independent data sets before any downstream application.

Mechanistic Insights

Each identified nutritional characteristic has plausible mechanisms by which it could enhance reinforcement and increase a food's addictive potential. Carbohydrates are evolutionarily salient energy sources that shaped the brain to find them especially rewarding.[2,3] Refined carbohydrates deliver concentrated, rapidly absorbed energy that produces robust glycemic and insulin responses, engaging reward-related brain areas.[16,18] Consistent with these mechanisms, foods higher in total and available carbohydrates were more strongly associated with perceived addictiveness, suggesting that carbohydrate dose and delivery rate are key drivers.

Foods that are more energy-dense deliver higher doses of carbohydrates and fat per bite, increasing their addictive potential.[24] Fat, the most energy-dense macronutrient improves texture, increases palatability and potentiates the sensory impact of carbohydrates.[25] When paired with refined carbohydrates, fat produces supra-additive activation of reward-related brain regions, indicating a possible synergistic interaction.[26] Beyond total fat, saturated fats (particularly palmitic acid) and trans fat contributed to perceived addictiveness, consistent with evidence linking saturated fat intake to reduced dopamine transporter function in reward-related striatal brain regions.[27] Iron, protein, and potassium exhibited small protective associations. These nutrients are more common in MPFs,[28] and protein may modestly reduce addictive potential by enhancing satiety or stabilizing blood glucose.[29] However, their effects were small compared with those observed for energy, carbohydrates, and fat. For instance, UPFs high in protein still promote overconsumption.[30] Although fortification and enrichment practices are valuable for preventing micronutrient deficiencies, our findings suggest that simply adding iron, protein, or potassium to energy-dense foods may not mitigate addictive potential. Front-of-package health claims based on nutrient addition may therefore mislead consumers about the overall healthfulness of such products, a phenomenon known as health-washing.[31]

Unexpectedly, sodium showed a small protective effect after adjusting for other nutrients. Although salt is a powerful flavor enhancer,[32] its reward value in isolation is likely limited. For example, salt added to steamed vegetables may increase palatability without driving overconsumption, whereas salt combined with carbohydrates and fat, as in potato chips, acts as a reward amplifier. Sodium's contribution to food addictiveness therefore appears context-dependent and may emerge primarily through synergy with other reinforcing ingredients. Water content was also associated with lower addictiveness ratings, likely reflecting reduced energy density[33] and concentration of rewarding nutrients.

Thresholds and Heterogeneity

Examining the distribution of nutrient characteristics revealed that the relationships between nutrients and perceived addictiveness were not purely linear. Instead, distinct elbows, or thresholds, emerged beyond which the likelihood of a food being rated as addictive increased sharply. We identified these thresholds preliminarily, but future work should include a robust estimation of these thresholds, which could be used to capture nutrient tipping points where reinforcing properties become especially salient.

The nutrient composition of MPFs were quantifiably different from those of many UPFs.[34] Examining our preliminary thresholds, it appears that some MPFs may exceed 1 threshold, but it is rare for an MPF to meet multiple thresholds. By contrast, in our data set, UPFs frequently exceeded several thresholds at once. This ability to combine multiple reinforcing features, including high energy density, rapidly available carbohydrates, and fat, may explain their dominance in the top addictiveness tertile, and it mirrors patterns seen with other addictive substances, where dose and delivery speed interact to heighten reinforcement.

Whereas 74.4% of foods in our stimulus set were classified as UPFs, over 90% of foods in the highest addictiveness tertile were UPFs. At the same time, not all UPFs share the same nutrient signature. Foods exceeding multiple preliminary nutrient thresholds were consistently rated as most addictive, whereas UPFs that did not reach these combinations tended to fall into the lowest tertile (i.e., low likelihood of addictive intake). Consistent with this pattern, UPFs were also represented among foods with lower addictive potential, indicating that processing status alone does not adequately capture addictive potential. Although some forms of food processing confer important benefits, such as improved safety or fortification, it appears to be the combination of industrial processing and the specific nutrient configurations that such processing enables that poses the greatest risk for addictive-like intake.

Our findings also highlight a potential spectrum of risk related to overconsumption within UPF classification. Our data add to the growing body of literature suggesting that UPFs, as opposed to MPFs, are more likely to contain the nutrient composition that confers risk for problematic eating behaviors. Despite this, it will be important for future studies to consider whether UPFs with lower addictive potential may still pose health risks. Such products should not be considered harmless, but they may be less likely to drive compulsive overconsumption.

Individual Differences

As reported in the Results section, individuals meeting criteria for clinically significant food addiction rated highly addictive foods as markedly more problematic than did those without food addiction. For example, the top 10 foods averaged over 72 on a 100-point scale among participants with food addiction, compared with 48 among those without. This pattern mirrors other addictive substances, such as alcohol, where most users experience limited problems but those with diagnosed addiction experience substantially greater harm.[10] Importantly, this difference was specific to the most addictive foods; both groups rated MPFs as the least addictive foods. Individuals with food addiction do not report heightened problems across all foods but specifically those that are ultraprocessed, energy-dense, and high in refined carbohydrates and fats.

Public Health Implications

These findings advance an evidence-based understanding of addictive potential in the modern food supply. Historically, when products are recognized as both harmful and capable of driving compulsive use, policy responses have shifted toward industry accountability and environmental change rather than reliance on individual choice alone, as occurred with cigarettes.[5] Identifying nutrient thresholds associated with compulsive intake offers a framework for informing reformulation, labeling, and marketing policies, with particular attention to high energy density, rapidly available carbohydrates, and added fats, analogous to how tobacco and alcohol policies target high-risk formulations. Although any policy application would require further validation and careful ethical and regulatory consideration, this approach aligns with emerging policy efforts, such as California's 2025 bill restricting UPFs in school meals, which explicitly references food addiction as a mechanism of harm. As addictiveness increasingly enters policy discussions, empirically grounded methods to operationalize this construct may inform standards for children's food environments, institutional procurement, marketing to minors, and integration into dietary guidance, clinical counseling, and public education.

Strengths and Limitations

Strengths include a large, demographically diverse US sample, broad coverage of foods across Nova categories, and evaluation of 166 nutritional characteristics. Limitations include reliance on self-report (a standard approach in abuse liability research when no biological marker exists), a food set that was broad but not exhaustive, and a high proportion of Nova 4 items that may have influenced results. Although quota sampling approximated US Census distributions for age, sex, and race/ethnicity, other aspects of representativeness were not captured, and a survey error prevented assessment of ethnicity and dietary restrictions. Replication is needed in more culturally diverse samples, with expanded Nova 1–3 representation, beverages, and products containing nonnutritive sweeteners. Future work should test how nutrient profiles interact with food matrix integrity, processing-related acceleration of nutrient delivery, sensory amplification, and additives, and how dietary patterns and food combinations shape addictive-like intake. Finally, extending this work to children and adolescents is a priority given developmental vulnerability and high UPF exposure.[35] AJPH

ABOUT THE AUTHORS

Ashley N. Gearhardt is with the Department of Psychology, University of Michigan, Ann Arbor. Zach Hutelin, Mary Elizabeth Baugh, and Alexandra G. DiFeliceantonio are with the Fralin Biomedical Research Institute, Virginia Tech Carilion, Roanoke. Emmanuel Nartey and Monica L. Ahrens are with the Center for Biostatistics and Health Data Science, Department of Statistics, Virginia Tech, Blacksburg. Tera L. Fazzino is with the Department of Psychology, University of Kansas, Lawrence. Erica M. LaFata is with the Oregon Research Institute, Eugene. Kendrin R. Sonneville is with the Department of Nutritional Sciences, University of Michigan School of Public Health, Ann Arbor.

CORRESPONDENCE

Correspondence should be sent to Ashley Gearhardt, 1305 Arborview Blvd, Ann Arbor MI 48103 (e-mail: agearhar@umich.edu). Reprints can be ordered at https://www.ajph.org by clicking the "Reprints" link.

PUBLICATION INFORMATION

Full Citation: Gearhardt AN, Hutelin Z, Nartey E, et al. Nutritional characteristics of foods with addictive potential: a machine-learning approach. *Am J Public Health*. 2026;116(7):950–959.

Acceptance Date: February 13, 2026

DOI: https://doi.org/10.2105/AJPH.2026.308500

ORCID iDs:
Ashley N. Gearhardt https://orcid.org/0000-0003-3843-5731

Zach Hutelin https://orcid.org/0000-0002-6179-5332

Mary Elizabeth Baugh https://orcid.org/0000-0002-3469-7040

Erica M. LaFata https://orcid.org/0000-0002-8505-6366

Kendrin R. Sonneville https://orcid.org/0000-0002-0359-3919

Alexandra G. DiFeliceantonio https://orcid.org/0000-0002-7155-6060

CONTRIBUTORS

A. N. Gearhardt, T. L. Fazzino, K. R. Sonneville, E. M. LaFata, A. G. DiFeliceantonio conceptualized and designed the study. Z. Hutelin and M. E. Baugh assisted with data conceptualization and coding. E. Nartey and M. L. Ahrens conducted the statistical and machine-learning analyses. All authors interpreted the data, contributed to the initial draft, revised the article critically for intellectual content, and approved the version to be published.

ACKNOWLEDGMENTS

This study was supported by Ardevora Asset Management, the Dohmen Company Foundation, and a grant from the National Institute on Drug Abuse (R01DA054750; principal investigator: A. N. Gearhardt).

Note. The funders had no role in study design, data collection and analysis, decision to publish, or preparation of the manuscript.

CONFLICTS OF INTEREST

A. N. Gearhardt has received speaking honoraria from academic organizations and health related nonprofits, consulting fees from health-related nonprofits and a law firm and receives royalties from Oxford University Press. A. N. Gearhardt is also a consultant for Dohmen Company Foundation (a funder of this study), unrelated to this research. T. L. Fazzino has received speaking honoraria from academic organizations and health-related nonprofits. E. M. LaFata has received speaking honoraria from academic organizations and health-related nonprofits and consulting fees from a law firm. A. G. DiFeliceantonio has received speaking honoraria from academic organizations and health-related nonprofits, consulting fees from health-related nonprofits. All other authors declare no competing interests.

HUMAN PARTICIPANT PROTECTION

This study was approved by the Virginia Tech institutional review board (#23-804).

REFERENCES

1. Hu FB. Obesity in the USA: diet and lifestyle key to prevention. *Lancet Diabetes Endocrinol.* 2023; 11(9):642–643. https://doi.org/10.1016/S2213-8587(23)00194-8
2. Gómez-Pinilla F. Brain foods: the effects of nutrients on brain function. *Nat Rev Neurosci.* 2008;9(7):568–578. https://doi.org/10.1038/nrn2421
3. Armelagos GJ. Brain evolution, the determinates of food choice, and the omnivore's dilemma. *Crit Rev Food Sci Nutr.* 2014;54(10):1330–1341. https://doi.org/10.1080/10408398.2011.635817
4. Monteiro CA, Louzada ML, Steele-Martinez E, et al. Ultra-processed foods and human health: the main thesis and the evidence. *Lancet.* 2025; 406(10520):2667–2684. https://doi.org/10.1016/S0140-6736(25)01565-X
5. Gearhardt AN, Brownell KD, Brandt AM. From tobacco to ultraprocessed food: how industry engineering fuels the epidemic of preventable disease. *Milbank Q.* 2026;104(1):76–115. https://doi.org/10.1111/1468-0009.70066
6. Schulte EM, Gearhardt AN. Development of the Modified Yale Food Addiction Scale Version 2.0. *Eur Eat Disord Rev.* 2017;25(4):302–308. https://doi.org/10.1002/erv.2515
7. Gearhardt AN, Corbin WR, Brownell KD. Development of the Yale Food Addiction Scale Version 2.0. *Psychol Addict Behav.* 2016;30(1):113–121. https://doi.org/10.1037/adb0000136
8. Praxedes DRS, Silva-Júnior AE, Macena ML, et al. Prevalence of food addiction determined by the Yale Food Addiction Scale and associated factors: a systematic review with meta-analysis. *Eur Eat Disord Rev.* 2022;30(2):85–95. https://doi.org/10.1002/erv.2878
9. Streck JM, Parker MA, Cruz R, et al. Prevalence and trends in cigarette smoking with and without tobacco use disorder among adults in the United States: 2010–2021. *J Clin Psychiatry.* 2024;85(3): 23m15086. https://doi.org/10.4088/JCP.23m15086
10. Grant BF, Goldstein RB, Saha TD, et al. Epidemiology of DSM-5 alcohol use disorder: results from the National Epidemiologic Survey on Alcohol and Related Conditions III. *JAMA Psychiatry.* 2015;72(8):757–766. https://doi.org/10.1001/jamapsychiatry.2015.0584
11. Loch LK, Kirch M, Singer DC, et al. Ultra-processed food addiction in a nationally representative sample of older adults in the USA. *Addiction.* 2026;121(3): 510–521. https://doi.org/10.1111/add.70186
12. Horsager C, Bruun JM, Færk E, Hagstrøm S, Lauritsen MB, Østergaard SD. Food addiction is strongly associated with type 2 diabetes. *Clin Nutr.* 2023;42(5):717–721. https://doi.org/10.1016/j.clnu.2023.03.014
13. Gearhardt AN, Corbin WR, Brownell KD. Preliminary validation of the Yale Food Addiction Scale. *Appetite.* 2009;52(2):430–436. https://doi.org/10.1016/j.appet.2008.12.003
14. Leung CW, Parnarouskis L, Slotnick MJ, Gearhardt AN. Food insecurity and food addiction in a large, national sample of lower-income adults. *Curr Dev Nutr.* 2023;7(12):102036. https://doi.org/10.1016/j.cdnut.2023.102036
15. Pursey KM, Collins CE, Stanwell P, Burrows TL. Foods and dietary profiles associated with "food addiction" in young adults. *Addict Behav Rep.* 2015;2:41–48. https://doi.org/10.1016/j.abrep.2015.05.007
16. Schulte EM, Avena NM, Gearhardt AN. Which foods may be addictive? The roles of processing, fat content, and glycemic load. *PLoS One.* 2015; 10(2):e0117959. https://doi.org/10.1371/journal.pone.0117959
17. Schulte EM, Smeal JK, Gearhardt AN. Foods are differentially associated with subjective effect report questions of abuse liability. *PLoS One.* 2017;12(8):e0184220. https://doi.org/10.1371/journal.pone.0184220
18. Schulte EM, Sonneville KR, Gearhardt AN. Subjective experiences of highly processed food consumption in individuals with food addiction. *Psychol Addict Behav.* 2019;33(2):144–153. https://doi.org/10.1037/adb0000441
19. US Dept of Agriculture, Agricultural Research Service. USDA Food and Nutrient Database for Dietary Studies 2021–2023. 2024. Available at: http://www.ars.usda.gov/nea/bhnrc/fsrg. Accessed July 28, 2025.
20. Schakel SF. Maintaining a nutrient database in a changing marketplace: keeping pace with changing food products—a research perspective. *J Food Compost Anal.* 2001;14(3):315–322. https://doi.org/10.1006/jfca.2001.0992
21. Vansickel A, Baxter S, Sherwood N, Kong M, Campbell L. Human abuse liability assessment of tobacco and nicotine products: approaches for meeting current regulatory recommendations. *Nicotine Tob Res.* 2022;24(3):295–305. https://doi.org/10.1093/ntr/ntab183
22. Eaton TA, Comer SD, Revicki DA, et al. Determining the clinically important difference in visual analog scale scores in abuse liability studies evaluating novel opioid formulations. *Qual Life Res.* 2012;21(6):975–981. https://doi.org/10.1007/s11136-011-0012-7
23. Adler NE, Epel ES, Castellazzo G, Ickovics JR. Relationship of subjective and objective social status with psychological and physiological functioning: preliminary data in healthy white women. *Health Psychol.* 2000;19(6):586–592. https://doi.org/10.1037//0278-6133.19.6.586
24. Fazzino TL, Courville AB, Guo J, Hall KD. Ad libitum meal energy intake is positively influenced by energy density, eating rate and hyper-palatable food across four dietary patterns. *Nat Food.* 2023;4(2):144–147. https://doi.org/10.1038/s43016-022-00688-4
25. Singh P, Kesharwani RK, Keservani RK. 6 - Protein, carbohydrates, and fats: energy metabolism. In: Bagchi D, ed. *Sustained Energy for Enhanced Human Functions and Activity.* London, UK: Academic Press; 2017:103–115. https://doi.org/10.1016/B978-0-12-805413-0.00006-5
26. DiFeliceantonio AG, Coppin G, Rigoux L, et al. Supra-additive effects of combining fat and carbohydrate on food reward. *Cell Metab.* 2018;28(1):33–44.e3. https://doi.org/10.1016/j.cmet.2018.05.018
27. Barnes CN, Wallace CW, Jacobowitz BS, Fordahl SC. Reduced phasic dopamine release and slowed dopamine uptake occur in the nucleus accumbens after a diet high in saturated but not unsaturated fat. *Nutr Neurosci.* 2022;25(1):33–45. https://doi.org/10.1080/1028415X.2019.1707421
28. Martini D, Godos J, Bonaccio M, Vitaglione P, Grosso G. Ultra-processed foods and nutritional dietary profile: a meta-analysis of nationally representative samples. *Nutrients.* 2021;13(10):3390. https://doi.org/10.3390/nu13103390
29. Veldhorst M, Smeets A, Soenen S, et al. Protein-induced satiety: effects and mechanisms of different proteins. *Physiol Behav.* 2008;94(2): 300–307. https://doi.org/10.1016/j.physbeh.2008.01.003
30. Hägele FA, Herpich C, Koop J, et al. Short-term effects of high-protein, lower-carbohydrate ultra-processed foods on human energy balance. *Nat Metab.* 2025;7(4):704–713. https://doi.org/10.1038/s42255-025-01247-4
31. Ares G, Natero V, Gugliucci V, et al. Health-washing of ultraprocessed products on Instagram: prevalence and strategies in an emerging market. *J Nutr Educ Behav.* 2023;55(11):815–822. https://doi.org/10.1016/j.jneb.2023.09.001
32. Breslin PA, Beauchamp GK. Salt enhances flavour by suppressing bitterness. *Nature.* 1997;387(6633): 563–563. https://doi.org/10.1038/42388
33. Klos B, Cook J, Crepaz L, Weiland A, Zipfel S, Mack I. Impact of energy density on energy intake in children and adults: a systematic review and meta-analysis of randomized controlled trials. *Eur J Nutr.* 2023;62(3):1059–1076. https://doi.org/10.1007/s00394-022-03054-z
34. Menichetti G, Barabási AL. Nutrient concentrations in food display universal behaviour. *Nat Food.* 2022;3(5):375–382. https://doi.org/10.1038/s43016-022-00511-0
35. Wang L, Martínez Steele E, Du M, et al. Trends in consumption of ultraprocessed foods among US youths aged 2–19 years, 1999-2018. *JAMA.* 2021; 326(6):519–530. https://doi.org/10.1001/jama.2021.10238

Public Awareness and Support for Governmental Intervention to Address Harms Associated With Consumption of Ultraprocessed Foods: A National Survey, United States, June 2025

Jeff Niederdeppe, PhD, Colleen L. Barry, PhD, MPP, Sarah E. Gollust, PhD, Norman Porticella, PhD, Kelly D. Brownell, PhD, and Ashley N. Gearhardt, PhD

See also Ultraprocessed Food, pp. 898–1029.

AJPH July 2026, Vol. 116, No. 7

Objectives. To assess public understanding of ultraprocessed foods (UPFs), support for governmental intervention to address UPF harms, and potential differences in understanding and support by political party.

Methods. We partnered with YouGov on a web-based survey of 2000 adults weighted to be nationally representative in the United States to assess awareness and confidence in explaining UPFs, beliefs about UPF harms and UPF companies, responsibility for addressing UPF harms, and support for governmental actions to regulate UPF products and companies. We stratified results by political party.

Results. Many Americans have heard of UPFs (58.1%), but fewer are confident in their understanding (32.8%). There is widespread recognition of UPF harms to physical health but less awareness of mental health harms. There is broad support among Democrats, Independents, and Republicans for several public policy and legal strategies designed to reduce UPF consumption.

Conclusions. There is robust and bipartisan support for addressing UPF harms through many specific legal and policy interventions. (*Am J Public Health*. 2026;116(7):960–970. https://doi.org/10.2105/AJPH.2026.308498)

Ultraprocessed foods (UPFs)—"formulations of ingredients, mostly of exclusive industrial use, that result from a series of industrial processes"[1(p937)]—now constitute a majority of calories consumed in the United States.[1,2] A growing body of evidence links high UPF consumption to cardiovascular disease, type 2 diabetes, obesity, depression, cognitive decline, and premature mortality.[3] Concerns are also emerging about their potential to promote addictive intake patterns through product engineering that heightens reward and craving.[4]

The dominance of UPFs in the US diet reflects deliberate corporate product design and marketing strategies. Companies deploy processing technologies that enhance sensory appeal and accelerate absorption, and invest heavily in child-focused marketing, product placement, and political lobbying.[5] This mirrors tactics used by tobacco and alcohol industries to normalize daily use, shape perception of harm, and delay regulation and litigation. The public health stakes are clear: these products are now major drivers of chronic disease and diminished well-being.[3]

Policymakers across the ideological spectrum have begun to respond. The

US Department of Health and Human Services (HHS) has prioritized diet-related chronic disease prevention, and hundreds of state bills have been introduced to address UPFs or related harms.[6] State attorneys general have launched investigations into company practices.[7] In October 2025, California became the first state to target UPFs for restrictions in school meals,[8] and in July 2025, the US Food and Drug Administration issued a Request for Information to inform regulatory definitions of UPFs.[9] Meanwhile, the HHS secretary and federally commissioned *Make America Healthy Again* report characterized UPFs as key contributors to the nation's metabolic and mental health crisis,[6] and the revised *Dietary Guidelines for Americans* newly recommends that people "limit highly processed foods."[10(p4)]

Despite this growing activity, we know little about what the American public believes or wants regarding UPFs. Historical precedent underscores the importance of public opinion: in tobacco control, shifts in public perception preceded—and enabled—successful litigation and regulatory reform.[11] While several European polls have examined UPF awareness and concern,[12,13] US polling remains extremely limited. A recent survey found that most people in the United States view processed foods as unhealthy but purchase them anyway, suggesting ambivalence rather than apathy.[14]

A more detailed understanding of where people in the United States stand is essential for guiding effective and politically feasible public health action. We fielded a US national opinion survey in June 2025 to better understand public awareness of UPFs, beliefs about UPF harms and UPF companies, perceived responsibility for addressing UPF harms, and support for governmental actions to regulate UPF products and companies. We analyzed overall patterns and gauged whether beliefs about UPFs differ by partisan identification.

METHODS

We conducted a web-based survey via YouGov Panel from June 6 to 16, 2025, among a national sample of 2000 adults aged 18 years or older and living in the United States. YouGov maintains a panel of Americans who periodically agree to take part in surveys. Adults living in the United States who have internet access are eligible to join the panel. Panel members are recruited through advertising and partnerships with a variety of websites. In exchange for taking surveys, respondents receive points that can be exchanged for credit at various vendors.

Study participants provided informed consent and then proceeded to the survey. We first assessed unaided awareness of UPFs and confidence in explaining UPFs (see Appendix A, available as a supplement to the online version of this article at https://ajph.org, for survey wording for all analyzed items). Next, we provided respondents with a short definition of UPFs (available throughout the rest of the survey). Respondents then answered blocks of questions about their support for various public policy and litigation strategies, beliefs about UPF harms and UPF companies, perceptions of blame and responsibility toward various actors, and demographic items that were not part of the previously collected panel profile variables provided by YouGov. Survey items were randomized within blocks. In the absence of validated measures on UPF-related awareness beliefs, we wrote survey items informed by studies in other related domains (e.g., sugary drinks and obesity).[15–18] The final sample (n = 2000; chosen to provide a margin of error of ± 2.4 percentage points for the overall sample) was weighted to be nationally representative of US adults (see Table A, available as a supplement to the online version of this article at https://ajph.org, for sample demographics).

Measures

To gauge awareness of UPFs, we asked, "Have you ever heard of ultraprocessed foods?" (dichotomized to 1 = yes vs 0 = no or unsure). Those who answered "yes" or "unsure" were then asked, "If you were asked to do so, how confident are you that you could explain to someone else what ultraprocessed foods are?" (1 = not at all confident to 5 = extremely confident). We dichotomized responses to 1 = somewhat, very, or extremely confident versus 0 = not at all or a little confident.

Informed by previous work,[15–18] we measured perceived responsibility for addressing the poor quality of American diets as follows: "Please indicate how much responsibility you think each of the following groups has for addressing the poor quality of American diets: [e.g., ultraprocessed food companies; individuals and their own dietary choices; the US government]" (1 = none at all to 5 = a great deal). We dichotomized these responses to 1 = a lot or a great deal versus 0 = a moderate amount, a little, or none.

To measure beliefs about UPF harms and impact (14 items), respondents were asked, "Please indicate your level of agreement with the following statements: [e.g., Ultraprocessed foods are addictive]" (1 = strongly disagree;

AJPH July 2026, Vol. 116, No. 7

5 = strongly agree). These items included both evidence-based harms and false claims made in public discourse. We dichotomized responses to 1 = agree or strongly agree versus 0 = neutral, disagree, or strongly disagree. We asked a parallel set of questions (13 items) with the same basic prompt and response categories to gauge a range of beliefs about UPF companies.

Also informed by previous work,[15–18] we asked about the harms of UPFs relative to a variety of other products as follows: "In general, how harmful do you feel each of the following is to the health of people who use or consume them? [e.g., cigarettes; alcoholic beverages; ultraprocessed foods]" (1 = not at all harmful to 5 = extremely harmful). We dichotomized these responses to 1 = very or extremely harmful versus 0 = somewhat, a little, or not at all harmful.

To measure support for public policy and litigation strategies (14 items), respondents were asked, "To what extent do you support or oppose the following policies: [e.g., Banning artificial food dyes (coloring) from all products]?" (1 = strongly oppose; 5 = strongly support). These items included strategies that have been discussed in the context of UPFs and other product categories. We dichotomized responses to 1 = support or strongly support versus 0 = neutral, oppose, or strongly oppose.

Political party identification was measured by asking, "Generally speaking, do you usually think of yourself as a Democrat, a Republican, an Independent, or another party?" We report results both overall (in the Appendix and text where relevant) and stratified by political party: Democrats (n = 666), Independents (n = 542), and Republicans (n = 583).

Data Analysis

We assessed the survey-weighted proportion of dichotomized item responses and calculated 95% confidence intervals (CIs) around these estimates overall and by political party. Figures show results stratified by political party, while Table B (available as a supplement to the online version of this article at https://ajph.org) provides overall and party-specific percentage and 95% CI estimates for all variables reported in the article. We ran logistic regressions to predict agreement or support for each item by political party; we report on differences between partisan groups only when political party was a significant ($P < .05$) predictor of awareness or support (group differences are noted in Table B). We conducted analyses using weighted data in SPSS version 29.[19]

RESULTS

More than half (58.1%; 95% CI = 56.0, 60.3) of respondents had heard of UPFs, but only 32.8% (95% CI = 30.8, 34.0) felt at least somewhat confident they could explain UPFs to someone else. Results were similar by political party.

Figure 1 presents sample percentages for awareness of UPFs, confidence in explaining them, and perceived responsibility for addressing UPF harms, stratified by political party. Respondents across political groups perceived individuals and their own dietary choices and parents of unhealthy children as the groups with the highest level of responsibility for addressing UPF harms (all > 63%), with Republicans and Independents ascribing more responsibility to both groups than Democrats. UPF companies were the next highest for all political groups (all > 52%), with Democrats assigning greater responsibility than Republicans or Independents. Respondents overall rated the US government at roughly the same level of responsibility as fast food and soda companies, with Democrats more likely to assign responsibility to federal actors than Republicans and Independents. State and local governments and schools were perceived as having the lowest responsibility.

Figure 2 presents sample percentages for beliefs about the harms of UPFs, stratified by political party. Across partisan identities, Americans widely agreed that UPFs are a major cause of obesity, are addictive, and cause type-2 diabetes and cardiovascular disease (each > 60% agreement). Fewer Americans agreed that UPFs cause vulnerability to mental health issues including depression, anxiety, and attention-deficit/hyperactivity disorder (each < 40%). Very few respondents agreed that the harms are overblown or that UPFs are healthy (both < 20%). Partisan differences emerged for agreement with several items. Republicans were more likely than Democrats to agree that UPFs are not what God intended, are a major cause of cancer, and cause vulnerability to attention-deficit/hyperactivity disorder and autism. Democrats were more likely than Independents to agree that UPFs are addictive, that we do not know enough about UPF harms, and that effects are overblown. Democrats were also more likely than both Republicans and Independents to agree that UPFs are bad for the environment and that they are healthy.

Additional analyses (Figure A, available as a supplement to the online version of this article at https://ajph.org) compared beliefs about the harms of UPFs to beliefs about the harms of other products (e.g., illegal opioid drugs, cigarettes, cannabis). More than half of

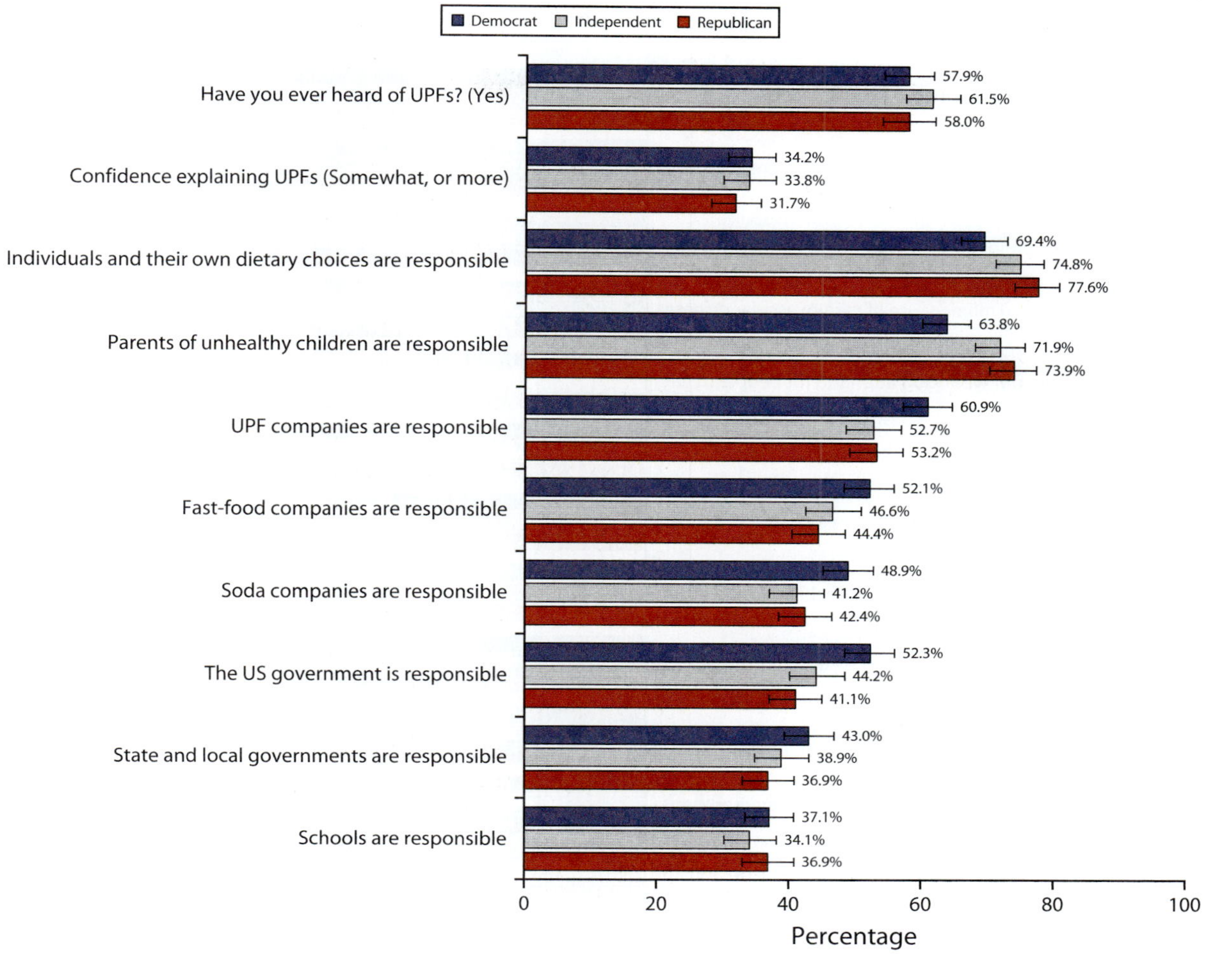

FIGURE 1— Awareness of Ultraprocessed Foods (UPFs), Confidence in Explaining It, and Perceived Responsibility for Addressing UPF Harms, Stratified by Political Party: United States, June 2025

Note. We measured perceived responsibility for addressing the quality of American diets as follows, "Please indicate how much **responsibility** you think each of the following groups has **for addressing the poor quality of American diets**: [example actors] ultraprocessed food companies; individuals and their own dietary choices; the US government" (1 = none at all to 5 = a great deal). We dichotomized these responses to 1 = a lot or a great deal versus 0 = a moderate amount, a little, or none. Error bars represent 95% confidence intervals.
Source. Survey fielded June 9–19, 2025, using the YouGov panel.

Democrats, Independents, and Republicans (each between 53.8% and 55.5%) thought that UPFs were very or extremely harmful. Across all political groups, perceived harms were lower than opioids, cigarettes, and e-cigarettes but similar to alcohol and higher than sugar-sweetened beverages, fast foods, and cannabis.

Figure 3 presents sample percentages for beliefs about UPF companies, stratified by political party. Respondents expressed broad cynicism around the motives and behaviors of the UPF industry, with greater than 60% overall agreeing with items related to profit motives and designing or marketing UPFs for overconsumption and addiction among children. With few exceptions, beliefs were similar by political party. Exceptions pertained to beliefs about targeting marginalized populations (Democrats agreed more than Independents or Republicans), UPF company rights to market their products (Republicans agreed more than Democrats), and 3 items where Independents but not Republicans differed from Democrats (tobacco industry strategies, testing chemicals for safety, and trust to make food products healthy).

Figure 4 presents sample percentages for support of governmental intervention to address the harms of UPFs, stratified by political party. Respondents expressed broad support

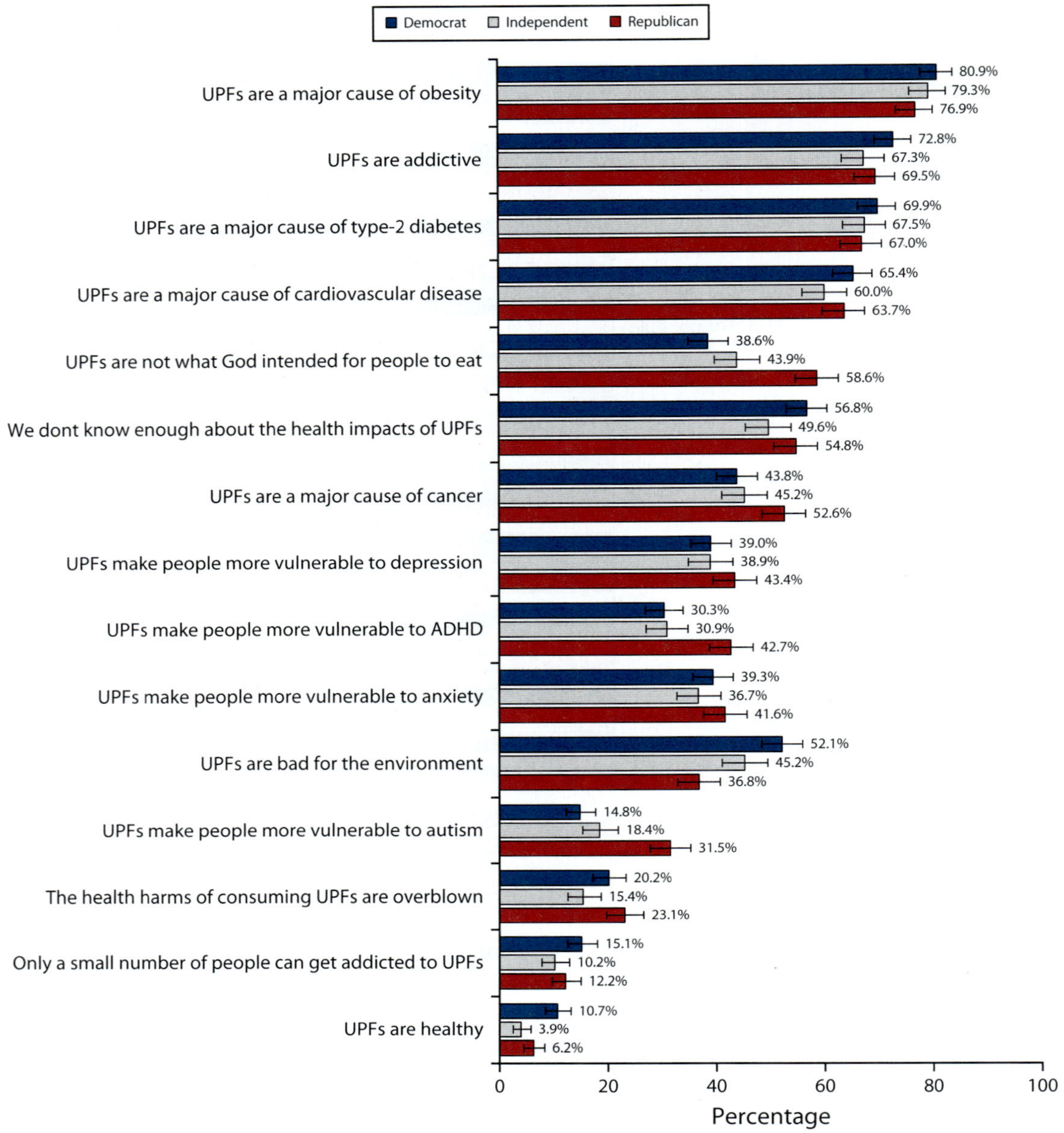

FIGURE 2— Beliefs About Harms of Ultraprocessed Foods (UPFs), Stratified by Political Party: United States, June 2025

Note. Respondents were asked, "Please indicate your level of agreement with the following statements: [example item] Ultraprocessed foods are addictive" (1 = strongly disagree; 5 = strongly agree). We dichotomized responses to 1 = agree or strongly agree versus 0 = neutral, disagree, or strongly disagree. Error bars represent 95% confidence intervals.
Source. Survey fielded June 9–19, 2025, using the YouGov panel.

for a variety of public policies with potential to reduce UPF consumption. Support was highest (83.1%; 95% CI = 81.4, 84.7) for requiring the government to test laboratory-made chemicals for safety before use in food products, but more than 64% of respondents overall also supported national education campaigns, restricting UPF advertising to children, banning dyes, and warning labels on products and ads. While modest differences by political party (8–15 percentage point differences) were found for 10 of 14 items (e.g., taxes, restricting placement at grocery stores, bringing lawsuits against UPF companies, requiring payments to a healthy food advertising fund), rank ordering of policy

AJPH July 2026, Vol. 116, No. 7

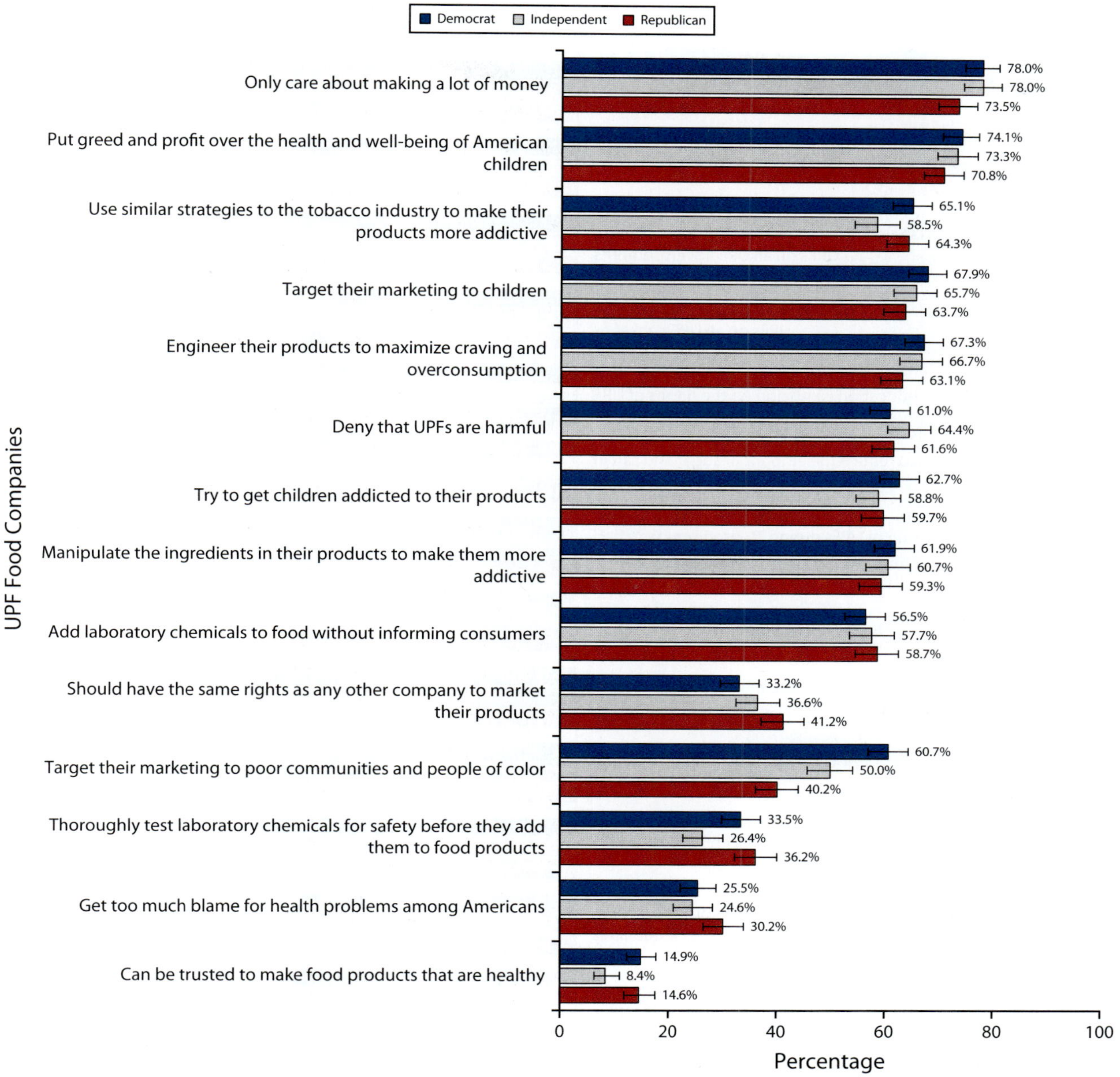

FIGURE 3— **Beliefs About Ultraprocessed Food (UPF) Companies, Stratified by Political Party: United States, June 2025**

Note. Respondents were asked, "Please indicate your level of agreement with the following statements: [example item] Ultraprocessed foods companies add laboratory chemicals to food without informing consumers" (1 = strongly disagree; 5 = strongly agree). We dichotomized responses to 1 = agree or strongly agree versus 0 = neutral, disagree, or strongly disagree. Error bars represent 95% confidence intervals.
Source. Survey fielded June 9–19, 2025, using the YouGov panel.

support was strikingly consistent across partisan groups. It is also notable (Figure B, available as a supplement to the online version of this article at https://ajph.org) that for almost all items, more respondents answered "neutral" than "oppose" (e.g., 30% of respondents were neutral about bringing lawsuits against UPF companies), suggesting greater ambivalence than opposition.

DISCUSSION

To our knowledge, this survey provides the first comprehensive assessment of how people in the United States

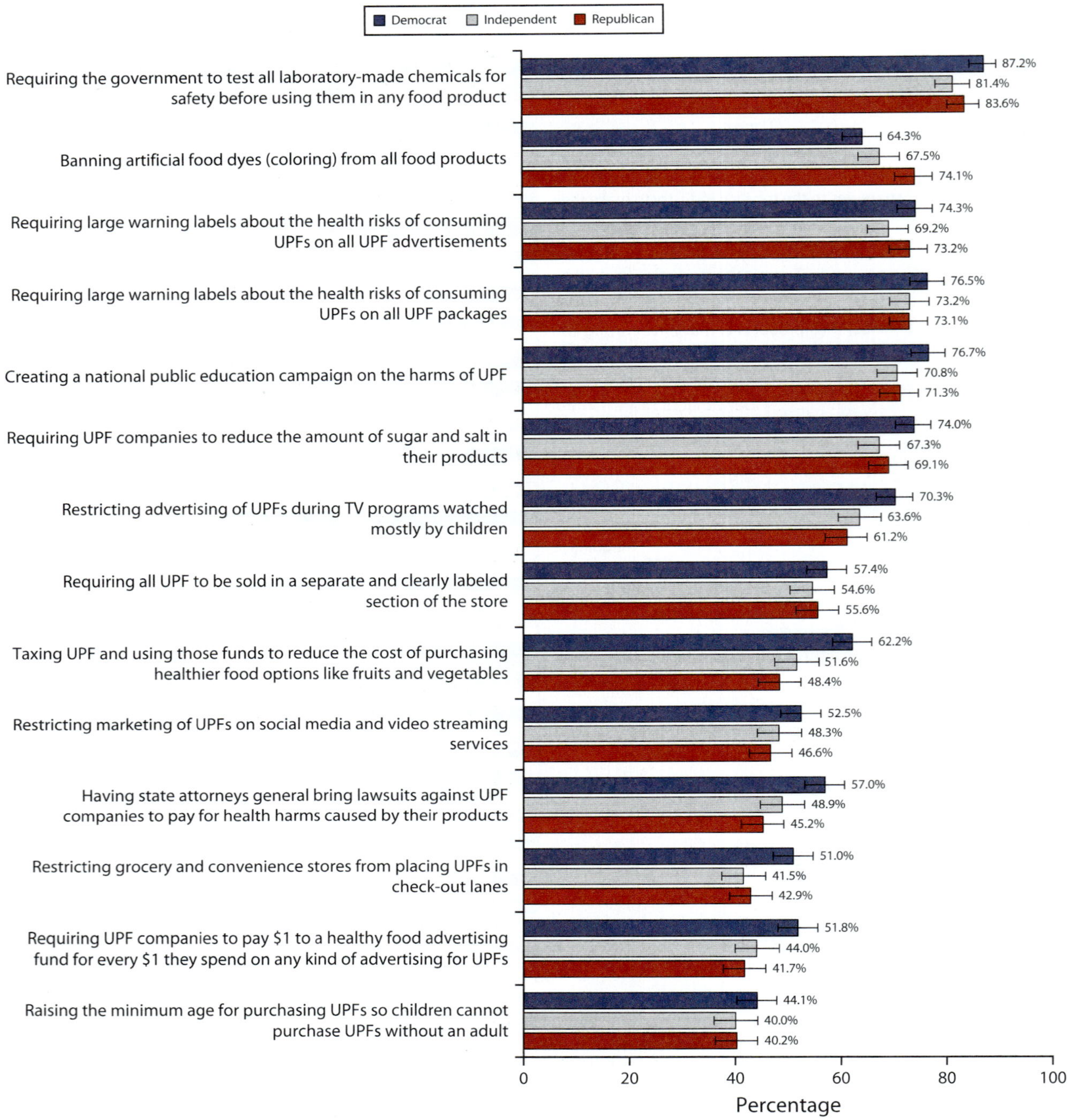

FIGURE 4— Support for Governmental Intervention to Address the Harms of Ultraprocessed Foods (UPFs), Stratified by Political Party: United States, June 2025

Note. Policy support was assessed using a 5-point Likert Scale, using the question, "To what extent do you support or oppose the following policies: [specific item wording shown in figure]" (1 = strongly oppose; 5 = strongly support). We dichotomized responses to 1 = agree or strongly agree versus 0 = neutral, disagree, or strongly disagree. Error bars represent 95% confidence intervals.
Source. Survey fielded June 9–19, 2025, using the YouGov panel.

understand and perceive UPFs and their regulation. More than half of adults had heard of UPFs, yet only one third felt confident explaining what UPFs are—revealing that public exposure to the term is expanding faster than comprehension. This underscores the need to build consensus around a clear and scientifically supported definition of UPFs for use in both (1) US regulatory policy (at both federal and state levels) and (2) health communication campaigns to increase public understanding and agency in addressing UPF harms.

Despite this limited understanding, Americans broadly recognize UPFs as harmful and assign responsibility for addressing their harms across individuals, parents, UPF companies, and (to a lesser extent) government. That distribution of perceived responsibility suggests the need for messaging that emphasizes the ways that the food environment, including the production and marketing of products that are engineered to promote craving and addiction, may undermine personal choice and agency and, thus, increase recognition of a need for more robust governmental intervention. The public appears to understand that dietary patterns are shaped not solely by individual willpower but by corporate and regulatory forces. As history with tobacco and other health threats demonstrates, voluntary reform by industry is rare; robust regulation is typically required to align profit incentives with public health.[11]

Perceived harms of UPFs were widespread and substantial. People in the United States rated them as less harmful than opioids or cigarettes but more harmful than cannabis and roughly equivalent to alcohol. This finding underscores that UPFs have entered public consciousness as a major health hazard—surpassing the perceived risk of individual product categories such as soda or fast food, which are themselves subsets of UPFs. Support for addressing UPFs as a category appears higher than for previous, more narrowly defined efforts such as soda regulation,[15] indicating that the public may be more receptive now to broader policy approaches. The consensus contrasts sharply with previous debates over obesity prevention and soda taxes, which were politically polarizing and framed as government overreach.[15–17]

Bipartisan Alignment and Political Shifts

Perhaps the most striking finding is the degree of bipartisan convergence. Republicans and Democrats expressed similar levels of concern about UPF harms and similar patterns of support for specific government regulations. Earlier national polls consistently found that conservatives or Republicans were less supportive of obesity-related or soda-tax policies, often citing concerns about personal freedom or paternalism.[15,18] Our results indicate that UPFs are breaking through this ideological barrier.

Recent polling among parents provides corroborating evidence. A 2025 KFF and *Washington Post* survey found that more than 80% of US parents, regardless of party affiliation, support stronger government regulation of dyes, additives, and highly processed foods—mirroring the levels of support observed in the current study.[20]

This alignment represents a pivotal political shift. Recent US governmental reports have reframed chronic disease as a bipartisan issue rooted in industrial food practices rather than individual failure.[6] Our data suggest that message is resonating. Republicans—long skeptical of nutrition regulation—now exhibit comparable, and in a few cases greater, concern about UPFs than Democrats. Such cross-party agreement is exceedingly rare in contemporary public health and may create a durable foundation for policy change.

Addiction and Industry Influence

Nearly 70% of Americans believe UPFs are addictive—a level of agreement that mirrors growing recognition among scientists, policymakers, and former FDA officials.[4] This public perception aligns with emerging evidence that UPFs can produce addiction-like patterns of intake and neurobiological adaptations similar to those seen with nicotine and alcohol.[5] The convergence of scientific and public understanding underscores a broader systems problem: the same multinational conglomerates that built global empires on tobacco and alcohol have expanded into UPFs, using shared expertise in product engineering, branding, and political influence to sustain consumption and deflect accountability.[21,22] Overlapping corporate ownership and coordinated lobbying link these sectors, all of which rely on the commercialization of addictive, high-margin products.[21,22] Beliefs about addiction and child-targeted marketing were among the most strongly endorsed items in our survey, reflecting widespread recognition of these corporate tactics. Recognizing these cross-industry linkages highlights the need for regulatory strategies that transcend food policy and address the wider addiction-industrial complex.

AJPH July 2026, Vol. 116, No. 7

Communication Opportunities

While most respondents acknowledged the physical harms of UPFs, far fewer recognized their connection to mental health or environmental sustainability. This represents both a gap and an opportunity. Emerging scientific evidence demonstrates consistent associations between higher UPF consumption and elevated risk of depression, anxiety, and psychological distress,[3] and there is emerging evidence on the broad environmental toll of UPF production and consumption.[23] Communicating the mental health consequences of UPF exposure could strengthen engagement across ideological lines, as concern for children's mental health ranks among the most unifying issues in the United States today.[20] Communicating the environmental consequences of producing and consuming UPFs, while potentially more politically divisive, may engage a different and larger set of issue interests.

Litigation, Regulation, and Advocacy

Study results reveal broad skepticism toward the UPF industry and high levels of support for specific policy and legal solutions that go beyond personal action. A large majority of people in the United States favor government testing of chemicals before they are added to food, mandatory reformulation to reduce sugar and salt, restrictions on child-directed advertising, and national education campaigns. Notably, public support is not limited to educational approaches: a majority also favors litigation or accountability measures targeting UPF companies.

These findings expose a critical gap between public expectations and current regulations. Although 83% of respondents support federal testing of food chemicals for safety, the FDA's Generally Recognized as Safe (GRAS) exemption allows companies to self-certify new ingredients without agency review.[24] Polling data from other sources similarly reveal that while most people in the United States strongly support the government's role in ensuring the safety of the food supply, public confidence in that supply has reached an all-time low amid perceptions that profits are being prioritized over safety.[25] Closing the GRAS loophole would not only align regulation with public expectations but also represent a tangible step toward rebuilding trust in food governance.

Litigation has historically played a pivotal role in advancing public health—most notably in tobacco control, where coordinated lawsuits by state attorneys general led to landmark settlements, industry disclosures, and major regulatory reforms.[11,21] Until recently, public support for such legal action in the food domain appeared minimal. For example, a 2003 Health Pulse of America poll found that only 6% of respondents believed parents should be able to sue major snack companies for contributing to childhood obesity, and 84% felt the government should pass laws to prevent such suits.[26] In stark contrast, our current findings reveal that 57% of Democrats, 49% of Independents, and 45% of Republicans now support state attorneys general bringing lawsuits against UPF companies for health harms caused by their products. The remaining respondents were largely neutral rather than opposed, suggesting openness to this avenue of accountability and an opportunity for additional mobilization. This shift marks a dramatic change in public sentiment over the course of 2 decades and signals growing readiness for legal strategies to hold UPF companies accountable for deceptive marketing and product engineering.

Overall, the parallels to tobacco control are striking. In both cases, widespread industry deception, targeted marketing to children, and escalating chronic disease burdens preceded decisive litigation and regulatory action.[27] Public opinion played a catalytic role in the success of antitobacco litigation and regulation, as rising awareness of corporate misconduct eroded the industry's political power.[11] UPFs may be approaching a similar inflection point. People in the United States view the industry with suspicion and favor government intervention to ensure safety and accountability.

Limitations

Several limitations should be noted. First, because awareness of UPFs remains modest, some participants were evaluating new information; their responses may not yet reflect stable beliefs. Second, the order of survey items could have introduced priming effects, though policy questions were presented before attitudinal items and all items were randomized within blocks to minimize this risk. Third, in the absence of previous surveys of UPF awareness and beliefs, we were largely unable to use previously validated measures. Fourth, while the sample was weighted to match national demographics, it was drawn from a nonprobability panel. Finally, these data capture a single point in time during a rapidly changing policy environment; continued monitoring will be essential as media coverage and political discourse evolve.

Public Health Implications

From a public health perspective, these findings are both timely and encouraging. People in the United States broadly believe that UPFs are harmful and addictive and are aligned in support of a variety of potential regulations. This perspective spans the political spectrum, signaling a rare moment of alignment that public health practitioners can leverage. Importantly, these attitudes coincide with mounting scientific consensus that certain UPFs possess addictive properties[4] and with increasing evidence that their consumption worsens both physical and mental health outcomes.[3]

The convergence of public belief, bipartisan support, and scientific evidence creates a critical window for policy action. Americans appear ready for stronger safeguards, ranging from additive testing to marketing restrictions. Public health communication strategies that highlight corporate engineering of addictive products and connect UPFs exposure to chronic disease, mental health, and environmental outcomes may hold strong promise. Like historical successes in reframing tobacco from a matter of personal failure to corporate manipulation,[28,29] a similar shift in narrative seems poised to accelerate momentum for reform around UPFs. Ongoing surveillance of public attitudes will be crucial as awareness of UPFs expands and policy debates evolve.

Ultimately, results suggest that the US public is not a barrier to progress—it may be the catalyst. With strong bipartisan concern, limited trust in industry, and high readiness for policy intervention, the conditions are ripe for transformative action to reduce the dominance of UPFs and improve public health. AJPH

ABOUT THE AUTHORS

Jeff Niederdeppe is with the College of Agriculture and Life Sciences, the Cornell Jeb E. Brooks School of Public Policy, and the Cornell Health Policy Center at Cornell University, Ithaca, NY. Colleen L. Barry is with the Cornell Jeb E. Brooks School of Public Policy and the Cornell Health Policy Center. Sarah E. Gollust is with the Division of Health Policy and Management at the University of Minnesota School of Public Health, Minneapolis. Norman Porticella is with the Department of Communication at Cornell University. Kelly D. Brownell is with the Sanford School of Public Policy at Duke University, Durham, NC. Ashley N. Gearhardt is with the Department of Psychology at the University of Michigan, Ann Arbor.

CORRESPONDENCE

Correspondence should be sent to Jeff Niederdeppe, PhD, 489B Mann Library Building, Cornell University, Ithaca, NY 14850 (e-mail: jdn56@cornell.edu). Reprints can be ordered at https://www.ajph.org by clicking the "Reprints" link.

PUBLICATION INFORMATION

Full Citation: Niederdeppe J, Barry CL, Gollust SE, Porticella N, Brownell KD, Gearhardt AN. Public awareness and support for governmental intervention to address harms associated with consumption of ultraprocessed foods: a national survey, United States, June 2025. *Am J Public Health*. 2026;116(7):960–970.

Acceptance Date: February 12, 2026.

DOI: https://doi.org/10.2105/AJPH.2026.308498

ORCID iDs:

Jeff Niederdeppe https://orcid.org/0000-0001-7686-1526

Sarah E. Gollust https://orcid.org/0000-0001-6109-5953

Norman Porticella https://orcid.org/0000-0002-1763-2472

Kelly D. Brownell https://orcid.org/0000-0003-4117-726X

Ashley N. Gearhardt https://orcid.org/0000-0003-3843-5731

CONTRIBUTORS

J. Niederdeppe, C. L. Barry, S. E. Gollust, N. Porticella, and A. N. Gearhardt conceptualized and designed the study. N. Porticella conducted the analyses. All authors interpreted the data, contributed to the initial draft, revised the article critically for intellectual content, and approved the version to be published.

ACKNOWLEDGMENTS

This research was supported by a grant from the Dohmen Company Foundation.

Note. The views expressed here do not necessarily reflect the views of the Dohmen Company Foundation.

CONFLICTS OF INTEREST

J. Niederdeppe and A. N. Gearhardt have received speaking honoraria from academic organizations and health-related nonprofits. A. N. Gearhardt has received consulting fees from health-related nonprofits and a law firm and receives royalties from Oxford University Press. S. E. Gollust, K. D. Brownell, and A. N. Gearhardt have served as consultants for Dohmen Company Foundation (a funder of this study).

HUMAN PARTICIPANT PROTECTION

The project was deemed exempt from human participation review by the institutional review board at Cornell University. All respondents provided informed consent before proceeding with the survey.

REFERENCES

1. Monteiro CA, Cannon G, Levy RB, et al. Ultra-processed foods: what they are and how to identify them. *Public Health Nutr*. 2019;22(5):936–941. https://doi.org/10.1017/S1368980018003762
2. Williams AM, Couch CA, Emmerich SD, Ogburn DF. Ultra-processed food consumption in youth and adults: United States, August 2021–August 2023. *NCHS Data Brief*. 2025(536):1–11. https://doi.org/10.15620/cdc/174612
3. Lane MM, Gamage E, Du S, et al. Ultra-processed food exposure and adverse health outcomes: umbrella review of epidemiological meta-analyses. *BMJ*. 2024;384:e077310. https://doi.org/10.1136/bmj-2023-077310
4. LaFata EM, Moran AJ, Volkow ND, Gearhardt AN. Now is the time to recognize and respond to addiction to ultra-processed foods. *Nat Med*. 2025;31(11):3586–3587. https://doi.org/10.1038/s41591-025-03858-6
5. Gearhardt AN, Bueno NB, DiFeliceantonio AG, et al. Social, clinical, and policy implications of ultra-processed food addiction. *BMJ*. 2023;383:e075354. https://doi.org/10.1136/bmj-2023-075354
6. Make America Healthy Again Commission. *Make Our Children Healthy Again: Assessment on Childhood Chronic Disease Drivers*. US Department of Health and Human Services. May 22, 2025. Available at: https://www.whitehouse.gov/wp-content/uploads/2025/05/MAHA-Report-The-White-House.pdf. Accessed October 18, 2025.
7. Stempel J. Texas probes M&M maker Mars' resistance to removing synthetic dyes. *Reuters*. July 16, 2025. Available at: https://www.reuters.com/legal/government/texas-probes-mm-maker-mars-resistance-removing-synthetic-dyes-2025-07-16. Accessed October 22, 2025.
8. Bendix A. California becomes the first state to phase ultraprocessed food out of school meals. *NBC News*. October 8, 2025. Available at: https://www.nbcnews.com/health/health-news/california-phase-ultraprocessed-food-school-meals-rcna236506. Accessed October 23, 2025.

9. USDA Food and Nutrition Service, US Department of Agriculture. Request for information: ultra-processed foods. September 19, 2025. Available at: https://www.fns.usda.gov/usda/fr-072525. Accessed October 23, 2025.

10. US Department of Agriculture, US Department of Health and Human Services. Dietary Guidelines for Americans, 2025–2030. 10th ed. January 2026. Available at: https://www.dietaryguidelines.gov. Accessed April 10, 2026.

11. Brandt AM. *The Cigarette Century: The Rise, Fall, and Deadly Persistence of the Product That Defined America.* New York, NY: Basic Books; 2007.

12. Robinson E, Cummings JR, Gough T, et al. Consumer awareness, perceptions and avoidance of ultra-processed foods: a study of UK adults in 2024. *Foods.* 2024;13(15):2317. https://doi.org/10.3390/foods13152317

13. EIT Food. Consumer perceptions unwrapped: ultra-processed foods (UPF). February 14, 2024. Available at: https://www.eitfood.eu/consumer-perceptions-unwrapped-ultra-processed-foods. Accessed June 21, 2025.

14. Balagtas J, Bryant E. Consumer food insights, volume 4, issue 2. Center for Food Demand Analysis and Sustainability, College of Agriculture, Purdue University. March 12, 2025. Available at: https://ag.purdue.edu/cfdas/wp-content/uploads/2025/03/Report_202502.pdf. Accessed October 23, 2025.

15. Gollust SE, Barry CL, Niederdeppe J. Americans' opinions about policies to reduce consumption of sugar-sweetened beverages. *Prev Med.* 2014;63:52–57. https://doi.org/10.1016/j.ypmed.2014.03.002

16. Wolfson JA, Gollust SE, Niederdeppe J, Barry CL. The role of parents in public views of strategies to address childhood obesity in the United States. *Milbank Q.* 2015;93(1):73–111. https://doi.org/10.1111/1468-0009.12106

17. Pew Research Center. Public agrees on obesity's impact, not government's role. November 12, 2013. Available at: https://www.pewresearch.org/politics/2013/11/12/public-agrees-on-obesitys-impact-not-governments-role. Accessed October 23, 2025.

18. Gollust SE, Niederdeppe J, Barry CL. Framing the consequences of childhood obesity to increase public support for obesity prevention policy. *Am J Public Health.* 2013;103(11):e96–e102. https://doi.org/10.2105/AJPH.2013.301271

19. IBM SPSS Statistics for Windows, Version 29.0. Armonk, NY: IBM Corp; 2024.

20. Kearney A, Valdes I, Montero A, et al. KFF/the *Washington Post* survey of parents: polling insights on the MAHA movement. Kaiser Family Foundation. October 15, 2025. Available at: https://www.kff.org/public-opinion/kff-the-washington-post-survey-of-parents-polling-insights-on-the-maha-movement. Accessed October 18, 2025.

21. Nguyen KH, Glantz SA, Palmer CN, Schmidt LA. Tobacco industry involvement in children's sugary drinks market. *BMJ.* 2019;364:l736. https://doi.org/10.1136/bmj.l736

22. Gearhardt AN, Brownell KD, Brandt AM. From tobacco to ultraprocessed food: how industry engineering fuels the epidemic of preventable disease. *Milbank Q.* 2026;104(1):76–115. https://doi.org/10.1111/1468-0009.70066

23. Kesse-Guyot E, Allès B, Brunin J, et al. Environmental impacts along the value chain from the consumption of ultra-processed foods. *Nat Sustain.* 2022;6(2):192–202. https://doi.org/10.1038/s41893-022-01013-4

24. Dragich M. GRAS-fed Americans: sick of lax regulation of food additives. *Ind Law Rev Arch.* 2016;49(2):305. https://doi.org/10.18060/4806.0069

25. International Food Information Council. 2025 IFIC food & health survey: a focus on food & ingredient safety. July 28, 2025. Available at: https://ific.org/research/2025-ific-food-health-survey. Accessed October 21, 2025.

26. Stony Brook University Center for Survey Research. Stony Brook poll #2003-HLTHA: Health Pulse of America, 2003 (Version 2). Ithaca, NY: Roper Center for Public Opinion Research; 2003. https://doi.org/10.25940/ROPER-31097945

27. Brownell KD, Warner KE. The perils of ignoring history: Big Tobacco played dirty and millions died. How similar is Big Food? *Milbank Q.* 2009;87(1):259–294. https://doi.org/10.1111/j.1468-0009.2009.00555.x

28. Farrelly MC, Davis KC, Haviland ML, et al. Evidence of a dose–response relationship between "truth" antismoking ads and youth smoking prevalence. *Am J Public Health.* 2005;95(3):425–431. https://doi.org/10.2105/AJPH.2004.049692

29. Niederdeppe J, Kellogg M, Skurka C, et al. Market-level exposure to state antismoking media campaigns and public support for tobacco control policy in the United States, 2001–2002. *Tob Control.* 2017;27(2):177–184. https://doi.org/10.1136/tobaccocontrol-2016-053506

Associations Between Household Food Insecurity and Participation in Nutrition Assistance Programs, and Ultraprocessed Food Consumption and Diet Quality Among Pregnant Women in NHANES, 2001–2018

Cristina R. Fernández, MD, MPH, Sandra H. Kahwaji, MPH, Pamela A. Koch, EdD, RDN, Randi L. Wolf, PhD, MPH, Eurídice Martínez-Steele, PhD, and Jennifer W. Cadenhead, PhD, RDN

See also Ultraprocessed Food, pp. 898–1029.

AJPH July 2026, Vol. 116, No. 7

Objectives. To examine associations between (1) food insecurity and participation in the Special Supplemental Nutrition Program for Women, Infants, and Children (WIC) and Supplemental Nutrition Assistance Program (SNAP), and (2) ultraprocessed food (UPF) consumption and Healthy Eating Index–2020 (HEI) score among US pregnant women.

Methods. We analyzed data from pregnant women (n = 1286) across 9 waves of National Health and Nutrition Examination Surveys, from 2001 to 2018. We assessed UPF consumption, as percentage of energy from Nova Group 4 classification, and HEI. Multivariable regressions estimated associations of food insecurity and WIC or SNAP participation with UPF consumption and HEI.

Results. Food insecurity affected 20% of women and was associated with lower HEI (B = −3.8; SE = 1.4; *P* = .01) but not UPF consumption. UPF consumption did not differ by WIC or SNAP participation status (*P* > .05). WIC participants had higher HEI while SNAP participants had lower HEI (*P* = .01).

Conclusions. Food insecurity was linked to lower prenatal HEI but not UPF consumption. WIC may improve otherwise low prenatal HEI; unchanged UPF consumption, irrespective of nutrition assistance beneficiary status, warrants public health and nutrition education strategies to reduce UPF consumption and scale access to affordable, less-processed, nutritious foods. (*Am J Public Health*. 2026;116(7): 971–980. https://doi.org/10.2105/AJPH.2026.308507)

Nutrition during pregnancy is a modifiable factor that can have an impact on long-term health outcomes for mothers and offspring. Insufficient intake of micronutrients and overconsumption of low-nutrient foods are associated with pregnancy complications, including excessive gestational weight gain, and adverse child health outcomes, like preterm birth.[1,2]

Pregnant women with lower socioeconomic status are particularly vulnerable to food insecurity, defined as a concern or inability to acquire sufficient, nutritionally adequate food.[3] The US Department of Agriculture (USDA) defines food security as high, marginal, low, or very low at its most severe; low and very low food security are indicative of reduced dietary quality and reduced food intake, respectively.[3] Though the national food insecurity rate among US pregnant women is unknown, available estimates suggest a range between 7% and 11%.[4,5] Food insecurity is associated with increased consumption of less nutritious, energy-dense foods among nonpregnant adults.[6] Increasing levels of food insecurity severity are associated with increasing consumption of industrially formulated, highly palatable, and typically energy-dense, nutritionally imbalanced ultraprocessed foods (UPFs) among nonpregnant adults.[7] Although not all UPF are equally unhealthy, particularly in terms of nutrient content, higher energy intake from UPF has been associated with excessive energy increases in added sugars, saturated fats, and refined carbohydrates, with increased risk for obesity and cardiovascular disease.[8,9] UPF constitutes more than 60% of total daily energy consumption among US adults, yet UPF consumption during pregnancy has not yet been examined in depth.[8] Among the few studies measuring UPF consumption during pregnancy, UPFs accounted for more than 50% of total daily energy consumed; however, these studies were limited by small sample sizes and limited representation across groups.[10,11]

The Special Supplemental Nutrition Program for Women, Infants, and Children (WIC) provides food packages to low-income pregnant women designed to support a healthy pregnancy and fetal development, with nutritional counseling by registered dietitians. The Supplemental Nutrition Assistance Program (SNAP) supports low-income adults with a monthly cash benefit for supplemental food purchases. However, studies among US pregnant women receiving WIC, SNAP, or both benefits are mixed, with unclear association of these nutrition assistance programs on the quality of the resulting diets.[12–15]

Better understanding of dietary patterns of US pregnant women with food insecurity and with participation in the WIC and SNAP programs can inform targeted public health policies and programs for pregnant women and their infants to advance health and nutrition equity. Our primary objective was to determine the association between food insecurity and prenatal UPF consumption and the Healthy Eating Index–2020 (HEI). Our secondary objective was to determine the association between WIC and SNAP participation and prenatal UPF consumption and HEI. We hypothesized that women with food insecurity would consume more UPF and have lower HEI compared with food-secure women. In addition, we hypothesized that WIC and SNAP participants would have lower UPF consumption and higher HEI compared with eligible nonparticipants.

METHODS

We conducted a secondary analysis of the publicly available, de-identified, individual-level cross-sectional data from 9 consecutive 2-year cycles of the National Health and Nutrition Examination Survey (NHANES) from 2001 to 2018. Protocols for NHANES have been previously explained.[16] Briefly, it is an ongoing, multilayered, stratified survey designed to be representative of the noninstitutionalized US population mirroring US Census data using 5000 participants annually; written and informed consent or assent, as appropriate, is required before participation.[16]

We selected NHANES cycles from 2001 to 2018 based on methodological consistency, data completeness, and alignment with NHANES analytic guidance, which states that pooling multiple cycles from more than 4 complete years enhances statistical power and representativeness, particularly for small subgroups such as pregnant women. NHANES standardized its dietary intake and food insecurity assessment protocols across 2001–2018 cycles, and the measures can be considered valid and reliable across pooled data without adjusting for methodology, as differences are unlikely to reflect changes in measurement. Notably, NHANES oversampled pregnant women from 2001 to 2006. We compared earlier and later analytical samples to rule out differences attributable to temporality. We elected not to include the 2019–2020 and 2021–2022 cycles because of data collection disruptions caused by the COVID-19 pandemic resulting in a potentially biased sample and because of introduced methodological changes in dietary recall collection and weighting procedures in postpandemic cycles. To maintain analytic validity and consistency across years, we restricted our sample to prepandemic cycles.

Our study accessed demographic, socioeconomic, and nutrition data of pregnant women with a self-reported pregnancy or valid urine pregnancy test at the NHANES mobile examination center. They were excluded if within NHANES datafiles their dietary recall was considered unreliable (from NHANES codes DR1DRSTZ or DR2DRSTZ), food insecurity status was not reported, or energy intake was greater than 2.5 standard deviations above the mean (Figure 1).

Measures

Our primary outcome measures were percentage of energy from UPF consumption and diet quality during pregnancy. NHANES nutrition data, excluding dietary supplements, followed the USDA Automated Multi-Pass Method with 24-hour recalls.[17] NHANES scheduled two 24-hour recalls approximately 3 to 10 days apart, covering a weekday and a weekend, with most participants having a combination of week and weekend days.[16] Where only one 24-hour recall

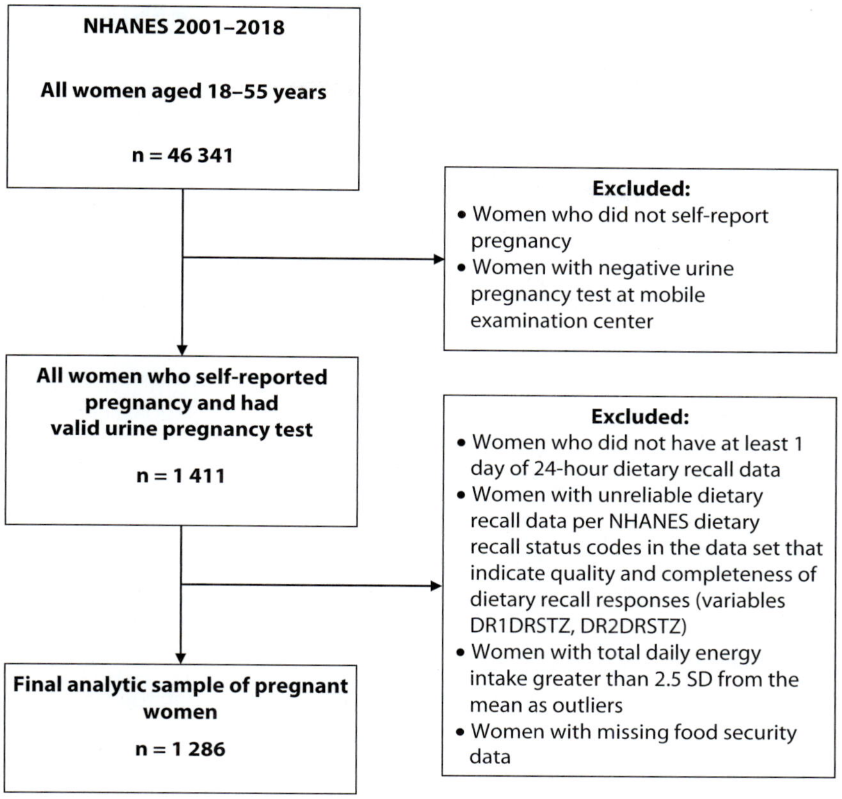

FIGURE 1— **Flow Chart Illustrating the Selection of the Final Analytic Sample of Pregnant Women With 24-Hour Dietary Recall Data and Food Security Data From the National Health and Nutrition Examination Survey (NHANES), United States, 2001–2018 Waves**

was available, the single 24-hour recall was used (~20%); otherwise, the averages of the two 24-hour recalls were used with special dietary weights provided by NHANES to ensure appropriate representation of weekday and weekend consumption at the population level and adjust for population weight.

UPF energy proportion was assessed using the Nova classification system applied to NHANES nutrition data. Nova categorizes foods based on the extent and purpose of processing into 4 groups: minimally processed foods (e.g., meat); processed culinary ingredients (e.g., oils); processed foods—minimally processed foods combined with processed culinary ingredients (e.g., canned fruit); and UPFs, industrial formulations using extracted substances (oils, starches) with additives like emulsifiers, colors, and flavorings to enhance taste and eating experience (e.g., packaged snacks).[18] With permission, the UPF classification for each food was taken from an existing, preclassified data set from the team that developed Nova.[19] In that data set, Nova classifications were based on the main food description and underlying Food and Nutrient Database for Dietary Studies ingredient codes.

Diet quality was assessed using the most current version of the HEI, which measures adherence to the 2020–2025 US Dietary Guidelines (DGAs). HEI has 13 components, with total scoring of 0 to 100, where higher scores indicate greater adherence. Suggested descriptive HEI grade cut points are "A," 90 to 100, decreasing by 10-point increments to "F," less than or equal to 59.[20] We used the simple method algorithm developed by the National Cancer Institute to program HEI scoring from NHANES data, modified for use from SAS to Stata (Box A, available as a supplement to the online version of this article at https://ajph.org).

The main exposures were food insecurity and WIC and SNAP participation. Food insecurity status was measured with the validated 18-item USDA Food Security Survey Module.[21] We categorized food insecurity high (score 0) or marginal (score 1–2) as "food secure" versus low (score 3–7) or very low food security (score 8–18) as "food insecure" per USDA convention. Using US poverty guidelines specific to the survey year and reported household income to calculate family income-to-poverty ratios, we identified women as WIC eligible: monthly gross income less than or equal to 185% of the US Department of Health and Human Services (HHS) poverty guidelines; and SNAP eligible: monthly gross income less than or equal to 130% of the HHS poverty guidelines. We measured WIC participation with affirmation of either: "In the last 12 mo, did {you/you or any member of your household} receive benefits from the WIC program?" or, for women with young children, "Did {you/survey participant} personally receive benefits from WIC in the past 12 mo?" Women who answered "No" to both were categorized as WIC-eligible nonparticipants. We measured SNAP participation from the question "In the last 12 mo, did {you/you or any member of your household} receive SNAP or Food Stamp benefits?" Women who answered "No" were categorized as SNAP-eligible nonparticipants.

We selected covariates as potential confounders based on a priori associations with dietary patterns and food insecurity, including age, race, ethnicity, nativity, education attainment, marital status, and household size. Race and ethnicity in the United States can be system-level proxies for access barriers to high-quality health care, food, housing, and other health-related needs. We also adjusted for survey cycle as a categorical covariate to account for temporal trends in dietary patterns, public health initiatives, policy changes, and food environment shifts, reducing potential confounding by calendar time.

Statistical Analyses

Survey weights were constructed and applied in accordance with NHANES analytic guidelines to account for NHANES's multistage sampling design, including stratification, cluster design, and weighting, enabling nationally representative estimates of the noninstitutionalized US population.[16] For pooled analyses across multiple NHANES cycles, the appropriate 2-year examination, interview, or dietary weights were rescaled by dividing each cycle's weight by the total number of combined cycles. Sensitivity analyses using a time period–based variable were consistent with results from fully pooled models, supporting the assumption of temporal stability (Table A, available as a supplement to the online version of this article at https://ajph.org). Survey design variables were retained as provided by NHANES, and all analyses incorporated Taylor series linearization for variance estimation.[16] Parametric and nonparametric tests compared sociodemographic characteristics and WIC and SNAP participation between pregnant women with food insecurity and those who were food secure. Associations between household food insecurity, WIC and SNAP participation, and UPF consumption and HEI outcomes were subsequently estimated using unadjusted and multivariable survey-weighted linear regression models. WIC and SNAP participation were then used as predictors of HEI and UPF consumption among those eligible for the programs by income level by comparing participants to eligible nonparticipants within each program. Unadjusted and adjusted means of UPF consumption and overall HEI were computed using least squared means in the respective linear regression models. All statistical tests were 2-sided and evaluated at the $\alpha = .05$ significance level. All statistical analyses were performed by using Stata version 17.0 (StataCorp LP, College Station, TX).

RESULTS

A detailed summary of descriptive characteristics of 1286 pregnant women is described in Table 1. Approximately 20% of the sample reported food insecurity. The weighted mean percentage of energy from UPF consumption was 57.1, and mean HEI score was 55.1 out of a total score of 100, suggesting misalignment between average prenatal diets and federal dietary guidelines (Table 1).

There was no significant difference in UPF consumption between pregnant women with food insecurity and those who were food secure on unadjusted models (60.1 ± 0.02 vs 56.4 ± 0.01: $P = .12$). After adjusting for covariates of age, race, nativity, education, marital status, household size, WIC and SNAP participation, and survey cycle to fit a more plausible and pragmatic model, food insecurity was not significantly predictive of percentage of daily energy from UPF consumption (B = 0.03; SE = 0.02; $t = 1.5$; 95% confidence interval [CI] = −0.01, 0.07; $P = .06$). HEI was significantly lower among pregnant women with food insecurity compared with those who were food secure on unadjusted models (51.1 ± 0.2 vs 56.0 ± 0.7; $P < .001$). After adjusting for covariates, the regression model predicted those who were food insecure would have significantly lower HEI (B = −3.8; SE = 1.4; $t = -2.8$; 95% CI = −6.4, −1.1; $P = .01$).

The adjusted percentage of energy from UPF consumption was not significantly different between WIC participants and WIC-eligible nonparticipants (57.6 vs 57.7; $P = .96$; Table 2). There were also no statistically significant differences in UPF consumption for SNAP participants compared with SNAP-eligible nonparticipants (59.5 vs 57.4, respectively; $P = .89$) or for participants

TABLE 1— Sociodemographic Characteristics of Pregnant Women in the US National Health and Nutrition Examination Survey (NHANES), 2001–2018, by Food Security Status

Variable	Total (n = 1286)	Food Secure (n = 1030)	Food Insecure (n = 256)	P
Weighted %	100.0	80.1	19.9	.27
Age, y, weighted mean	28.3	27.7	28.4	.45
Age category, y, no. (weighted %)				.03
≤ 20	191 (8.6)	140 (8.0)	51 (10.9)	
21–29	651 (50.7)	524 (49.8)	127 (54.4)	
30–39	422 (37.1)	353 (39.6)	69 (26.6)	
≥ 40	22 (3.6)	13 (2.6)	9 (8.1)	
Education, no. (weighted %)				< .001
< high school	376 (20.6)	250 (16.7)	126 (37.4)	
High school or GED	283 (18.8)	219 (16.8)	64 (27.6)	
≥ college	627 (60.6)	561 (66.6)	66 (35.1)	
Nativity, no. (weighted %)				.11
US-born	923 (76.9)	793 (79.2)	130 (67.3)	
Foreign-born	363 (23.1)	237 (20.8)	126 (32.7)	
Race/ethnicity, no. (weighted %)				< .001
Hispanic	409 (20.0)	270 (16.4)	139 (35.1)	
Non-Hispanic White	532 (53.5)	485 (58.0)	47 (34.9)	
Non-Hispanic Black	237 (16.2)	183 (15.2)	54 (20.6)	
Other (includes multiracial, Asian)	108 (10.3)	92 (10.5)	16 (9.5)	
Marital status, no. (weighted %)				.001
Unpartnered	318 (22.5)	229 (20.0)	89 (33.1)	
Married or partnered	966 (77.4)	800 (80.0)	166 (66.6)	
Household size, no. (weighted %)				.01
1–3 people	652 (55.8)	564 (58.8)	88 (42.9)	
4–7 people	634 (44.2)	466 (41.2)	168 (57.1)	
Income-eligible for WIC, no. (weighted %)				< .001
Yes	618 (42.2)	411 (33.4)	207 (79.5)	
No	604 (57.8)	570 (66.6)	34 (20.5)	
WIC participation in the last 12 mo (mother and household level), no. (weighted %)				< .001
Yes	562 (35.0)	391 (29.2)	171 (59.6)	
No	719 (65.0)	635 (70.8)	84 (40.4)	
Income-eligible for SNAP, no. (weighted %)				< .001
Yes	460 (29.0)	296 (22.1)	164 (58.4)	
No	762 (71.0)	685 (77.9)	77 (41.6)	
SNAP participation in the last 12 mo (mother and household level), no. (weighted %)				< .001
Yes	307 (43.3)	198 (36.5)	109 (62.8)	
No	511 (56.5)	427 (63.2)	84 (37.0)	
Refused, don't know	4 (0.3)	3 (0.3)	1 (0.2)	
Both WIC and SNAP participation in the last 12 mo (mother and household level) , no. (weighted %)				< .001
Yes	228 (22.3)	151 (17.2)	77 (54.6)	
No	644 (77.7)	591 (82.8)	53 (45.4)	

Continued

TABLE 1— Continued

Variable	Total (n = 1286)	Food Secure (n = 1030)	Food Insecure (n = 256)	P
Percentage of energy intake from ultraprocessed food[a] (SE)	57.1 (0.01)	56.4 (0.01)	60.1 (0.02)	.12
Healthy Eating Index–2020 score[a] (SE)	55.1 (0.6)	56.0 (0.7)	51.1 (1.2)	<.001

Note. GED = general educational development; SNAP = Supplemental Nutrition Assistance Program; WIC = Supplemental Nutrition Program for Women, Infants, and Children.
[a]Weighted mean values reported from the analytic sample of pregnant women with at least one 24-hour dietary recall, with reliable dietary recall data as determined by NHANES dietary recall status code in the data set indicative of quality and completeness of dietary recall responses (variables DR1DRSTZ, DR2DRSTZ), with total daily energy intake ≤ 2.5 standard deviations of the mean, and with food security data (n = 1286).

in both WIC and SNAP programs compared with income-eligible nonparticipants (57.6 vs 54.5; $P = .38$).

Adjusted mean HEI was significantly higher for WIC participants compared with WIC-eligible nonparticipants (54.4 vs 49.8; $P = .01$) and significantly lower for SNAP participants compared with SNAP-eligible nonparticipants (50.0 vs 56.8; $P = .01$; Table 2). There was no significant difference in adjusted mean HEI among pregnant women participating in both WIC and SNAP programs compared with benefits-eligible nonparticipants (51.9 vs 51.3; $P = .77$).

DISCUSSION

To the best of our knowledge, we present the first US nationally representative study of pregnant women, food insecurity, nutrition assistance program participation, and the associations with UPF and HEI. We were most surprised by the ubiquity of high amounts of UPF consumed but encouraged by the association of food programs and improved HEI when pregnant women were food insecure.

Food insecurity was associated with lower overall HEI in pregnancy, despite controlling for confounders or participation in the WIC and SNAP programs. However, no association was observed between food insecurity and UPF consumption. Although the association between food insecurity and lower HEI is similar to results seen in other US adult nonpregnant populations,[22] our findings contrast with results specific to prenatal diet quality from other cross-sectional studies with small cohorts and nationally representative samples of US pregnant women.[23–25] Our use of HEI, which measures adherence to DGAs, versus Alternative Healthy Eating Index–Pregnancy,

TABLE 2— Associations Between WIC and SNAP Eligibility and Participation Status and Ultraprocessed Food Intake and Overall Diet Quality in Pregnancy: US National Health and Nutrition Examination Survey (NHANES), 2001–2018

US Nutrition Assistance Program	HEI-2020			Nova UPF Group 4 Foods Intake		
	Weighted No.	Score[a]	P	Weighted No.	Percentage of Daily Energy Intake[a]	P
WIC-eligible						
Participants	424	54.4	.01	427	57.6	.96
Non-participants (Ref)	197	49.8		199	57.7	
SNAP-eligible						
Participants	238	50.0	.01	238	59.5	.89
Non-participants (Ref)	132	56.8		132	57.4	
Both WIC- and SNAP-eligible						
Participants in both	197	51.9	.77	197	57.6	.38
Nonparticipants in both (Ref)	127	51.3		12	54.5	

Note. HEI = Healthy Eating Index; SNAP = Supplemental Nutrition Assistance Program; UPF = ultraprocessed food; WIC = Supplemental Nutrition Program for Women, Infants, and Children. The sample size was n = 1286. Multivariable linear regression models were adjusted for potential confounders with a priori associations with dietary intake patterns in the general population: age, race, nativity, education, marital status, food security status, household size, and NHANES survey cycle year.
[a]Weighted mean values.

which measures different food group components, likely contributed to these differences.

Our findings suggest that supplemental support from nutrition assistance programs may not be enough to overcome potentially structural and policy-related challenges that pregnant women with food insecurity navigate to maintain diet quality. Such challenges include having limited affordable nutritious food locally available and instead relying on affordable, nutritionally imbalanced, shelf-stable food, with transportation instability limiting ability to seek alternative food.[26,27] A qualitative study found that food-insecure pregnant women chose cheaper, more convenient, less nutrient-dense food as a strategy to address a limited food budget, pregnancy symptoms, and stress.[27]

The adjusted mean percentage of energy from UPF consumption was not statistically different between pregnant women with food insecurity and pregnant women who were food secure. This finding contrasts with that of Leung et al., who found more severe food insecurity was associated with higher UPF consumption among all nonpregnant adults in the 2007–2016 NHANES waves.[7] The lack of significant difference in UPF consumption between the food-secure and food-insecure groups may have been attributable to insufficient statistical power. However, it also is suggestive of the ubiquity of UPF and limited nutrition education on what constitutes UPF. In addition, we combined high and marginal food security levels together, which may have increased the average UPF consumption of the combined "food secure" group and potentially masked small but meaningful differences in UPF consumption, as adults with marginal food security can experience suboptimal coping behaviors in response to anxiety around adequate food access.[28]

Similar to findings between food-secure and food-insecure women, there was no statistically significant difference in the UPF consumption between WIC participants and WIC-eligible nonparticipants, SNAP participants and SNAP-eligible nonparticipants, and SNAP and WIC participants compared with income-eligible nonparticipants. Our findings are different from the report by Leung et al. of greater UPF consumption among SNAP nonpregnant adult participants in NHANES data from all nonpregnant adults from 2007 to 2016.[7] Although WIC and SNAP participation can alleviate food insecurity and increase overall food consumption, low-income pregnant women who qualify for WIC or SNAP may experience additional challenges to optimal dietary intake quality, regardless of whether they have nutrition assistance benefts.[14] As suggested previously, historical and structural barriers in low-income neighborhoods can limit access to nutritious, affordable food in urban and rural areas, exacerbated by transportation challenges.[29] Pregnant women with very low income participating in both WIC and SNAP may purchase WIC-approved products—which must meet specific nutritional requirements by approved retailers—that are the longest-lasting to support their additional nutrient needs in pregnancy in the setting of limited economic resources. The Nova Group 4 classification includes some UPFs that contain adequate amounts of macro- and micronutrients per the DGAs, even with a high level of processing, such as whole-grain breads.[30]

WIC participants had significantly higher HEI score compared with WIC-eligible nonparticipants, likely attributable to the facts that (1) WIC is the only federal nutrition assistance program with legislative and regulatory requirements to provide targeted nutrition education and counseling to participants, and (2) WIC requires participating retailers to carry specific nutrient-dense products.[31] SNAP participants had lower HEI compared with SNAP-eligible nonparticipants, a similar pattern that has been widely reported in the literature as a reflection of increased economic vulnerability and the constraints on limited resources noted among low-income adults who actively apply for this nutrition benefit.[14] Despite the WIC participants having higher HEI compared with benefits-eligible nonparticipants, the overall mean total HEI score was an "F," suggesting an average diet quality least aligned with DGAs.[20]

Our findings are similar to other studies reporting that US pregnant women generally have better HEI than nonpregnant women, yet still fail to meet overall dietary guidelines, even with dietary supplements.[24,32] Variability in prenatal health care access, health care provider nutrition knowledge, experience with dietary counseling, and diet-related pregnancy conditions or complications may contribute to knowledge gaps for optimal prenatal nutritional needs. Pregnant women face numerous challenges besides access to affordable nutritious food in their neighborhood: financial pressures, time constraints with additional family and work responsibilities, cultural and societal expectations, social media misinformation, and other underacknowledged tasks that affect nutritious food consumption. Pregnant women, even in this study, had higher HEI than reported for nonpregnant women,[6] suggesting intentionality; yet the consistency of UPF levels across the groups of women is suggestive of high ubiquity of UPFs requiring policy shifts.

Strengths and Limitations

A strength of this study is the use of multiple waves of a large, nationally stratified and weighted representative sample allowing generalization to a US population. Restricting the analyses to the final completed cycle before the COVID-19 pandemic allowed consistent survey design, uniform diet and food security measurement, and standard multicycle weights, contributing to validity and reliability in the measures of interest. Our findings are also strengthened by model adjustment for NHANES survey cycle to account for temporal trends in associations attributable to external social and public health policy changes.

Limitations include the cross-sectional study design of NHANES, which precludes determining causality and temporality, and smaller sample size with focus on pregnant women. Food insecurity questions measure any risk in the last 12 months and do not differentiate previous food insecurity that has since resolved from the current active state when the questionnaire was completed. Dietary intake was self-reported with 24-hour recalls, which are subject to recall and social desirability bias because of under- or overreporting. However, given that our entire sample was pregnant women, where mean intake was compared, bias in recall of food intake because of pregnancy status is likely to be mitigated. Participants in the sample provided either one or two 24-hour recalls, potentially leading to variability in estimates of usual dietary intake for this population; however, given 80% reported 2 recall days, and all recalls used were deemed reliable by the NHANES collectors, variability is likely small. The standardized methods and approaches used by NHANES have been shown to produce accurate intake estimates with minimal measurement error or bias.[33]

The nutrition portion of NHANES was not specifically designed to assess the level of processing of foods, and this could lead to less accurate estimates of UPF consumption.[34] Yet the rigor of the USDA Automated Multi-Pass Method to collect 24-hour recall data makes the lack of food processing focus unlikely to substantially affect the tested associations.[34] As the WIC and SNAP models were restricted to participants who were eligible for the programs by income and had program participation data and dietary outcomes, the subgroup analyses used smaller samples than the primary analytic sample. This restriction may reduce precision and limit generalizability to all pregnant participants. Another limitation is the lack of detailed geographic information in the publicly available datafiles to enable analysis of urban and rural regional differences allowing context to public health implications.

Public Health Implications

Our findings suggest the ubiquity of UPFs such that selecting less processed options is unrealistic for pregnant women. Yet, nutrition assistance support is associated with greater adherence to federal dietary recommendations. UPF consumption was similar despite food insecurity status or nutrition program participation.[8] Food insecurity was associated with lower HEI, even after adjusting for WIC and SNAP participation, suggesting a need to optimize nutrition assistance programs for low-income pregnant women at risk for food insecurity.[8] WIC participation was also associated with higher HEI. Differences in overall HEI were small and may not denote clinically meaningful health differences. However, given the modest number of food items in the WIC package, its targeted nutrition education component, and retailer WIC package requirements, the potential influence of this program on HEI suggests that even small changes in dietary patterns from the WIC benefits may yield a positive public health impact.

These findings underscore the need for public health strategies to reduce UPF consumption and promote nutritious, less-processed alternatives across all communities. Policies for front-of-the package warning labels, banning UPF beverages in school food programs, banning UPF marketing in schools, and taxation based on sugar or salt volume have been effective in countries such as Chile, Brazil, and South Africa.[35] These approaches, where proposed in the United States, could meaningfully change the food environments underpinning UPF food purchase and consumption behaviors. In addition, there is a need to identify potential structural-level barriers to less-processed, nutritious food access, availability, and affordability by low-income pregnant women. Such barriers may contribute to sustained UPF consumption among this vulnerable population, regardless of public health and fiscal food policy changes. Future research incorporating geographic data and postpartum mother–infant nutrition may determine how urban–rural landscapes, timing of nutrition assistance program participation, and state-level food policies may relate to small observed differences in patterns of UPF consumption and diet quality across pregnancy and early childhood. AJPH

ABOUT THE AUTHORS

Cristina R. Fernández is with the Department of Pediatrics, Columbia University Vagelos College of Physicians and Surgeons, New York, NY. Sandra H. Kahwaji, Pamela A. Koch, and Randi L. Wolf are with the Laurie M. Tisch Center for Food, Education and Policy, Program in Nutrition, Department of Health Studies and Applied Educational Psychology, Teachers College, Columbia University, New York, NY. Eurídice Martínez-Steele is with the Department of Nutrition, Faculty of Public Health and Center for Epidemiological Studies in Health and Nutrition, University of São Paulo, São Paulo, Brazil. Jennifer W. Cadenhead was with the Laurie M. Tisch Center for Food, Education and Policy, Program in Nutrition, Department of Health Studies and Applied Educational Psychology, Teachers College, Columbia University, for part of the time with this study and is with the Department of Environmental, Occupational, and Geospatial Health Sciences, Graduate School of Public Health, City University of New York, New York, NY.

CORRESPONDENCE

Correspondence should be sent to Cristina R. Fernández, Columbia University Vagelos College of Physicians and Surgeons, 622 West 168th St, Department of Pediatrics, Vanderbilt Clinic 4-417, New York, NY 10032 (e-mail: crf2101@cumc.columbia.edu). Reprints can be ordered at https://www.ajph.org by clicking the "Reprints" link.

PUBLICATION INFORMATION

Full Citation: Fernández CR, Kahwaji SH, Koch PA, Wolf RL, Martínez-Steele E, Cadenhead JW. Associations between household food insecurity and participation in nutrition assistance programs, and ultraprocessed food consumption and diet quality among pregnant women in NHANES, 2001–2018. *Am J Public Health*. 2026;116(7): 971–980.

Acceptance Date: February 17, 2026.

DOI: https://doi.org/10.2105/AJPH.2026.308507

ORCID iDs:

Cristina R. Fernández https://orcid.org/0000-0003-1557-0041

Pamela A. Koch https://orcid.org/0000-0001-7300-908X

Randi L. Wolf https://orcid.org/0000-0002-8155-3082

Eurídice Martínez-Steele https://orcid.org/0000-0002-2907-3153

Jennifer W. Cadenhead https://orcid.org/0000-0002-5922-3597

CONTRIBUTORS

C. R. Fernández conceptualized the project and article with input from S. H. Kahwaji and J. W. Cadenhead. S. H. Kahwaji and J. W. Cadenhead abstracted the data. E. Martínez-Steele provided the National Health and Nutrition Examination Survey (NHANES) Nova code, and S. H. Kahwaji performed the analysis, with supervision from J. W. Cadenhead. C. R. Fernández wrote the first drafts. All authors reviewed and commented on subsequent drafts and revisions of the article, and all approve of and agree to be accountable for all content in the version to be published.

ACKNOWLEDGMENTS

C. R. Fernández was supported in part by the National Center for Advancing Translational Sciences, National Institutes of Health, through grant KL2TR001874, and by joint support from the Columbia University Vagelos College of Physicians and Surgeons, the Doris Duke Charitable Foundation COVID-19 Fund to Retain Clinical Scientists, and the American Heart Association grant 923718/Fernandez/2021. J. W. Cadenhead was supported by the Goldberg Family Foundation, the National Institute of Diabetes and Digestive and Kidney Diseases, National Institutes of Health, through grant U24DK132733, and start-up funding through the City University of New York, Graduate School of Public Health & Health Policy.

Note. The content is solely the responsibility of the authors and does not necessarily represent the official views of the National Institutes of Health.

CONFLICTS OF INTEREST

The authors have no potential conflicts of interest with respect to the research, authorship, or publication of this article.

HUMAN PARTICIPANT PROTECTION

This study was deemed exempt by the Columbia University Irving Medical Center institutional review board under federal regulation 45 CFR 46.101 because of the use of publicly available, de-identified, and aggregated NHANES data.

REFERENCES

1. Mousa A, Naqash A, Lim S. Macronutrient and micronutrient intake during pregnancy: an overview of recent evidence. *Nutrients*. 2019;11(2): 443. https://doi.org/10.3390/nu11020443
2. Raghavan R, Dreibelbis C, Kingshipp BL, et al. Dietary patterns before and during pregnancy and birth outcomes: a systematic review. *Am J Clin Nutr*. 2019;109(suppl 7):729S–756S. https://doi.org/10.1093/ajcn/nqy353
3. US Department of Agriculture, Economic Research Service. Food security in the U.S.—key statistics & graphics. Available at: https://www.ers.usda.gov/topics/food-nutrition-assistance/food-security-in-the-us/key-statistics-graphics. Accessed February 26, 2025.
4. Hinkle SN, Dolin CD, Keddem S, Kinsey EW. Patterns in food insecurity during pregnancy, 2004 to 2020. *JAMA Netw Open*. 2023;6(7): e2324005. https://doi.org/10.1001/jamanetworkopen.2023.24005
5. Ujah OI, Olaore P, Ogbu CE, Kirby RS. Trends, prevalence, and risk factors of food insecurity among pregnant and postpartum women in the United States: findings from the 2019–2021 National Health Interview Survey. *J Womens Health (Larchmt)*. 2023;32(10):1096–1103. https://doi.org/10.1089/jwh.2023.0250
6. Leung CW, Epel ES, Ritchie LD, Crawford PB, Laraia BA. Food insecurity is inversely associated with diet quality of lower-income adults. *J Acad Nutr Diet*. 2014;114(12):1943–1953.e2. https://doi.org/10.1016/j.jand.2014.06.353
7. Leung CW, Fulay AP, Parnarouskis L, Martinez-Steele E, Gearhardt AN, Wolfson JA. Food insecurity and ultra-processed food consumption: the modifying role of participation in the Supplemental Nutrition Assistance Program (SNAP). *Am J Clin Nutr*. 2022;116(1):197–205. https://doi.org/10.1093/ajcn/nqac049
8. Martínez Steele E, Popkin BM, Swinburn B, Monteiro CA. The share of ultra-processed foods and the overall nutritional quality of diets in the US: evidence from a nationally representative cross-sectional study. *Popul Health Metr*. 2017;15(1):6. https://doi.org/10.1186/s12963-017-0119-3
9. Hall KD, Ayuketah A, Brychta R, et al. Ultra-processed diets cause excess calorie intake and weight gain: an inpatient randomized controlled trial of ad libitum food intake. *Cell Metab*. 2019; 30(1):67–77.e3. https://doi.org/10.1016/j.cmet.2019.05.008
10. Rohatgi KW, Tinius RA, Cade WT, Steele EM, Cahill AG, Parra DC. Relationships between consumption of ultra-processed foods, gestational weight gain and neonatal outcomes in a sample of US pregnant women. *PeerJ*. 2017;5:e4091. https://doi.org/10.7717/peerj.4091
11. Cummings JR, Lipsky LM, Schwedhelm C, Liu A, Nansel TR. Associations of ultra-processed food intake with maternal weight change and cardiometabolic health and infant growth. *Int J Behav Nutr Phys Act*. 2022;19(1):61. https://doi.org/10.1186/s12966-022-01298-w
12. Rojhani A, Ouyang P, Gullon-Rivera A, Dale TM. Dietary quality of pregnant women participating in the Special Supplemental Nutrition Program for Women, Infants, and Children. *Int J Environ Res Public Health*. 2021;18(16):8370. https://doi.org/10.3390/ijerph18168370
13. Melo Herrera Y, Tovar A, Oaks BM, Quashie NT, Vadiveloo M. Associations between participation in the Special Supplemental Nutrition Program for Women, Infants, and Children (WIC) and maternal diet quality. *J Nutr*. 2023;153(11): 3317–3326. https://doi.org/10.1016/j.tjnut.2023.08.021
14. Andreyeva T, Tripp AS, Schwartz MB. Dietary quality of Americans by Supplemental Nutrition Assistance Program participation status: a systematic review. *Am J Prev Med*. 2015;49(4):594–604. https://doi.org/10.1016/j.amepre.2015.04.035
15. Murphy R, Marshall K, Zagorin S, Devarshi PP, Hazels Mitmesser S. Socioeconomic inequalities impact the ability of pregnant women and women of childbearing age to consume nutrients needed for neurodevelopment: an analysis of NHANES 2007–2018. *Nutrients*. 2022;14(18): 3823. https://doi.org/10.3390/nu14183823
16. Chen T, Clark J, Riddles M, Mohadjer L, Fakhouri T. National Health and Nutrition Examination Survey, 2015 – 2018: sample design and estimation procedures. Hyattsville, MD: National Center for Health Statistics; 2020.
17. US Centers for Disease Control and Prevention, National Center for Health Statistics. NHANES

questionnaires, datasets, and related documentation. Available at: https://wwwn.cdc.gov/nchs/nhanes/Default.aspx. Accessed February 25, 2025.

18. Monteiro CA, Cannon G, Levy RB, et al. Ultra-processed foods: what they are and how to identify them. *Public Health Nutr.* 2019;22(5):936–941. https://doi.org/10.1017/S1368980018003762

19. Martínez Steele E, Baraldi LG, da Costa Louzada ML, Moubarac JC, Mozaffarian D, Monteiro CA. Ultra-processed foods and added sugars in the US diet: evidence from a nationally representative cross-sectional study. *BMJ Open.* 2016;6(3):e009892. https://doi.org/10.1136/bmjopen-2015-009892

20. Krebs-Smith SM, Pannucci TE, Subar AF, et al. Update of the Healthy Eating Index: HEI-2015. *J Acad Nutr Diet.* 2018;118(9):1591–1602. https://doi.org/10.1016/j.jand.2018.05.021

21. Bickel G, Nord M, Price C, Hamilton W, Cook JT. *Guide to Measuring Household Food Security.* US Department of Agriculture, Food and Nutrition Service; 2000:82. Available at: https://www.fns.usda.gov/guide-measuring-household-food-security-revised-2000. Accessed August 20, 2016.

22. Leung CW, Tester JM. The association between food insecurity and diet quality varies by race/ethnicity: an analysis of National Health and Nutrition Examination Survey 2011–2014 results. *J Acad Nutr Diet.* 2019;119(10):1676–1686. https://doi.org/10.1016/j.jand.2018.10.011

23. Gonzalez-Nahm S, Ostbye T, Hoyo C, Kravitz RM, Benjamin-Neelon SE. Associations among food security, diet quality, and dietary intake during pregnancy in a predominantly African American group of women from North Carolina. *J Acad Nutr Diet.* 2022;122(3):565–572. https://doi.org/10.1016/j.jand.2021.08.110

24. Hill AM, Nunnery DL, Ammerman A, Dharod JM. Racial/ethnic differences in diet quality and eating habits among WIC pregnant women: implications for policy and practice. *Am J Health Promot.* 2020;34(2):169–176. https://doi.org/10.1177/0890117119883584

25. Gamba R, Leung CW, Guendelman S, Lahiff M, Laraia BA. Household food insecurity is not associated with overall diet quality among pregnant women in NHANES 1999–2008. *Matern Child Health J.* 2016;20(11):2348–2356. https://doi.org/10.1007/s10995-016-2058-1

26. Odoms-Young A, Brown AGM, Agurs-Collins T, Glanz K. Food insecurity, neighborhood food environment, and health disparities: state of the science, research gaps and opportunities. *Am J Clin Nutr.* 2024;119(3):850–861. https://doi.org/10.1016/j.ajcnut.2023.12.019

27. Zinga J, McKay FH, Lindberg R, van der Pligt P. Experiences of food-insecure pregnant women and factors influencing their food choices. *Matern Child Health J.* 2022;26(7):1434–1441. https://doi.org/10.1007/s10995-022-03440-3

28. Cook JT, Black M, Chilton M, et al. Are food insecurity's health impacts underestimated in the U.S. population? Marginal food security also predicts adverse health outcomes in young U.S. children and mothers. *Adv Nutr.* 2013;4(1):51–61. https://doi.org/10.3945/an.112.003228

29. de Brito JN, Loth KA, Fertig A, Trofholz AC, Tate A, Berge JM. Participant characteristics and dietary correlates of SNAP and other assistance programs among families with children from racially and ethnically diverse households. *Appetite.* 2022;174:106015. https://doi.org/10.1016/j.appet.2022.106015

30. Hess JM, Comeau ME, Casperson S, et al. Dietary guidelines meet Nova: developing a menu for a healthy dietary pattern using ultra-processed foods. *J Nutr.* 2023;153(8):2472–2481. https://doi.org/10.1016/j.tjnut.2023.06.028

31. US Department of Agriculture. WIC Nutrition Education Guidance. WIC Works Resource System. Available at: https://wicworks.fns.usda.gov/resources/wic-nutrition-education-guidance. Accessed February 26, 2025.

32. Bailey RL, Pac SG, Fulgoni VL, Reidy KC, Catalano PM. Estimation of total usual dietary intakes of pregnant women in the United States. *JAMA Netw Open.* 2019;2(6):e195967. https://doi.org/10.1001/jamanetworkopen.2019.5967

33. Blanton CA, Moshfegh AJ, Baer DJ, Kretsch MJ. The USDA Automated Multiple-Pass Method accurately estimates group total energy and nutrient intake. *J Nutr.* 2006;136(10):2594–2599. https://doi.org/10.1093/jn/136.10.2594

34. Steele EM, O'Connor LE, Juul F, et al. Identifying and estimating ultraprocessed food intake in the US NHANES according to the Nova classification system of food processing. *J Nutr.* 2023;153(1):225–241. https://doi.org/10.1016/j.tjnut.2022.09.001

35. Popkin BM, Barquera S, Corvalan C, et al. Toward unified and impactful policies for reducing ultra-processed food consumption and promoting healthier eating globally. *Lancet Diabetes Endocrinol.* 2021;9(7):462–470. https://doi.org/10.1016/S2213-8587(21)00078-4

Ultraprocessed Foods and the Risk of Cognitive Impairment and Dementia in Older US Adults: 2013–2020 Health and Retirement Study

Heejin Lee, PhD, Claire T. McEvoy, PhD, Euridice Martinez Steele, PhD, Neha Khandpur, ScD, Steven G. Heeringa, PhD, Lindsay H. Ryan, PhD, Kenneth M. Langa, MD, PhD, Julia A. Wolfson, PhD, MPP, and Cindy W. Leung, ScD, MPH

See also Ultraprocessed Food, pp. 898–1029.

Objectives. To examine associations between ultraprocessed food (UPF) consumption and risks of dementia, cognitive impairment with no dementia (CIND), and a composite outcome of CIND or dementia in a nationally representative longitudinal study of older US adults.

Methods. Participants were from the Health and Retirement Study (HRS 2013–2020; n = 5370). We assessed UPF intake via a semiquantitative food frequency questionnaire from the 2013 HRS Health Care and Nutrition Study. We defined cognitive impairment outcomes based on the validated Langa-Weir classification from biennial cognitive assessments (2014–2020). We used weighted Cox regression to examine associations.

Results. Compared with quintile 1, quintile 5 of UPF intake was associated with higher risks of dementia (hazard ratio [HR] = 1.58; 95% confidence interval [CI] = 1.003, 2.48; *P* for trend = .50), CIND (HR = 1.46; 95% CI = 1.13, 1.88; *P* for trend = .03), and CIND or dementia (HR = 1.47; 95% CI = 1.16, 1.87; *P* for trend = .02). Unprocessed or minimally processed food consumption was associated with lower risks of these outcomes.

Conclusions. Increased UPF consumption is associated with higher risks of dementia, CIND, and CIND or dementia among US older adults.

Public Health Implications. Our findings suggest a potential need to reduce UPF consumption for maintaining cognitive health among older adults. (*Am J Public Health*. 2026;116(7):981–992. https://doi.org/10.2105/AJPH.2026.308505)

AJPH July 2026, Vol. 116, No. 7

Ultraprocessed food (UPF) is industrially produced food and beverages to which chemical additives or chemically modified ingredients are added to enhance palatability, extend shelf life, or reduce cost.[1] Characteristics of UPFs, which are often high in saturated fat, sodium, sugar, and energy density and low in dietary fiber, include foods such as sugar-sweetened beverages, breakfast cereals, pizza, and other shelf-stable or ready-to-eat foods.[1,2] Given their widespread availability and convenience, UPF consumption contributes more than 50% of energy intake among US adults, with a concerning increase over time among older adults.[3,4]

Higher UPF consumption has been associated with a range of adverse health outcomes, including obesity,[5,6] diabetes,[7] cardiovascular disease,[8] and a higher risk of mortality.[9] Of particular relevance to healthy cognitive aging, a recent prospective cohort study of Brazilian adults found that UPF consumption was associated with a faster rate of decline in global cognition and executive function.[10] Similarly, higher UPF consumption was potentially associated with executive function impairment among US middle-aged and older adults.[11]

A recent meta-analysis showed that high UPF consumption was associated with an increased risk of all-cause dementia, whereas no association was observed with mild cognitive impairment.[12] Despite accumulating evidence on the link between UPF consumption and cognitive health, evidence from nationally representative studies among US older adults remains limited.[12,13] One US-based longitudinal study reported no significant association between UPFs and a composite outcome of cognitive impairment, combining cognitive impairment with no dementia (CIND) and dementia.[14] However, the previous study did not quantify UPF intake using energy-standardized measures, which may better reflect the overall dietary contribution of UPFs.[15] Evidence regarding the association between UPF consumption and individual cognitive outcomes, including dementia and CIND, remains limited. Diets high in UPFs often reflect poor diet quality, which may contribute to cognitive decline, underscoring the need for further investigation.

Thus, our primary objective was to examine the associations between UPF consumption and the risk of dementia, CIND, and a composite outcome of CIND or dementia using the longitudinal and nationally representative Health and Retirement Study (HRS) among adults aged 50 years or older. As a secondary objective, we examined the associations between unprocessed or minimally processed food (MPF) consumption and cognitive outcomes and assessed the extent to which gender, educational attainment, and social isolation modified the associations between UPF consumption and cognitive impairment. We hypothesized that adults with lower educational attainment and greater social isolation would be more susceptible to cognitive impairment and would show stronger associations. We examined gender differences in an exploratory manner.

METHODS

Participants were from the HRS, a US nationally representative longitudinal survey of adults aged 50 years and older and their spouse or partner. The HRS was initiated in 1992 and has since been conducted biennially (HRS Core).[16] The HRS is conducted by the University of Michigan. Briefly, the HRS adopts a stratified, multistage area probability sampling design, with oversampling of non-Hispanic Black and Hispanic individuals. In addition to its biennial Core survey, the HRS conducted the 2013 Health Care and Nutrition Study (HCNS) as a supplemental off-year survey on food purchases and dietary intake. Measures assessed in the HRS Core survey, such as socioeconomic, health, and lifestyle information, were not collected in the HCNS and were therefore drawn from the most recent previous HRS Core survey (2012).

We combined HRS Core data (2012–2020) with 2013 HCNS (n = 8073).[17,18] We included participants aged 50 years or older with UPF consumption data who had no previous Alzheimer's disease, dementia, or memory problems at baseline (2012) and who did not develop cognitive impairment within the first 2 years of follow-up (n = 1173) to mitigate the possibility of reverse causation. Additionally, we excluded participants with implausible energy intake (men: < 800 kcal/day or > 4000 kcal/day; women: < 500 kcal/day or > 3500 kcal/day; n = 348), nonpositive sampling weights (n = 157), or missing covariate information for whom data from earlier waves could not be carried forward (n = 183). This yielded 5370 participants for analysis (Figure A, available as a supplement to the online version of this article at http://www.ajph.org).

Dietary Assessment and Nova Classification

We collected dietary data using a validated semistructured food frequency questionnaire (FFQ), based on the Harvard FFQ, from the 2013 HCNS.[19] We linked dietary data to the Harvard food composition tables to estimate total energy and nutrient intake. UPF classifications followed the Nova system: MPFs (Nova 1), processed culinary ingredients (Nova 2), processed foods (Nova 3), and UPFs (Nova 4).[20] We categorized FFQ items for UPFs based on the approach previously applied in large US prospective cohorts.[21] Slight modifications to the Nova coding scheme included classifying hamburgers and chicken or turkey sandwiches as UPFs, because these foods were typically commercially prepared when the FFQ was administered. UPF and MPF items are listed in Tables A and B (available as a supplement to the online version of this article at http://www.ajph.org). We categorized UPFs into 13 mutually exclusive subgroups:

1. whole grains,
2. grains and derivatives,
3. dairy,
4. fats and oils,
5. processed meats,
6. processed fish,
7. snacks and sweets,
8. sweeteners,
9. sugar-sweetened beverages,
10. other beverages,
11. liquor,
12. sauces, and
13. mixed dishes.

We calculated energy-adjusted UPF or MPF intake (in grams) using the residual method and grouped it into gender-specific quintiles for analysis.[22]

Cognitive Impairment

We used the Langa-Weir classification of cognitive function, which has high sensitivity and specificity,[23] to define cognitive impairment. We included data through 2020, as the summary scores for the classifications were available up to 2020 in the data set distributed via the HRS website. The HRS Core interview included tests of serial 7s, backward counting, and immediate and delayed word recall to assess cognitive impairment at each wave, with a total score of 27. We classified participants as having dementia if they scored 6 or less, as having CIND if they scored 7 to 11, and as having normal cognitive function if they scored 12 to 27. We defined CIND or dementia as a score of 11 or less, encompassing both dementia and CIND as the composite outcome. We calculated person-years from the entry date to the date of first identification of outcome of interest or a censoring event (death, loss to follow-up, or end of follow-up in May 2021), whichever occurred first. For dementia analysis, we treated dementia onset as an event. For CIND, follow-up continued until CIND onset with dementia treated as an additional censoring event. For the composite CIND or dementia outcome, follow-up continued until CIND, dementia, or a censoring event.

Sociodemographic and Lifestyle Covariates

We selected demographic, socioeconomic, lifestyle, and health-related covariates as potential factors related to both UPF consumption and cognitive impairment. For race/ethnicity, the HRS assessed Hispanic/Latino ethnicity first, followed by self-reported race/ethnicity categories including non-Hispanic White, non-Hispanic Black/African American, non-Hispanic American Indian/Alaska Native, non-Hispanic Asian/Native Hawaiian/Pacific Islander, and other. We derived demographic covariates, including age (years, continuous), gender (men, women), and race/ethnicity (non-Hispanic White, non-Hispanic Black, Hispanic, and other), from the 2013 HCNS, and we drew other covariates from the baseline HRS Core (2012). If information on a covariate was missing, we carried data from earlier waves forward.

We used socioeconomic variables, including marital status (never married, married but spouse absent, separated, divorced, widowed; married or living with a partner), education (less than high school, high school graduate, some college/college graduate, postcollege), total net worth (tertiles), and household size (1, 2, ≥ 3). We calculated total net worth as the sum of all wealth components minus debts.[24] To account for cases in which debts exceeded assets, we added a small random constant. We then log-transformed the resulting values and categorized them into tertiles.

Lifestyle and health-related variables included vigorous activity (none, ≤ once/week, > once/week), smoking status (never, ever, current), alcohol consumption (nondrinker, < 5g/day, ≥ 5g/day), total energy intake (in kcal), body mass index (BMI = < 25, 25–29.9, or ≥ 30; defined as weight in kilograms divided by the square of height in meters), depressive symptoms at baseline (yes, no), and chronic disease history (yes, no). Participants reported the frequency of vigorous physical activity as every day, more than once per week, once per week, 1 to 3 times per month, or never. We assessed depressive symptoms using the 8-item Center for Epidemiologic Studies Depression Scale, with scores of 5 or higher indicating the presence of depressive symptoms. We defined chronic disease history based on self-reported physician-diagnosed diabetes, stroke, heart problems, cancer, or hypertension reported in 2 consecutive surveys.

For subgroup analyses by social isolation, we derived a social isolation index score based on the 2012 HRS Core items administered to approximately half of the participants:

1. unmarried or living alone;
2. contact with children less than once a month;
3. contact with family members other than children less than once a month;
4. contact with friends less than once a month; and
5. participation in groups, clubs, or other social organizations less than once a month.

We assigned 1 point for each condition met and summed the points across the 5 items (range = 0–5). We classified scores of 2 or more as socially isolated.[25,26]

Statistical Analysis

We applied attrition-adjusted sampling weights to account for the multistage area probability sampling design of the HRS and the analytic subsample. We estimated propensity scores using logistic regression to model the probability that HCNS respondents were eligible for the analytic subsample, adjusting for age, gender, race/ethnicity, and years of education. We multiplied decile-based reciprocals of the mean propensity score by the original HCNS full-sample weight to compute the adjusted sampling weight. For participant characteristics, we present continuous variables as weighted means and SEs and categorical variables as frequencies and weighted percentages.

We used weighted Cox proportional hazards models to examine the associations of UPF and MPF consumption with the risks of cognitive impairment, estimating hazard ratios (HRs) and 95% confidence intervals (CIs). The proportional hazards assumption was not violated based on Schoenfeld residuals. We adjusted models for age, gender, and race/ethnicity (Model 1). Model 2 additionally adjusted for marital status, educational attainment, total net worth, household size, total energy intake, vigorous physical activity, smoking, alcohol consumption, depressive symptoms, and chronic disease history. We assessed linear trends by including the median value of UPF consumption in each quintile as a continuous variable in the model. We used restricted cubic splines (4 knots) to assess possible nonlinearity between UPF consumption and cognitive impairment risk, after truncating the top 1% of UPF intake. In sensitivity analyses, we further adjusted for BMI and diet quality. We assessed diet quality using the Mediterranean diet score (Table C),[27] given its relevance to cognitive health, and we included BMI as a potential mediator. Because UPF intake units might affect the UPF–disease associations, we further modeled UPFs as percentage of total grams and percentage of total energy intake.

To test for effect modification by gender, education, and social isolation, we included multiplicative interaction terms in the model and assessed their statistical significance using the Wald test. We did not examine effect modification by social isolation for dementia owing to small case numbers in some strata. We also estimated the associations between each UPF category and the risk of cognitive impairment. We simultaneously included each UPF category in fully adjusted models and excluded total UPF intake from the models. We conducted all statistical analyses using SAS 9.4 (SAS Institute Inc., Cary, NC; we set significance level at $P < .05$).

RESULTS

In 2013, the weighted mean age was 64.5 years (SE = 0.3); 55.2% were women, and 81.7% were non-Hispanic White. Over 8.7 years of median follow-up, we identified 266 (5.0%) new cases of dementia, 1191 (22.2%) cases of CIND, and 1310 (24.4%) cases of CIND or dementia. On average, UPFs (Nova 4) accounted for 21.5% (SD = 13.8%) of total food intake (in grams), whereas MPF (Nova 1) accounted for 71.8% (SD = 15.0%). By energy, UPFs contributed 42.4% (SD = 12.3%) and MPF contributed 43.1% (SD = 11.7%) of total energy intake. The largest contributors to total UPF intake were sugar-sweetened beverages (31.2%), other beverages (22.2%), dairy (11.2%), snacks and sweets (9.7%), and grains and derivatives (6.2%) (Table D). Participants with higher UPF consumption, compared with those in the lowest quintile, were more likely to be men, non-Hispanic Black, never married, living in a single-person household, high school graduates, current smokers, nondrinkers, physically inactive and to have lower total net worth, obesity, depressive symptoms, history of chronic disease, and higher energy intake (Table 1).

Ultraprocessed Food and Cognitive Outcomes

The associations between UPF consumption and incident cognitive impairment are shown in Table 2. UPF consumption (quintile 5 vs quintile 1) was associated with a higher risk of dementia (HR = 1.58; 95% CI = 1.003, 2.48) after adjustment for socioeconomic, health, and lifestyle factors (model 2), although the linear trend across quintiles was not statistically significant (P for trend = .50). For CIND, compared with quintile 1, UPF consumption was associated with higher risk of CIND (quintile 5: HR = 1.46; 95% CI = 1.13, 1.88), with a significant linear trend (P for trend = .03). Greater UPF consumption was associated with a higher risk of CIND or dementia (quintile 5 vs quintile 1: HR = 1.47; 95% CI = 1.16, 1.87), with a significant linear trend (P for trend = .02). We observed no significant linear or nonlinear associations for dementia, CIND, or the composite outcome of CIND or dementia in spline models (Figure B, available as a supplement to the online version of this article at http://www.ajph.org).

Sensitivity Analysis

Further adjustment for BMI yielded similar results, and adjustment for the Mediterranean diet scores somewhat attenuated HRs for dementia (quintile 5: HR = 1.53; 95% CI = 0.96, 2.42), for CIND (quintile 5: HR = 1.39; 95% CI = 1.08, 1.80), and for CIND or dementia (quintile 5: HR = 1.43; 95% CI = 1.11, 1.83; Table E, available as a supplement to the online version of this article at http://www.ajph.org). When we used UPF percentage of

TABLE 1— Baseline Characteristics for Dementia Analysis by Quintile of Energy-Adjusted Ultraprocessed Food Intake: United States, Health and Retirement Study, 2013–2020

Baseline Characteristic	Energy-Adjusted Ultraprocessed Food Intake, No. (%) or Mean ±SE					
	Total	Quintile 1	Quintile 2	Quintile 3	Quintile 4	Quintile 5
Age, y	64.5 ±0.3	65.0 ±0.6	65.9 ±0.5	65.4 ±0.5	64.7 ±0.3	62.0 ±0.3
Gender = women	3185 (55.2)	637 (58.3)	637 (54.9)	637 (54.2)	637 (54.9)	637 (53.9)
Race/ethnicity						
Non-Hispanic White	3961 (81.7)	793 (80.5)	813 (82.4)	803 (82.5)	759 (79.0)	793 (83.6)
Non-Hispanic Black	721 (7.9)	102 (5.1)	140 (8.8)	135 (7.3)	190 (11.3)	154 (7.4)
Hispanic	540 (7.3)	130 (9.1)	98 (6.3)	111 (7.8)	94 (7.3)	107 (6.3)
Other	148 (3.1)	49 (5.3)	23 (2.6)	25 (2.4)	31 (2.4)	20 (2.7)
Marital status						
Never married[a]	1601 (29.2)	295 (26.9)	325 (29.8)	320 (29.3)	336 (31.2)	325 (29.1)
Married or living with a partner	3769 (70.8)	779 (73.1)	749 (70.2)	754 (70.8)	738 (68.9)	749 (70.9)
Total net worth						
Tertile 1 (low)	1789 (32.7)	298 (26.6)	310 (28.4)	308 (26.8)	394 (35.8)	479 (44.1)
Tertile 2 (medium)	1791 (32.9)	349 (31.7)	363 (33.0)	360 (34.5)	368 (34.5)	351 (31.0)
Tertile 3 (high)	1790 (34.5)	427 (41.7)	401 (38.6)	406 (38.7)	312 (29.7)	244 (25.0)
Household size						
1	1110 (20.9)	204 (19.8)	231 (21.5)	214 (20.0)	237 (21.5)	224 (21.5)
2	2964 (53.8)	629 (57.1)	587 (52.1)	620 (57.7)	585 (52.6)	543 (50.1)
≥3	1296 (25.3)	241 (23.2)	256 (26.4)	240 (22.3)	252 (26.0)	307 (28.4)
Education level						
< high school	676 (10.8)	125 (9.8)	128 (9.4)	130 (10.4)	136 (11.3)	157 (12.8)
High school graduate	1739 (31.4)	315 (26.8)	337 (31.8)	341 (30.4)	361 (32.7)	385 (35.1)
Some college/college graduate	2172 (42.3)	454 (44.4)	435 (43.1)	432 (41.8)	429 (41.5)	422 (40.8)
Postcollege	783 (15.5)	180 (19.0)	174 (15.7)	171 (17.5)	148 (14.6)	110 (11.4)
Smoking status						
Never smoker	2489 (46.8)	519 (48.3)	505 (45.5)	491 (47.5)	502 (48.3)	472 (44.6)
Ever smoker	2179 (38.4)	461 (41.1)	453 (42.0)	462 (40.1)	412 (35.1)	391 (34.3)
Current smoker	702 (14.8)	94 (10.6)	116 (12.5)	121 (12.4)	160 (16.6)	211 (21.2)
Alcohol consumption, g/d						
Nondrinker	1973 (34.2)	327 (27.3)	361 (30.4)	373 (32.3)	417 (36.9)	495 (43.0)
< 5	1912 (35.3)	361 (32.7)	369 (33.9)	414 (36.9)	399 (38.2)	369 (35.0)
≥ 5	1485 (30.5)	386 (40.1)	344 (35.8)	287 (30.8)	258 (25.0)	210 (22.0)
Vigorous activity						
None	2011 (35.5)	335 (30.5)	362 (32.1)	401 (33.9)	430 (38.3)	483 (42.0)
≤ once/wk	1258 (24.1)	215 (19.8)	240 (23.1)	288 (27.7)	269 (26.1)	246 (24.0)
> once/wk	2101 (40.4)	524 (49.7)	472 (44.8)	385 (38.4)	375 (35.6)	345 (34.0)
Body mass index,[b] kg/m^2						
< 25	1126 (21.3)	292 (29.7)	262 (25.0)	210 (19.2)	198 (18.3)	164 (14.9)
25–29.9	1839 (34.3)	397 (35.2)	365 (34.5)	407 (38.8)	333 (30.2)	337 (33.0)
≥ 30	2405 (44.4)	385 (35.2)	447 (40.5)	457 (42.1)	543 (51.5)	573 (52.1)

Continued

TABLE 1— Continued

Baseline Characteristic	Energy-Adjusted Ultraprocessed Food Intake, No. (%) or Mean ±SE					
	Total	Quintile 1	Quintile 2	Quintile 3	Quintile 4	Quintile 5
Has depressive symptoms[c]	363 (7.1)	66 (6.2)	52 (5.8)	72 (6.2)	80 (7.6)	93 (9.3)
Has history of chronic disease[d]	3882 (67.0)	740 (62.9)	785 (66.8)	774 (66.9)	806 (70.5)	777 (67.8)
Total energy intake, kcal/d	1629.8 ±9.6	1581.4 ±23.1	1642.9 ±23.6	1669.7 ±21.6	1658.8 ±21.3	1602.0 ±26.9

Note. Total participants = 5370; n = 1074 per quintile. Characteristics are presented for the baseline analytic sample used in the dementia analysis. We weighted all values using attrition-adjusted sampling weights. We defined quintiles as gender-specific categories of energy-adjusted ultraprocessed food intake.

[a]We included never married, married but spouse absent, separated, divorced, and widowed in this category.

[b]Body mass index is defined as weight in kilograms divided by the square of height in meters.

[c]We defined depressive symptoms as a Center for Epidemiologic Studies Depression Scale–8 items score of ≥ 5 at baseline.

[d]Chronic diseases included diabetes, stroke, heart problems, cancer, and hypertension.

total grams, the associations did not substantially change (Table F). Using UPF percentage of total energy intake, the associations were attenuated, with the association for dementia no longer statistically significant (Table G, available as a supplement to the online version of this article at http://www.ajph.org). Across UPF subgroups modeled simultaneously, only processed meat consumption was associated with a higher risk of dementia (quintile 5: HR = 2.25; 95% CI = 1.31, 3.87), for CIND (quintile 5: HR = 1.32; 95% CI = 1.02, 1.72), and for CIND or dementia (quintile 5: HR = 1.38; 95% CI = 1.09, 1.75; Table H, available as a supplement to the online version of this article at http://www.ajph.org). By contrast, MPF consumption was associated with lower risks of dementia (quintile 5: HR = 0.59; 95% CI = 0.32, 0.98), for CIND (quintile 5: HR = 0.76; 95% CI = 0.62, 0.93), and for CIND or dementia (quintile 5: HR = 0.74; 95% CI = 0.61, 0.90; Table I).

Subgroup Analysis

In subgroup analyses, higher UPF consumption was associated with increased risk of CIND (*P* for trend = .02) and CIND or dementia (*P* for trend = .02) among socially isolated participants (n = 525; 22.8%), whereas we observed no significant trends among nonsocially isolated participants (Table 3). However, we observed no statistically significant interactions, although results were suggestive (*P* for interaction = .08 for both outcomes). There was no significant interaction by gender (*P* for interaction = .99 for dementia, .71 for CIND, and .75 for CIND or dementia) or educational attainment (*P* for interaction = .87 for dementia, .62 for CIND, and .54 for CIND or dementia).

DISCUSSION

Increased UPF consumption was associated with higher risks of dementia, CIND, and CIND or dementia in a nationally representative longitudinal cohort of US older adults. Greater MPF consumption was associated with lower risks of these outcomes. Processed meat was the only UPF subgroup associated with increased risks of dementia, CIND, and CIND or dementia. The UPF-cognitive outcome associations did not differ by gender, education level, or social isolation.

Our findings build on previous research on UPF consumption and cognition. A meta-analysis[12] and prospective findings from the UK Biobank have reported that UPF consumption is associated with an increased risk of dementia,[28] and the Framingham Heart Study observed a higher risk of Alzheimer's disease.[29] Despite these studies, the research on UPF consumption and cognition remains mixed. A meta-analysis found no significant associations between UPF consumption and mild cognitive impairment.[12] Some included studies focused on selected UPF subgroups, such as processed meat and sugar-sweetened beverages, which may not capture the breadth of UPF intakes. Similarly, a study using the HRS observed no significant associations of UPF consumption with incident cognitive impairment, which encompassed both dementia and CIND.[14]

Extending previous research, our study quantified UPF intake using energy-adjusted measures (in grams) rather than daily servings (i.e., number of servings per day). Gram-based metrics may be particularly informative for certain UPF categories, such as artificially sweetened beverages, which can contribute substantial weight (in grams) but little or no energy.[30] Of note, previous FFQ validation studies of UPFs have shown that energy-adjusted values are

TABLE 2— Association Between Energy-Adjusted UPF Intake and Incident Dementia, CIND, and CIND or Dementia: United States, Health and Retirement Study, 2013–2020

Outcome	Quintile 1	Quintile 2	Quintile 3	Quintile 4	Quintile 5	*P* for Trend
Median (IQR) UPF intake, g/d[a]	222.7 (182.5–253.8)	328.4 (304.1–354.0)	434.0 (403.8–468.4)	596.1 (549.0–656.7)	972.6 (826.8–1284.4)	
Dementia						
No. of cases/person-years	39/8227	70/8167	56/8185	62/8193	39/8259	
Model 1,[b] HR (95% CI)	1 (Ref)	2.17 (1.38, 3.41)	1.80 (1.11, 2.93)	1.97 (1.33, 2.93)	1.86 (1.19, 2.91)	.07
Model 2,[c] HR (95% CI)	1 (Ref)	2.16 (1.42, 3.29)	1.74 (1.07, 2.83)	1.80 (1.20, 2.71)	1.58 (1.003, 2.48)	.5
CIND						
No. of cases/person-years	220/7571	264/7520	237/7563	230/7536	240/7586	
Model 1,[b] HR (95% CI)	1 (Ref)	1.44 (1.17, 1.78)	1.31 (1.04, 1.64)	1.28 (1.02, 1.61)	1.80 (1.40, 2.33)	≤.001
Model 2,[c] HR (95% CI)	1 (Ref)	1.41 (1.13, 1.74)	1.28 (0.97, 1.67)	1.15 (0.90, 1.45)	1.46 (1.13, 1.88)	.03
CIND or dementia						
No. of cases/person-years	238/7571	292/7520	261/7563	260/7536	259/7586	
Model 1,[b] HR (95% CI)	1 (Ref)	1.46 (1.19, 1.78)	1.32 (1.07, 1.62)	1.34 (1.07, 1.66)	1.81 (1.42, 2.30)	≤.001
Model 2,[c] HR (95% CI)	1 (Ref)	1.42 (1.16, 1.75)	1.28 (1.00, 1.64)	1.20 (0.95, 1.50)	1.47 (1.16, 1.87)	.02

Note. CI = confidence interval; CIND = cognitive impairment with no dementia; HR = hazard ratio; IQR = interquartile range; UPF = ultraprocessed food. Total participants = 5370.

[a]Values are presented as the energy-adjusted UPF intake (g/day) estimated using residual method, using gender-specific quintile.

[b]We adjusted models for age (continuous, years), gender (men, women), and race/ethnicity (non-Hispanic White, non-Hispanic Black, Hispanic, and other [Alaska Native/American Indian, Asian/Pacific Islander]).

[c]We further adjusted models for marital status (never married, married but spouse absent, separated, divorced, widowed; married or living with a partner), education (< high school, high school graduate, some college/college graduate, postcollege), total net worth (tertile), household size (1, 2, ≥ 3), energy intake (continuous, kcal/d), vigorous physical activity (none, ≤ once/week, > once/week), smoking (never smoker, ever smoker, current smoker), alcohol consumption (nondrinker, < 5g/d, ≥ 5g/d), baseline depressive symptom (yes or no; Center for Epidemiologic Studies Depression Scale–8 items score ≥ 5), and chronic disease history (yes or no; diseases included diabetes, stroke, heart problems, cancer, and hypertension). All models incorporated attrition-adjusted sampling weights and accounted for the complex sampling design.

TABLE 3— Associations Between Energy-Adjusted UPF Intake and Incident Dementia, CIND, and CIND or Dementia Stratified by Sociodemographic and Social Factors: United States, Health and Retirement Study, 2013–2020

Sociodemographic or Social Factor	No. Cases/ Person-Years	Quintile 1, HR (95% CI)	Quintile 2, HR (95% CI)	Quintile 3, HR (95% CI)	Quintile 4, HR (95% CI)	Quintile 5, HR (95% CI)	*P* for Trend	*P* for Interaction
Gender (n = 5 370)								
Dementia								.99
Men	113/16 574	1 (Ref)	2.10 (1.02, 4.34)	1.79 (0.80, 3.99)	1.53 (0.74, 3.19)	1.50 (0.68, 3.32)	.86	
Women	153/24 457	1 (Ref)	2.15 (1.15, 4.01)	1.75 (0.91, 3.36)	2.08 (1.25, 3.47)	1.70 (0.88, 3.28)	.4	
CIND								.71
Men	512/15 210	1 (Ref)	1.44 (1.03, 2.02)	1.37 (0.90, 2.09)	1.15 (0.78, 1.70)	1.55 (1.04, 2.32)	.11	
Women	679/22 566	1 (Ref)	1.37 (1.07, 1.75)	1.19 (0.87, 1.63)	1.15 (0.86, 1.53)	1.38 (1.03, 1.86)	.17	
CIND or dementia								.75
Men	563/15 210	1 (Ref)	1.47 (1.04, 2.06)	1.41 (0.95, 2.08)	1.23 (0.84, 1.79)	1.55 (1.05, 2.29)	.11	
Women	747/22 566	1 (Ref)	1.37 (1.10, 1.72)	1.18 (0.88, 1.58)	1.18 (0.89, 1.55)	1.41 (1.07, 1.87)	.11	
Educational level (n = 5 370)								
Dementia								.87
< high school	78/4 876	1 (Ref)	3.21 (1.62, 6.39)	2.95 (1.38, 6.32)	2.13 (1.03, 4.40)	2.62 (1.09, 6.32)	.34	
High school graduate	83/13 022	1 (Ref)	2.66 (1.17, 6.07)	1.57 (0.64, 3.81)	1.46 (0.63, 3.40)	1.29 (0.48, 3.46)	.5	
≥ college	105/23 133	1 (Ref)	1.66 (0.80, 3.45)	1.43 (0.70, 2.90)	2.39 (1.37, 4.17)	1.40 (0.64, 3.04)	.31	
CIND								.62
< high school	286/4 096	1 (Ref)	1.57 (0.99, 2.49)	0.94 (0.58, 1.53)	0.79 (0.47, 1.33)	1.37 (0.81, 2.32)	.5	
High school graduate	435/11 777	1 (Ref)	1.42 (0.98, 2.06)	1.14 (0.73, 1.77)	1.04 (0.70, 1.54)	1.19 (0.78, 1.81)	.99	
≥ college	470/21 903	1 (Ref)	1.24 (0.87, 1.75)	1.54 (1.12, 2.13)	1.38 (0.98, 1.93)	1.65 (1.05, 2.60)	.03	
CIND or dementia								.54
< high school	313/4 096	1 (Ref)	1.63 (1.06, 2.51)	1.08 (0.65, 1.78)	0.86 (0.52, 1.42)	1.46 (0.86, 2.48)	.4	
High school graduate	465/11 777	1 (Ref)	1.45 (1.03, 2.04)	1.17 (0.76, 1.78)	1.07 (0.74, 1.54)	1.20 (0.81, 1.78)	.98	
≥ college	532/21 903	1 (Ref)	1.26 (0.90, 1.78)	1.46 (1.10, 1.95)	1.45 (1.07, 1.97)	1.65 (1.07, 2.55)	.02	
Social isolation (n = 2 303)[a]								
CIND								.08
Nonsocially isolated	379/12 785	1 (Ref)	1.81 (1.30, 2.54)	1.49 (1.04, 2.14)	1.19 (0.77, 1.86)	1.08 (0.72, 1.61)	.22	
Socially isolated	151/3 450	1 (Ref)	0.57 (0.29, 1.13)	1.33 (0.62, 2.89)	0.61 (0.30, 1.21)	1.84 (0.90, 3.74)	.02	

Continued

TABLE 3— Continued

Sociodemographic or Social Factor	No. Cases/ Person-Years	Quintile 1, HR (95% CI)	Quintile 2, HR (95% CI)	Quintile 3, HR (95% CI)	Quintile 4, HR (95% CI)	Quintile 5, HR (95% CI)	*P* for Trend	*P* for Interaction
CIND or dementia								.08
Nonsocially isolated	418/12 785	1 (Ref)	1.80 (1.33, 2.44)	1.55 (1.09, 2.21)	1.23 (0.82, 1.85)	1.12 (0.77, 1.62)	.27	
Socially isolated	165/3 450	1 (Ref)	0.66 (0.35, 1.27)	1.38 (0.66, 2.86)	0.74 (0.38, 1.43)	1.82 (0.94, 3.53)	.02	

Note. CI = confidence interval; CIND = cognitive impairment with no dementia; HR = hazard ratio; UPF = ultraprocessed food. We incorporated attrition-adjusted sampling weights and accounted for the complex sampling design in all models. We adjusted models for age (continuous, years), gender (men, women), and race/ethnicity (non-Hispanic White, non-Hispanic Black, Hispanic, and other [Alaska Native/American Indian, Asian/Pacific Islander]), marital status (never married, married but spouse absent, separated, divorced, widowed; married or living with a partner), education (< high school, high school graduate, some college/college graduate, postcollege), total net worth (tertile), household size (1, 2, ≥ 3), energy intake (continuous, kcal/d), vigorous activity (none, ≤ once/week, > once/week), smoking (never smoker, ever smoker, current smoker), alcohol consumption (nondrinker, < 5g/day, ≥ 5g/day), baseline depressive symptom (yes or no; Center for Epidemiologic Studies Depression Scale–8 items score ≥ 5), and chronic disease history (yes or no; diseases include diabetes, stroke, heart problems, cancer, and hypertension). When testing effect modification by social isolation, we excluded marital status and household size because they were components of the social isolation measure.

[a]Because we observed fewer than 5 dementia cases in some UPF–social isolation subgroups (n = 525 socially isolated participants), we did not examine effect modification by social isolation in relation to dementia.

less biased in examining disease associations than are absolute intake measures.[15] Associations with dementia, CIND, and CIND or dementia combined were attenuated when UPFs were modeled as a percentage of energy intake, suggesting there should be careful consideration of UPF intake measures in cognitive health analyses.

Several possible mechanisms may underlie these associations, including gut microbiota alterations that may affect brain-derived neurotrophic factor signaling cascades and neuroplasticity.[31] UPFs may disrupt the gut–brain axis and reward system, leading to compulsive eating behaviors and biological dysfunctions. These effects may increase oxidative stress and chronic inflammation. Moreover, food additives (e.g., dietary emulsifiers and nonnutritive sweeteners) may alter antimicrobial activity, potentially increasing cognitive risks.[31–35] However, this evidence is largely based on animal models, and further studies in humans are needed.

UPFs represent a heterogeneous group, with health effects varying across UPF subcategories.[8,36] We observed adverse associations between processed meat consumption and cognitive outcomes. Our findings align with previous studies reporting that UPF animal products were associated with higher risk of cognitive impairment.[14] However, these subgroup-specific findings should be interpreted cautiously given potential limitations, including a limited range of intake levels and exposure misclassification.[37]

We found that the associations between UPF consumption and cognitive impairment tended to be stronger among socially isolated older adults, with a marginally significant interaction. Given that social isolation is a risk factor for dementia,[38] our findings indicate that greater attention is warranted in this subgroup. Screening for social isolation has been encouraged in the United States through initiatives from the Administration for Community Living,[39] and integrating such efforts into public health or clinical settings may help identify high-risk individuals, who could benefit from reducing UPF intake for healthier cognitive aging.

Limitations

This study has several strengths, including the use of a nationally representative longitudinal cohort, which allowed us to examine temporal associations. Assessing UPF intake in different units and sensitivity analyses demonstrated the robustness of our findings.

Several limitations should also be acknowledged. The FFQ was not specifically validated for UPF consumption and may have underestimated UPF intake. We observed that the average UPF consumption was 42% in our study population, lower than the 57% reported in the Centers for Disease Control and Prevention's National Health and Nutrition Examination Survey, which used 24-hour dietary recalls.[4] As FFQs are prone to underestimating UPF intake compared with 24-hour recalls,[40] such underestimation may have attenuated the associations toward the null. However, the Nova categorization applied to this FFQ has been associated with outcomes such as cardiovascular disease and type 2 diabetes,[7,8] supporting its use.

Second, dementia and CIND were not clinically diagnosed, which may have led to misclassification of cognitive outcomes. However, we defined the cognitive outcomes based on the validated Langa-Weir classification, which has been shown to have high sensitivity and specificity and incorporates proxy assessments that may improve ascertainment of cognitive impairment or dementia in population-based studies.[23]

Third, although we excluded cognitive impairment cases occurring within the first 2 years, we cannot entirely rule out reverse causation, as cognitive changes may influence dietary behaviors. Fourth, the potential for misclassification should be acknowledged. For example, yogurt was assessed as a single FFQ item in the HRS, grouping plain and artificially sweetened yogurt, and thus classifying it as a UPF in our analysis. However, a previous study using the Harvard FFQ reported that such ambiguous items accounted for less than 5% of the total FFQ items.[8,21]

Fifth, the observed associations may partly reflect poorer overall diet quality rather than ultraprocessing per se. However, adjustment for diet quality did not fully explain the higher risks of CIND and CIND or dementia observed with greater UPF intake. Lastly, we cannot rule out potential residual or unmeasured confounding. Future studies with longer follow-ups are needed to replicate our findings.

Public Health Implications

UPF consumption has increased among US older adults, and the intake of MPF has simultaneously decreased.[4,41] We observed that, among US older adults, UPF consumption was associated with higher risks of incident dementia, CIND, and CIND or dementia combined, whereas MPF consumption was associated with lower risks of these outcomes. These findings underscore the potential importance of lower UPF consumption and greater intake of MPF for healthy cognitive aging. Consistent with this perspective, the Dietary Guidelines for the Brazilian Population recommend avoiding UPFs while emphasizing a diet based on MPFs.[42] In addition, the 2025 US Dietary Guidelines Advisory Committee highlighted the need for further research on cognitive decline.[43] The Dietary Guidelines for Americans, 2025–2030 recommend "[avoiding] highly processed foods", although they do not explicitly reference UPFs.[44]

From a public health perspective, strategies to reduce UPF intake among older adults could include expanding community-based meal programs prioritizing MPFs and promoting simple food preparation skills to reduce reliance on convenient UPFs. However, policy- and industry-level action should be prioritized. Given UPFs' low cost, taxation may be warranted, as illustrated by Colombia's recent UPF tax.[45] Front-of-package labeling, warning labels, and advertising restrictions also merit consideration.[45] Regulation of health- or environment-related marketing claims is needed, as such messaging may lead to a misperception that all UPFs are acceptable.[39] As seen in tobacco control, these measures are most effective when implemented simultaneously,[46] suggesting that a similarly coordinated regulatory approach may be necessary to mitigate the growing burden of UPF consumption. Our findings may provide evidence to inform future dietary guidance aimed at limiting UPFs while encouraging greater intake of MPFs to support cognitive health. Future studies examining food-to-food replacement across different levels of food processing may help clarify the potential cognitive benefits. AJPH

ABOUT THE AUTHORS

Heejin Lee and Cindy W. Leung are with the Department of Nutrition, Harvard T. H. Chan School of Public Health, Boston, MA. Claire T. McEvoy is with the Centre for Public Health, Institute for Global Food Security, Queen's University Belfast, United Kingdom. Euridice Martinez Steele is with the Department of Nutrition, School of Public Health, University of São Paulo, São Paulo, Brazil. Neha Khandpur is with the Division of Human Nutrition and Health, Wageningen University, Netherlands. Steven G. Heeringa and Lindsay H. Ryan are with the Institute for Social Research, University of Michigan, Ann Arbor. Kenneth M. Langa is with the Department of Internal Medicine, University of Michigan, Ann Arbor. Julia A. Wolfson is with the Department of International Health, Johns Hopkins Bloomberg School of Public Health, Baltimore, MD.

CORRESPONDENCE

Correspondence should be sent to Heejin Lee, PhD, Department of Nutrition, Harvard T.H. Chan School of Public Health, Boston, MA 02115 (e-mail: heejinlee@hsph.harvard.edu). Reprints can be ordered at https://www.ajph.org by clicking the "Reprints" link.

PUBLICATION INFORMATION

Full Citation: Lee H, McEvoy CT, Steele EM, et al. Ultraprocessed foods and the risk of cognitive impairment and dementia in older US adults: 2013–2020 Health and Retirement Study. *Am J Public Health*. 2026;116(7):981–992.

Acceptance Date: February 16, 2026.

DOI: https://doi.org/10.2105/AJPH.2026.308505

ORCID iDs:

Heejin Lee https://orcid.org/0000-0002-6811-6726

Claire T. McEvoy https://orcid.org/0000-0001-8512-3293

Euridice Martinez Steele https://orcid.org/0000-0002-2907-3153

Neha Khandpur https://orcid.org/0000-0002-4766-8361

Steven G. Heeringa https://orcid.org/0000-0002-3920-8074

Lindsay H. Ryan https://orcid.org/0000-0001-8498-2539

Kenneth M. Langa https://orcid.org/0000-0002-2798-1836

Julia A. Wolfson https://orcid.org/0000-0001-9155-2609

Cindy W. Leung https://orcid.org/0000-0001-6718-3487

CONTRIBUTORS

H. Lee performed the data analysis and drafted the article. H. Lee and C. W. Leung conceptualized and designed the study. C. T. McEvoy, E. Martinez Steele, N. Khandpur, S. G. Heeringa, L. H. Ryan, K. M. Langa, J. A. Wolfson, and C. Leung provided critical revisions. E. Martinez Steele, N. Khandpur, S. G. Heeringa, L. H. Ryan, and K. M. Langa assisted with data analysis and provided analytic support. C. W. Leung supervised the study. All authors reviewed and approved the final article.

ACKNOWLEDGMENTS

This work was supported by the National Institutes of Health (NIH; grant R01AG0792786; primary investigator was C. W. L.). The Health and Retirement Study is sponsored by the National Institute on Aging (grant U01AG009740).

Note. The NIH had no role in study design, data collection, data analysis, article preparation, or the decision to submit the article for publication.

CONFLICTS OF INTEREST

N. Khandpur served as a consultant to United Nations Children's Fund and the Ministry of Health of the government of the Philippines, with no financial or other conflicts of interest to disclose with commercial or for-profit entities. S. G. Heeringa received grants from the NIH and was supported by a subaward to the University of Michigan from Harvard University. L. H. Ryan and J. A. Wolfson received grants from the NIH. K. M. Langa received grants from the NIH and the National Institute on Aging. The other authors have no conflicts of interest to declare.

HUMAN PARTICIPANT PROTECTION

This study was approved by the University of Michigan institutional review board. All participants provided verbal or written informed consent. The study data are publicly available at the Health and Retirement Study websites (https://hrsdata.isr.umich.edu).

REFERENCES

1. Monteiro CA, Cannon G, Levy RB, et al. Ultra-processed foods: what they are and how to identify them. *Public Health Nutr.* 2019;22(5):936–941. https://doi.org/10.1017/S1368980018003762
2. Monteiro CA, Louzada ML, Steele-Martinez E, et al. Ultra-processed foods and human health: the main thesis and the evidence. *Lancet.* 2025; 406(10520):2667–2684. https://doi.org/10.1016/S0140-6736(25)01565-X
3. Marino M, Puppo F, Del Bo C, et al. A systematic review of worldwide consumption of ultraprocessed foods: findings and criticisms. *Nutrients.* 2021;13(8):2778. https://doi.org/10.3390/nu13082778
4. Juul F, Parekh N, Martinez-Steele E, Monteiro CA, Chang VW. Ultra-processed food consumption among US adults from 2001 to 2018. *Am J Clin Nutr.* 2022;115(1):211–221. https://doi.org/10.1093/ajcn/nqab305
5. Pagliai G, Dinu M, Madarena MP, Bonaccio M, Iacoviello L, Sofi F. Consumption of ultra-processed foods and health status: a systematic review and meta-analysis. *Br J Nutr.* 2021;125(3): 308–318. https://doi.org/10.1017/S0007114520002688
6. Askari M, Heshmati J, Shahinfar H, Tripathi N, Daneshzad E. Ultra-processed food and the risk of overweight and obesity: a systematic review and meta-analysis of observational studies. *Int J Obes (Lond).* 2020;44(10):2080–2091. https://doi.org/10.1038/s41366-020-00650-z
7. Chen Z, Khandpur N, Desjardins C, et al. Ultra-processed food consumption and risk of type 2 diabetes: three large prospective US cohort studies. *Diabetes Care.* 2023;46(7):1335–1344. https://doi.org/10.2337/dc22-1993
8. Mendoza K, Smith-Warner SA, Rossato SL, et al. Ultra-processed foods and cardiovascular disease: analysis of three large US prospective cohorts and a systematic review and meta-analysis of prospective cohort studies. *Lancet Reg Health Am.* 2024;37:100859. https://doi.org/10.1016/j.lana.2024.100859
9. Taneri PE, Wehrli F, Roa-Diaz ZM, et al. Association between ultraprocessed food intake and all-cause mortality: a systematic review and meta-analysis. *Am J Epidemiol.* 2022;191(7):1323–1335. https://doi.org/10.1093/aje/kwac039
10. Gomes Goncalves N, Vidal Ferreira N, Khandpur N, et al. Association between consumption of ultraprocessed foods and cognitive decline. *JAMA Neurol.* 2023;80(2):142–150. https://doi.org/10.1001/jamaneurol.2022.4397
11. Lee H, Ludwig-Borycz E, McEvoy CT, et al. Ultra-processed food intake and impairment across multiple cognitive domains in nationally representative older US adults. *Front Public Health.* 2025;13:1695540. https://doi.org/10.3389/fpubh.2025.1695540
12. Henney AE, Gillespie CS, Alam U, Hydes TJ, Mackay CE, Cuthbertson DJ. High intake of ultra-processed food is associated with dementia in adults: a systematic review and meta-analysis of observational studies. *J Neurol.* 2024;271(1): 198–210. https://doi.org/10.1007/s00415-023-12033-1
13. Shahatah FA, Hill TR, Fairley A, Watson AW. Ultra-processed food intakes and health outcomes in adults older than 60 years: a systematic review. *Nutr Rev.* 2025;83(9):1711–1724. https://doi.org/10.1093/nutrit/nuae223
14. Seago ER, Rego ML, Davy BM, Katz B. Differential association of ultraprocessed food categories with risk of developing cognitive impairment in middle-aged and older adults in a longitudinal panel study. *Am J Clin Nutr.* 2025;121(5):965–971. https://doi.org/10.1016/j.ajcnut.2025.02.008
15. Loftfield E, Zhang P, O'Connell CP, et al. Performance of a food frequency questionnaire for estimating ultraprocessed food intake according to the Nova classification system in the United States NIH-AARP Diet and Health Study. *J Nutr.* 2025;155(7):2376–2384. https://doi.org/10.1016/j.tjnut.2025.04.029
16. Sonnega A, Faul JD, Ofstedal MB, Langa KM, Phillips JW, Weir DR. Cohort profile: the Health and Retirement Study (HRS). *Int J Epidemiol.* 2014;43(2):576–585. https://doi.org/10.1093/ije/dyu067
17. Health and Retirement Study (HRS Core 2012–2020) dataset. Ann Arbor, MI: University of Michigan; 2023. Available at: https://hrsdata.isr.umich.edu/sites/default/files/documentation/data-descriptions/1686078541/h20dd.pdf. Accessed April 27, 2026.
18. Health and Retirement Study (2013 Health Care and Nutrition Study (HCNS)) data set. Ann Arbor, MI: University of Michigan; 2018. Available at: https://hrsdata.isr.umich.edu/data-products/2013-health-care-and-nutrition-study-hcns?_ga=2.139958

836.667444908.1777333578-1859204428.1777333227. Accessed April 27, 2026.

19. Willett WC, Sampson L, Stampfer MJ, et al. Reproducibility and validity of a semiquantitative food frequency questionnaire. *Am J Epidemiol.* 1985;122(1):51–65. https://doi.org/10.1093/oxfordjournals.aje.a114086

20. Monteiro CA, Cannon G, Moubarac JC, Levy RB, Louzada MLC, Jaime PC. The UN decade of nutrition, the Nova food classification and the trouble with ultra-processing. *Public Health Nutr.* 2018;21(1):5–17. https://doi.org/10.1017/S1368980017000234

21. Khandpur N, Rossato S, Drouin-Chartier JP, et al. Categorising ultra-processed foods in large-scale cohort studies: evidence from the Nurses' Health Studies, the Health Professionals Follow-up Study, and the Growing Up Today Study. *J Nutr Sci.* 2021;10:e77. https://doi.org/10.1017/jns.2021.72

22. Willett WC, Howe GR, Kushi LH. Adjustment for total energy intake in epidemiologic studies. *Am J Clin Nutr.* 1997;65(4 suppl):1220S–1228S. https://doi.org/10.1093/ajcn/65.4.1220S

23. Crimmins EM, Kim JK, Langa KM, Weir DR. Assessment of cognition using surveys and neuropsychological assessment: the Health and Retirement Study and the Aging, Demographics, and Memory Study. *J Gerontol B Psychol Sci Soc Sci.* 2011;66(suppl 1):i162–i171. https://doi.org/10.1093/geronb/gbr048

24. RAND Center for the Study of Aging. RAND HRS longitudinal file 2020 (V2). Santa Monica, CA: RAND Corporation; 2024. Available at: https://www.rand.org/pubs/tools/TLA2097-1-v3.html. Accessed April 27, 2026.

25. Lyu C, Siu K, Xu I, Osman I, Zhong J. Social isolation changes and long-term outcomes among older adults. *JAMA Netw Open.* 2024;7(7):e2424519. https://doi.org/10.1001/jamanetworkopen.2024.24519

26. Steptoe A, Shankar A, Demakakos P, Wardle J. Social isolation, loneliness, and all-cause mortality in older men and women. *Proc Natl Acad Sci U S A.* 2013;110(15):5797–5801. https://doi.org/10.1073/pnas.1219686110

27. McEvoy CT, Guyer H, Langa KM, Yaffe K. Neuroprotective diets are associated with better cognitive function: the Health and Retirement Study. *J Am Geriatr Soc.* 2017;65(8):1857–1862. https://doi.org/10.1111/jgs.14922

28. Li H, Li S, Yang H, et al. Association of ultraprocessed food consumption with risk of dementia: a prospective cohort study. *Neurology.* 2022;99(10):e1056–e1066. https://doi.org/10.1212/WNL.0000000000200871

29. Weinstein G, Kojis D, Banerjee A, Seshadri S, Walker M, Beiser AS. Ultra-processed food consumption and risk of dementia and Alzheimer's disease: the Framingham Heart Study. *J Prev Alzheimers Dis.* 2025;12(2):100042. https://doi.org/10.1016/j.tjpad.2024.100042

30. Levy RB, Rauber F, Chang K, et al. Ultra-processed food consumption and type 2 diabetes incidence: a prospective cohort study. *Clin Nutr.* 2021;40(5):3608–3614. https://doi.org/10.1016/j.clnu.2020.12.018

31. Mottis G, Kandasamey P, Peleg-Raibstein D. The consequences of ultra-processed foods on brain development during prenatal, adolescent and adult stages. *Front Public Health.* 2025;13:1590083. https://doi.org/10.3389/fpubh.2025.1590083

32. Ionescu-Tucker A, Cotman CW. Emerging roles of oxidative stress in brain aging and Alzheimer's disease. *Neurobiol Aging.* 2021;107:86–95. https://doi.org/10.1016/j.neurobiolaging.2021.07.014

33. Maki KA, Sack MN, Hall KD. Ultra-processed foods: increasing the risk of inflammation and immune dysregulation? *Nat Rev Immunol.* 2024;24(7):453–454. https://doi.org/10.1038/s41577-024-01049-x

34. Roca-Saavedra P, Mendez-Vilabrille V, Miranda JM, et al. Food additives, contaminants and other minor components: effects on human gut microbiota—a review. *J Physiol Biochem.* 2018;74(1):69–83. https://doi.org/10.1007/s13105-017-0564-2

35. Chassaing B, Compher C, Bonhomme B, et al. Randomized controlled-feeding study of dietary emulsifier carboxymethylcellulose reveals detrimental impacts on the gut microbiota and metabolome. *Gastroenterology.* 2022;162(3):743–756. https://doi.org/10.1053/j.gastro.2021.11.006

36. Cordova R, Kliemann N, Huybrechts I, et al. Consumption of ultra-processed foods associated with weight gain and obesity in adults: a multinational cohort study. *Clin Nutr.* 2021;40(9):5079–5088. https://doi.org/10.1016/j.clnu.2021.08.009

37. Rezende LFM, Martinez-Steele E, da Costa Louzada ML, Levy RB, Monteiro CA. Misleading narrative of "healthy" ultraprocessed foods. *BMJ.* 2026;392:e087538. https://doi.org/10.1136/bmj-2025-087538

38. Shen C, Rolls ET, Cheng W, et al. Associations of social isolation and loneliness with later dementia. *Neurology.* 2022;99(2):e164–e175. https://doi.org/10.1212/WNL.0000000000200583

39. US Department of Health and Human Services. Helping older adults take charge of their social well-being. 2025. Available at: https://odphp.health.gov/news/202509/helping-older-adults-take-charge-their-social-well-being. Accessed September 30, 2025.

40. Thompson FE, Kipnis V, Midthune D, et al. Performance of a food-frequency questionnaire in the US NIH-AARP Diet and Health Study. *Public Health Nutr.* 2008;11(2):183–195. https://doi.org/10.1017/S1368980007000419

41. Wolfson JA, Tucker AC, Leung CW, Rebholz CM, Garcia-Larsen V, Martinez-Steele E. Trends in adults' intake of unprocessed/minimally processed and ultra-processed foods at home and away from home in the United States from 2003–2018. *J Nutr.* 2025;155(1):280–292. https://doi.org/10.1016/j.tjnut.2024.10.048

42. Food and Agriculture Organization of the United Nations. Food-based dietary guidelines—Brazil. 2014. Available at: https://www.fao.org/nutrition/education/food-dietary-guidelines/regions/countries/brazil/en. Accessed September 29, 2025.

43. Department of Health and Human Services. Scientific report of the 2025 Dietary Guidelines Advisory Committee. 2024. Available at: https://www.dietaryguidelines.gov/2025-advisory-committee-report. Accessed April 27, 2026.

44. US Department of Agriculture. Dietary Guidelines for Americans, 2025–2030. 2026. Available at: https://cdn.realfood.gov/DGA.pdf. Accessed February 5, 2026.

45. Scrinis G, Popkin BM, Corvalan C, et al. Policies to halt and reverse the rise in ultra-processed food production, marketing, and consumption. *Lancet.* 2025;406(10520):2685–2702. https://doi.org/10.1016/S0140-6736(25)01566-1

46. Flor LS, Reitsma MB, Gupta V, Ng M, Gakidou E. The effects of tobacco control policies on global smoking prevalence. *Nat Med.* 2021;27(2):239–243. https://doi.org/10.1038/s41591-020-01210-8

The Intersection of Diet Quality and Ultraprocessed Food Intake: Using Evidence-Based Categories to Characterize Differences in Cardiometabolic Profiles

Elise Sheinberg, MPH, RDN, Laura A. Schmidt, PhD, MSW, MPH, Jerold R. Mande, MPH, Euridice Martinez-Steele, PhD, Deirdre K. Tobias, ScD, and Cindy W. Leung, ScD, MPH

See also Ultraprocessed Food, pp. 898–1029.

Objectives. To examine how ultraprocessed food (UPF) consumption and diet quality jointly relate to cardiometabolic health.

Methods. This serial cross-sectional study used data from 15 760 US adults (aged ≥ 20 years) in the 2009–2018 National Health and Nutrition Examination Surveys. Participants completed two 24-hour recalls and did not have a chronic disease. Diet quality was categorized using Healthy Eating Index–2020 (HEI) scores as high (70 to 100), moderate (60 to < 70), low (50 to < 60), and very low (0 to < 50). UPF consumption, determined by Nova classification, was categorized as high (≥ 40% energy intake) and low (< 40% energy intake). Joint HEI–UPF categories combined these variables. We examined unadjusted and adjusted associations between joint HEI–UPF category and anthropometric and cardiometabolic biomarkers.

Results. Among US adults, only 0.3% had high HEI–low UPF consumption, while 45.3% had very low HEI–high UPF consumption. Those with very low HEI–high UPF intake had the least favorable metabolic profiles, including the highest mean body mass index (29.6, defined as weight in kilograms divided by the square of height in meters) and fasting glucose (106.2 milligrams per deciliter).

Conclusions. Diet quality was more consistently associated with cardiometabolic health than UPF intake.

Public Health Implications. Overall diet quality is a strong predictor of cardiometabolic health, even with varying UPF consumption. (*Am J Public Health*. 2026;116(7):993–1003. https://doi.org/10.2105/AJPH.2026.308494)

AJPH July 2026, Vol. 116, No. 7

Poor diet quality is a risk factor for chronic diseases, including obesity, diabetes, cardiovascular disease, stroke, and some cancers.[1–3] Diet quality is often measured with nutrient and food-based indices, such as the Healthy Eating Index (HEI), which assesses how well consumption aligns with the *Dietary Guidelines for Americans*. The average HEI–2020 score for adults is 58 out of 100, reflecting suboptimal adherence to dietary recommendations.[4] Low-quality diets are driven by low intake of fruits, vegetables, whole grains, seafood, and plant proteins and high intake of refined grains and foods high in saturated fat, added sugar, and sodium. This dietary pattern is associated with an increased likelihood of adiposity, insulin resistance, and adverse lipid profiles, which contribute to chronic disease risk.[1–3]

There is growing evidence of the negative health impacts of ultraprocessed foods (UPFs), defined as "formulations of industrial food ingredients that are created from industrial processes, including added colors, flavors, and other additives."[5(p937)] UPFs account for more than half of the daily energy intake of children and adults in the United States.[6] Higher UPF consumption is associated with obesity, hypertension, dyslipidemia, and type 2 diabetes.[7–9] Several mechanisms between UPF consumption and poor health outcomes have been proposed, including UPF's poorer nutrient profile, higher glycemic load, displacement of whole foods, and hyperpalatable taste that increases consumption, as well as the effects of processing on satiety, gut microbiota, and metabolic regulation.[10,11]

This study used nationally representative data from the National Health and Nutrition Examination Survey (NHANES) to evaluate the combined associations of diet quality and UPF consumption with cardiometabolic health outcomes. Our objective was to examine differences in anthropometric measures, lipid profiles, and glycemic outcomes by joint HEI–2020 score and UPF consumption.

METHODS

We conducted our analyses using data from the 2009–2018 NHANES. NHANES is an ongoing multistage, nationally representative survey conducted by the National Center for Health Statistics. NHANES data were limited to 2009 to 2018 because Nova classification codes for more recent cycles were not available to the research team at the time of analysis. Adults with preexisting congestive heart failure, angina or angina pectoris, heart attack, stroke, liver condition, diabetes, and cancer were excluded. The analytic sample included 15 760 adults aged 20 years or older with 2 valid 24-hour recalls. There were 8487 participants in the fasting sample. Data collection was approved by the National Center for Health Statistics ethics review board, and all participants provided written consent.

Dietary Assessment and Healthy Eating Index–2020

Dietary intake was assessed via two 24-hour dietary recalls administered by trained interviewers using the US Department of Agriculture Automated Multi-Pass Method.[12] One 24-hour recall is collected in person, and a second recall is completed by telephone 3 to 10 days later. Methods and validation studies for conducting 24-hour recalls have been previously published.[13] Data from the two 24-hour recalls were converted into standard food groups and food pattern components using the Food Patterns Equivalents Database to calculate individual HEI–2020 scores.

Participants' HEI–2020 scores per day were first calculated using the simple HEI scoring algorithm method. Then, we used the National Cancer Institute (NCI) SAS Macros (version 2.1) to estimate usual intake to account for the within-person variability of dietary intake and to estimate predicted HEI scores (i.e., usual HEI).[14] Specifically, we used the MIXTRAN macro to generate parameter estimates for dietary intake accounting for all sociodemographic covariates (as described subsequently), and we used the INDIVINT macro to predict individual intakes using the previously generated parameter estimates. More information about this method can be found here: https://epi.grants.cancer.gov/diet/usualintakes/macros_single.html.

Healthy Eating Index–2020 Categories

The determination of the cut points used to define HEI–2020 categories was informed on multiple criteria. First, we considered NCI's suggested HEI cut-points and corresponding grade.[15] Because less than 1% of the population had an HEI score of 80 or above, corresponding to an A or B grade, we comprehensively reviewed previous findings from prospective observational studies that examined HEI scores in relation to major chronic disease outcomes (Table A, available as a supplement to the online version of this article at https://ajph.org).[2] Most studies derived population-specific quintiles of HEI scores as the exposure, and individuals in the highest HEI quintile consistently had lower risks of cardiovascular disease, cancer, type 2 diabetes, and all-cause mortality compared with individuals in the lowest quintile.[2] Finally, we examined the distributions of HEI scores in NHANES to understand the extent to which US adults aligned with the cut points in the studies in Table A. Collectively, this evidence informed the following category definitions: high HEI score (70 to 100), moderate HEI score (60 to < 70), low HEI score (50 to < 60), and very low HEI score (0 to < 50). High HEI score indicates a higher adherence to the DGA and where the greatest risk reduction of morbidity and mortality from diet-related chronic diseases has been observed.[2,16] In contrast, very low HEI score indicates lower adherence to the DGA and is associated with the highest risks of morbidity and mortality from diet-related chronic diseases.[2,16] Moderate and low HEI scores are intermediate risk levels.

Ultraprocessed Food Intake

The Nova classification has 4 categories: unprocessed or minimally processed foods, processed culinary ingredients, processed foods, and ultraprocessed foods.[5] We used an established methodology and data set to code foods by Nova category that is supported by the NCI.[17,18] Briefly, NHANES 24-hour diet recalls were linked to the Food and Nutrient Database for Dietary Studies, where each food was mapped to its underlying food code and standard reference codes. For mixed dishes and homemade foods, Food and Nutrient Database for Dietary Studies recipe files were used to decompose items into their standard reference components, which were individually classified into the corresponding Nova category. Food codes were broken into their component standard reference codes, which were classified according to Nova and used to derive daily intake for each Nova category.[17] In this analysis, we focused on Nova category 4, ultraprocessed foods, because groups 2 (culinary ingredients) and 3 (processed foods) are a much lower percentage of total energy intake, and UPFs are of greater health concern.[19] Similar to the approach for HEI–2020 scores, we used the NCI MIXTRAN and INDIVINT SAS macros to estimate usual UPF intake as a percentage of total energy (% kilocalories [kcal]) from UPFs, consistent with methods used in other NHANES studies of UPF and health outcomes.[20,21] UPF food consumption was then dichotomized as follows: high UPF consumption was defined as 40% or more of total energy intake (% kcal), and low UPF consumption as less than 40% of total energy intake (% kcal). This cut point was selected because it corresponds to the top quartile of UPF consumption that has been previously associated with poor health outcomes in this sample.[21,22]

Joint Diet and Food Processing Categories

We combined the 4-category usual HEI–2020 variable and the 2-category usual UPF intake variable to create an 8-level categorical variable representing all combinations of usual HEI score and usual UPF consumption, where high HEI score (70 to 100), moderate HEI score (60 to < 70), low HEI score (50 to < 60), and very low HEI score (0 to < 50) and high UPF consumption was 40% or more of total energy intake and low UPF consumption was less than 40% of total energy intake. This variable is referred to as the joint HEI–UPF category. The reference group is very low HEI–high UPF.

Cardiometabolic Health Outcomes

Height, weight, and waist circumference were measured by trained personnel in the Mobile Examination Center.[23] Body mass index (BMI) was calculated as weight in kilograms divided by the square of height in meters (kg/m^2). Obesity was defined as a BMI greater than or equal to 30 kg/m^2.[24] High waist circumference was defined as greater than 88 centimeters for females and greater than 102 centimeters for males.[24]

Other biomarker outcomes include blood levels of total cholesterol (milligrams per deciliter [mg/dL]), high-density lipoprotein cholesterol (HDL; mg/dL), fasting low-density lipoprotein cholesterol (LDL; mg/dL), fasting triglycerides (mg/dL), hemoglobin A1c (HbA1c), and fasting glucose (mg/dL). Low HDL cholesterol was defined as less than 40 mg/dL and elevated LDL cholesterol was defined as greater than or equal to 100 mg/dL.[25] Elevated triglycerides were defined as greater than or equal to 150 mg/dL.[26] Elevated HbA1c was defined as greater than or equal to 5.7%, and elevated fasting glucose was defined as greater than 100 mg/dL.[27] Blood samples were collected by NHANES medical personnel following standardized phlebotomy protocols and analyzed at the National Center for Environmental Health laboratories.

Sociodemographic Characteristics

We included characteristics associated with diet quality and UPF consumption in previous research as covariates.[21,22,28] Sociodemographic variables were ascertained at the NHANES interview, including self-reported age, gender, race and ethnicity, place of birth, educational attainment, employment status, marital status, family income to poverty ratio, and food security status. We derived household food security status by using the 18-item US Food Security Survey Module.

Statistical Analysis

We performed all statistical analyses with SAS version 9.4 (SAS Institute Inc, Cary, NC). Per NHANES guidelines, we recalculated complex dietary (WTDR2D) and fasting subsample (WTSAF2YR) sampling weights by dividing by 5 to reflect the probability of being sampled across the 10-year period. In SAS, we

AJPH July 2026, Vol. 116, No. 7

used SURVEYMEANS, SURVEYFREQ, SURVEYREG, and SURVEYLOGISTIC procedures with strata (SDMVSTRA), cluster (SDMVPSU), and weight statements to account for the complex sampling scheme and to make nationally representative inferences. We applied dietary weights to all analyses, with the exception of analyses involving LDL cholesterol, triglycerides, and fasting glucose, which used the fasting subsample weights because the fasting subsample has a smaller number of respondents than the dietary subsample.

We evaluated survey-weighted differences in sociodemographic characteristics by joint HEI–UPF categories using the Rao–Scott χ-square test. Next, we estimated unadjusted means and proportions of cardiometabolic characteristics by joint HEI–UPF categories. Then, we used survey-weighted multivariable linear and logistic regression models to examine differences in cardiometabolic outcomes by joint HEI–UPF categories, with the reference category of very low HEI–high UPF. These models adjusted for all sociodemographic characteristics and usual total energy intake (following the same approach as HEI-2020 scores and UPF intake). We report least squared means (for continuous outcomes) and predicted probabilities (for categorical outcomes) of the 8 HEI–UPF categories. We used pairwise differences to evaluate differences within HEI category and by UPF consumption category.

RESULTS

Among US adults, 46.0% had a very low usual HEI score (< 50), 40.6% had a low usual HEI score (50 to < 60), 12.6% had a moderate usual HEI score (60 to < 70), and 0.8% had a high usual HEI score (≥ 70). High usual UPF consumption (≥ 40% kcal) was observed among 93.7% of US adults, and 6.3% had low usual UPF consumption (< 40% kcal). When examining joint HEI–high UPF categories, 45.3% of US adults had very low HEI–high UPF consumption, 37.5% had low HEI–high UPF consumption, 10.3% had moderate HEI–high UPF consumption, and 0.6% had high HEI–high UPF consumption (Figure 1). When examining joint HEI–low UPF consumption, 0.7% US adults had very low HEI–low UPF consumption, 3.1% had low HEI–low UPF, 2.3% had moderate HEI–low UPF, and 0.3% had high HEI–low UPF.

There were significant differences in joint HEI–UPF categories by all sociodemographic characteristics except employment status (Table 1, *P* linear trend < .01). Very low HEI–high UPF consumption was more prevalent among individuals who were younger, male, non-Hispanic Black, born in the United States, high-school educated or less, single, lower income, and food insecure.

Unadjusted Differences vs Reference Group

In unadjusted analyses (Table 2), there were consistent differences in anthropometric measures across joint HEI–UPF categories. The reference group, very low HEI–high UPF consumption, had the highest mean BMI (29.6 kg/m^2), percentage with obesity (41.6%), mean waist circumference (100.0 cm), and percentage with high waist circumference (55.4%) compared with the other joint HEI–UPF categories. There were inconsistent patterns for cardiometabolic biomarkers. HDL cholesterol tended to be higher among categories with higher HEI scores. Unadjusted means for total cholesterol and LDL cholesterol were higher

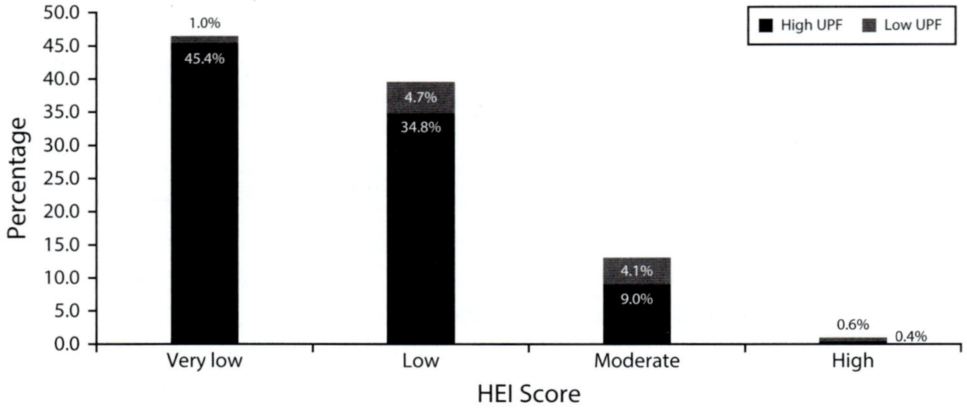

FIGURE 1— Proportion of High Versus Low Ultraprocessed Food (UPF) Consumption by Healthy Eating Index (HEI) Score Category: United States, National Health and Nutrition Examination Survey, 2009–2018

TABLE 1— Sociodemographic Characteristics of US Adults (Aged ≥ 20 Years) Stratified by Joint Healthy Eating Index (HEI) Score Categories and Ultraprocessed Food (UPF) Consumption Using Usual Intake: National Health and Nutrition Examination Survey, 2009–2018

		Very Low HEI (< 50)		Low HEI (50 to < 60)		Moderate HEI (60 to < 70)		High HEI (≥ 70)		
	Overall	High UPF, No. (Weighted %) (n = 7152 [45.3])	Low UPF, No. (Weighted %) (n = 165 [0.7])	High UPF, No. (Weighted %) (n = 5483 [37.5])	Low UPF, No. (Weighted %) (n = 747 [3.1])	High UPF, No. (Weighted %) (n = 1422 [10.3])	Low UPF, No. (Weighted %) (n = 639 [2.3])	High UPF, No. (Weighted %) (n = 64 [0.6])	Low UPF, No. (Weighted %) (n = 88 [0.3%])	P
Age, y										< .001
≤ 30	3 752 (26.1)	2 337 (61.6)	42 (0.8)	1 024 (29.1)	116 (2.3)	171 (5.1)	59 (1.0)	1 (0.04)	2 (0.03)	
31–50	6 319 (40.7)	2 988 (45.9)	68 (0.8)	2 206 (38.1)	304 (3.4)	496 (9.3)	216 (2.0)	19 (0.3)	22 (0.2)	
≥ 51	5 689 (33.3)	1 827 (31.8)	55 (0.4)	2 253 (43.4)	327 (3.3)	755 (15.5)	364 (3.8)	44 (1.2)	64 (0.6)	
Gender										< .001
Male	7 288 (47.8)	3 831 (53.0)	104 (0.8)	2 246 (33.4)	347 (2.9)	475 (7.7)	239 (1.7)	16 (0.3)	30 (0.2)	
Female	8 472 (52.2)	3 321 (38.2)	61 (0.5)	3 237 (41.3)	400 (3.2)	947 (12.6)	400 (3.0)	48 (0.8)	58 (0.3)	
Race and ethnicity										< .001
Hispanic	3 931 (15.6)	1 613 (46.4)	38 (0.6)	1 514 (37.5)	245 (5.1)	313 (6.5)	176 (3.0)	9 (0.4)	23 (0.5)	
Non-Hispanic Black	3 459 (11.6)	2 016 (61.6)	20 (0.6)	1 056 (28.8)	85 (2.6)	205 (4.8)	56 (1.2)	10 (0.2)	11 (0.2)	
Non-Hispanic White	6 186 (63.8)	2 992 (44.4)	18 (0.2)	2 335 (40.8)	57 (1.0)	689 (12.1)	56 (0.9)	32 (0.7)	7 (0.04)	
Other[a]	2 184 (9.0)	531 (28.9)	89 (3.9)	578 (26.1)	360 (15.1)	215 (11.1)	351 (13.0)	13 (0.4)	47 (1.6)	
Birthplace										< .001
United States	11 538 (82.7)	6 303 (50.0)	30 (0.2)	4 040 (37.9)	76 (0.7)	984 (10.1)	54 (0.5)	42 (0.6)	9 (0.02)	
Outside of the United States	4 222 (17.3)	849 (22.8)	135 (2.8)	1 443 (35.6)	671 (14.5)	438 (10.9)	585 (11.3)	22 (0.6)	79 (1.5)	
Educational attainment										< .001
High school education or less	6 567 (35.3)	3 866 (62.8)	78 (0.8)	1 877 (27.7)	271 (2.7)	300 (4.5)	158 (1.4)	4 (0.1)	13 (0.1)	
Any college or college graduate	9 193 (64.7)	3 286 (35.8)	87 (0.6)	3 606 (42.9)	476 (3.3)	1 122 (13.4)	481 (2.9)	60 (0.8)	75 (0.4)	
Employment status										.61
Employed	10 054 (68.8)	4 581 (45.5)	108 (0.7)	3 499 (37.7)	488 (3.0)	906 (10.3)	386 (2.2)	34 (0.5)	52 (0.2)	
Not employed	5 706 (31.2)	2 571 (45.0)	57 (0.6)	1 984 (37.2)	259 (3.2)	516 (10.2)	253 (2.6)	30 (0.7)	36 (0.3)	
Marital status										< .001
Married or living with partner	9 460 (62.8)	3 862 (40.9)	97 (0.6)	3 411 (39.5)	557 (3.5)	937 (11.6)	477 (2.8)	47 (0.7)	72 (0.4)	
Single	6 300 (37.2)	3 290 (52.7)	68 (0.7)	2 072 (34.2)	190 (2.2)	485 (8.1)	162 (1.7)	17 (0.3)	16 (0.1)	

Continued

TABLE 1— Continued

	Overall	Very Low HEI (<50) High UPF, No. (Weighted %) (n = 7152 [45.3])	Very Low HEI (<50) Low UPF, No. (Weighted %) (n = 165 [0.7])	Low HEI (50 to <60) High UPF, No. (Weighted %) (n = 5483 [37.5])	Low HEI (50 to <60) Low UPF, No. (Weighted %) (n = 747 [3.1])	Moderate HEI (60 to <70) High UPF, No. (Weighted %) (n = 1422 [10.3])	Moderate HEI (60 to <70) Low UPF, No. (Weighted %) (n = 639 [2.3])	High HEI (≥70) High UPF, No. (Weighted %) (n = 64 [0.6])	High HEI (≥70) Low UPF, No. (Weighted %) (n = 88 [0.3%])	P
Household income[b]										<.001
≤200% federal poverty level	6740 (32.2)	3835 (59.3)	84 (1.1)	2001 (29.4)	275 (3.3)	347 (5.2)	172 (1.5)	11 (0.2)	15 (0.1)	
>200% federal poverty level	9020 (67.8)	3317 (38.7)	81 (0.4)	3482 (41.4)	472 (3.0)	1075 (12.7)	467 (2.8)	53 (0.7)	73 (0.3)	
Household food security[c]										NA
High or marginal food security	12 488 (84.5)	5065 (41.1)	121 (0.6)	4634 (39.9)	632 (3.2)	1309 (11.6)	581 (2.6)	64 (0.7)	82 (0.3)	
Low or very low food security	3272 (15.5)	2087 (68.2)	44 (1.1)	849 (24.5)	115 (2.2)	113 (3.1)	58 (0.9)	0	6 (0.1)	

Note. High UPF ≥ 40% kcal; low UPF < 40% kcal; NA = not available.
[a]Other included American Indian or Alaskan Native, Asian, Native Hawaiian or Pacific Islander, and other.
[b]As defined by the US Department of Health and Human Services.
[c]Household food security assessed using the US Household Food Security Survey Module.

among categories with higher HEI scores. There were no differences in fasting glucose levels compared with the reference category.

Unadjusted Differences Within Diet Categories

Within each HEI category, there were few differences in unadjusted anthropometric and cardiometabolic markers between low and high UPF consumption. Among participants with low and very low HEI scores, those with low UPF consumption had lower mean BMI, obesity prevalence, mean waist circumference, and prevalence of high waist circumference. In the low HEI group, mean HDL cholesterol was lower in the low UPF group (54.6 mg/dL) compared with the high UPF group (56.3 mg/dL). In the moderate HEI category, fasting glucose was higher for the low UPF consumption (100.7 mg/dL vs 98.3 mg/dL), while in the high HEI category, low UPF was associated with lower HDL (57.6 mg/dL vs 74.1 mg/dL) and higher triglyceride levels (126.5 mg/dL vs 82.8 mg/dL) compared with the high UPF group.

Adjusted Differences vs Reference Group

After we adjusted for sociodemographic covariates, there were consistent differences in anthropometric measures between the very low HEI–high UPF and the other joint HEI–UPF categories (Table 3). The very low HEI–high UPF category had a mean BMI of 29.6 kg/m^2 compared with 23.8 kg/m^2 in the high HEI–high UPF category (P < .001). Obesity prevalence was lower in all categories compared with the reference category, where 40.9% had obesity, compared with 7.4% in the high HEI–high UPF category (P = .004). Only

TABLE 2— Unadjusted Anthropometric and Cardiometabolic Markers Stratified by Joint Healthy Eating Index (HEI)–Ultraprocessed Food (UPF) Category: United States, National Health and Nutrition Examination Survey, 2009–2018

	Very Low HEI (<50)		Low HEI (50 to <60)		Moderate HEI (60 to <70)		High HEI (≥70)	
	High UPF	Low UPF	High UPF	Low UPF	High UPF	Low UPF	High UPF	Low UPF
BMI								
Mean (95% CI), kg/m^2	29.6 (29.4, 29.9)	27.1 (25.3, 28.8)	28.5 (28.2, 28.8)	26.6 (26.1, 27.2)	27.0 (26.6, 27.5)	26.4 (25.8, 27.0)	24.1 (22.1, 26.1)	25.7 (24.5, 26.8)
% with obesity (95% CI)	41.6 (39.8, 43.6)	26.6 (18.3, 37.0)	34.2 (23.1, 36.4)	24.7 (20.7, 29.1)	22.4 (19.6, 25.6)	23.1 (18.8, 28.0)	8.1 (2.1, 26.8)	16.0 (8.0, 29.4)
Waist circumference								
Mean (95% CI), cm	100.0 (99.4, 100.6)	93.6 (89.6, 97.7)	97.2 (96.5, 97.9)	92.1 (90.7, 93.4)	93.7 (92.5, 95.0)	91.4 (89.9, 92.9)	85.8 (81.1, 90.5)	91.1 (88.9, 93.3)
% with high waist circumference (95% CI)	55.4 (53.4, 57.4)	34.1 (24.9, 44.7)	54.6 (51.8, 57.5)	41.1 (35.6, 46.9)	47.8 (43.5, 52.1)	39.5 (34.4, 45.0)	27.6 (14.5, 46.3)	40.9 (53.4, 57.4)
Total cholesterol								
Mean (95% CI), mg/dL	192.0 (190.5, 193.6)	198.6 (185.5, 211.7)	197.2 (195.3, 199.1)	199.3 (193.7, 204.9)	199.0 (195.9, 202.1)	196.1 (191.9, 200.3)	202.9 (184.6, 221.2)	203.2 (193.0, 213.4)
% ≥ 200 mg/dL (95% CI)	38.6 (37.0, 40.4)	44.8 (34.1, 56.0)	44.0 (41.8, 46.2)	44.4 (38.7, 50.2)	46.4 (42.9, 50.0)	47.1 (39.7, 54.6)	49.5 (31.4, 67.7)	56.0 (41.7, 69.3)
HDL cholesterol								
Mean (95% CI), mg/dL	50.8 (50.2, 51.3)	52.6 (47.8, 57.5)	56.3 (55.6, 57.0)	54.6 (53.0, 56.2)	60.1 (58.8, 61.4)	58.5 (56.4, 60.5)	74.1 (61.9, 86.3)	57.6 (51.7, 63.5)
% < 40 mg/dL (95% CI)	22.0 (20.5, 23.5)	19.7 (12.3, 29.9)	13.3 (12.0, 14.7)	14.9 (11.5, 19.1)	9.5 (7.3, 12.3)	12.8 (9.2, 17.6)	5.2 (0.7, 29.5)	10.9 (4.8, 22.9)
LDL cholesterol								
Mean (95% CI), mg/dL	114.4 (112.9, 115.8)	120.6 (111.1, 130.1)	116.5 (114.5, 118.1)	122.2 (117.1, 127.3)	115.6 (111.7, 119.6)	120.8 (116.8, 124.8)	112.1 (95.3, 128.9)	120.7 (106.6, 134.8)
% ≥ 100 mg/dL (95% CI)	64.1 (61.8, 66.3)	61.7 (47.8, 73.9)	68.2 (65.8, 70.6)	68.0 (61.7, 73.7)	66.5 (61.5, 71.0)	72.8 (67.0, 77.9)	58.6 (35.0, 78.8)	72.9 (53.2, 86.5)
Triglycerides								
Mean (95% CI), mg/dL	117.6 (113.5, 121.7)	160.8 (111.1, 210.4)	114.1 (109.2, 119.1)	116.1 (106.0, 126.1)	104.7 (97.5, 112.0)	102.9 (90.6, 115.2)	82.8 (72.0, 93.6)	126.5 (102.3, 150.6)
% ≥ 150 mg/dL (95% CI)	21.8 (20.0, 23.7)	27.2 (17.5, 39.6)	20.2 (18.0, 22.6)	24.0 (19.0, 29.9)	16.3 (13.0, 20.3)	14.0 (9.5, 20.0)	1.9 (0.2, 13.1)	30.2 (17.9, 46.2)
Hemoglobin A1c								
Mean (95% CI), %	5.42 (5.40, 5.44)	5.44 (5.24, 5.64)	5.43 (5.40, 5.46)	5.48 (5.42, 5.54)	5.41 (5.38, 5.45)	5.59 (5.52, 5.65)	5.40 (5.26, 5.53)	5.61 (5.53, 5.69)
% ≥ 5.7% (95% CI)	23.8 (22.2, 25.4)	23.6 (17.2, 31.5)	23.8 (22.1, 25.7)	26.5 (21.9, 31.8)	21.9 (18.5, 25.8)	35.0 (30.0, 40.4)	26.7 (14.4, 43.7)	39.2 (27.1, 52.8)
Fasting glucose								
Mean (95% CI), mg/dL	100.5 (99.8, 101.2)	102.0 (99.8, 101.2)	100.4 (99.6, 101.2)	102.1 (100.3, 103.9)	98.3 (97.0, 99.6)	100.7 (98.9, 102.4)	95.6 (92.3, 98.8)	102.6 (95.5, 109.7)
% > 100 mg/dL (95% CI)	36.8 (33.0, 40.7)	50.5 (23.4, 77.3)	35.8 (32.0, 39.7)	30.9 (23.0, 40.0)	34.7 (27.6, 42.5)	42.5 (31.2, 54.7)	37.1 (20.1, 58.0)	57.6 (24.4, 85.1)

Note. BMI = body mass index (defined as weight in kilograms divided by the square of height in meters); CI = confidence interval; high UPF ≥ 40% kcal; low UPF < 40% kcal.

TABLE 3— Multivariable-Adjusted Anthropometrics and Cardiometabolic Markers Stratified by Joint Healthy Eating Index (HEI)–Ultraprocessed Food (UPF) Category, United States, National Health and Nutrition Examination Survey, 2009–2018

	Very Low HEI (<50)		Low HEI (50 to <60)		Moderate HEI (60 to <70)		High HEI (≥70)	
	High UPF	Low UPF	High UPF	Low UPF	High UPF	Low UPF	High UPF	Low UPF
BMI								
Mean (95% CI), kg/m^2	29.6 (29.3, 29.8)	27.6 (25.7, 29.5)[a,b]	28.4 (28.1, 28.7)[a]	27.1 (26.5, 27.7)[a,b]	26.9 (26.5, 27.4)[a]	26.8 (26.0, 27.5)[a]	23.8 (21.8, 25.8)[a]	25.9 (24.6, 27.2)[a]
% with obesity (95% CI)	40.9 (38.9, 43.0)	29.9 (20.6, 41.3)	33.3 (31.2, 35.5)[a]	27.6 (23.0, 32.6)[a,b]	21.6 (18.7, 24.7)[a]	25.3 (20.2, 31.2)[a]	7.4 (1.8, 25.4)[a]	17.1 (8.3, 31.6)[a]
Waist circumference								
Mean (95% CI), cm	99.2 (98.6, 99.8)	95.3 (90.9, 99.6)	96.3 (95.5, 97.0)[a]	93.4 (91.9, 94.9)[a,b]	92.6 (91.4, 93.8)[a]	92.6 (90.8, 94.3)[a]	83.8 (78.8, 88.8)[a]	91.3 (88.8, 93.9)[a,b]
% with high waist circumference (95% CI)	58.3 (56.1, 60.4)	42.5 (30.4, 55.6)[a,b]	50.5 (47.5, 53.4)[a]	42.5 (36.8, 48.6)[a,b]	39.3 (34.9, 43.9)[a]	35.1 (29.1, 41.6)[a]	15.1 (6.6, 30.8)[a]	33.9 (22.3, 47.8)[a,b]
Total cholesterol								
Mean (95% CI), mg/dL	193.6 (192.1, 195.1)	198.8 (187.0, 210.7)	193.1 (191.4, 194.8)	194.3 (188.6, 199.9)	191.9 (189.0, 194.8)	187.4 (183.1, 191.6)[a]	190.6 (173.3, 207.9)	189.8, (180.4, 199.2)
% ≥ 200 mg/dL (95% CI)	39.3 (37.4, 41.3)	44.7 (34.4, 55.5)	38.7 (36.6, 40.8)	38.4 (32.2, 45.0)	37.9 (34.6, 41.2)	37.1 (30.1, 44.7)	35.6 (21.2, 53.2)	40.8 (27.4, 55.7)
HDL cholesterol								
Mean (95% CI), mg/dL	51.7 (51.1, 52.3)	55.6 (51.6, 59.6)	55.0 (54.4, 55.6)[a]	55.7 (54.0, 57.4)[a]	57.3 (56.1, 58.5)[a]	57.5 (55.3, 59.6)[a]	69.1 (57.5, 80.8)[a]	56.4 (50.7, 62.2)
% < 40 mg/dL (95% CI)	17.7 (16.2, 19.3)	13.3 (7.8, 21.8)	12.6 (11.3, 14.1)[a]	11.7 (8.7, 15.6)[a]	10.5 (8.0, 13.8)[a]	12.5 (8.4, 18.3)	7.6 (1.0, 40.2)	11.1 (4.4, 25.2)
LDL cholesterol								
Mean (95% CI), mg/dL	115.6 (114.1, 117.0)	117.9 (109.1, 126.6)	114.1 (112.4, 115.8)	117.5 (112.0, 123.1)	111.5 (107.8, 115.1)	114.4 (110.2, 118.6)	105.6 (88.4, 122.7)	110.4 (96.5, 124.3)
% ≥ 100 mg/dL (95% CI)	67.1 (64.7, 69.4)	57.4 (42.6, 70.9)	66.5 (63.8, 69.0)	61.9 (54.1, 69.1)	62.0 (56.9, 66.9)	65.0 (58.4, 71.0)	50.2 (27.2, 73.1)	58.8 (37.0, 77.8)[b]
Triglycerides								
Mean (95% CI), mg/dL	115.5 (111.4, 119.6)	154.2 (103.9, 204.4)	112.0 (107.7, 116.4)	111.4 (101.0, 121.9)	103.0 (95.9, 110.1)[a]	101.4 (88.9, 114.0)[a]	81.1 (66.4, 95.8)[a]	112.5 (96.8, 148.2)
% ≥ 150 mg/dL (95% CI)	19.8 (18.0, 21.8)	23.0 (13.4, 36.5)	18.3 (16.3, 20.5)	20.9 (16.3, 26.5)	14.9 (11.7, 18.7)[a]	12.6 (8.5, 18.3)[a]	1.7 (0.2, 11.7)[a]	27.2 (14.6, 45.1)[b]
Hemoglobin A1c								
Mean (95% CI), %	5.49 (5.47, 5.51)	5.36 (5.16, 5.57)[a]	5.45 (5.43, 5.48)[a]	5.36 (5.31, 5.42)[a,b]	5.40 (5.37, 5.43)[a]	5.41 (5.35, 5.47)[a]	5.31 (5.19, 5.43)[a]	5.33 (5.24, 5.43)[a]
% ≥ 5.7% (95% CI)	31.9 (29.8, 34.1)	19.1 (13.8, 25.8)[a,b]	27.8 (26.0, 29.7)[a]	17.2 (13.7, 21.4)[a,b]	24.0 (21.1, 27.2)[a]	25.0 (20.4, 30.4)[a]	20.9 (12.1, 33.6)	21.2 (13.5, 31.7)
Fasting glucose								
Mean (95% CI), mg/dL	106.2 (105.2, 107.2)	101.2 (97.8, 104.5)[a,b]	105.1 (103.8, 106.3)	101.5 (99.1, 103.8)[a,b]	99.8 (98.4, 101.3)[a]	103.3 (98.7, 107.9)	98.3 (91.1, 105.5)[a]	96.4 (89.3, 103.5)[a]
% > 100 mg/dL (95% CI)	36.6 (32.5, 40.9)	43.7 (17.2, 74.4)	33.6 (29.3, 38.3)	26.3 (17.2, 38.0)	29.0 (23.1, 35.7)	37.9 (27.1, 50.1)	31.5 (13.6, 57.4)	43.8 (12.1, 81.5)

Note. BMI = body mass index (defined as weight in kilograms divided by the square of height in meters); CI = confidence interval; high UPF ≥ 40% kcal; low UPF < 40% kcal. Values adjusted for age, sex, race and ethnicity, birthplace, educational attainment, employment status, marital status, household income, household food security, and usual total energy intake (kilocalories). Fasting sample n = 8487.

[a]Significantly different from the reference group, very low HEI–high UPF.

[b]Significantly different from high UPF group within the same HEI score category.

the moderate HEI–low UPF category had lower total cholesterol (187.4 mg/dL; $P = .01$) compared with the reference category (193.6 mg/dL). Mean HDL cholesterol was 51.7 mg/dL in the very low HEI–high UPF category compared with 69.1 mg/dL in the high HEI–high UPF category ($P < .001$). LDL cholesterol did not differ between categories. Mean triglycerides were lower for the moderate HEI–high UPF (103.0 mg/dL; $P = .005$), the moderate HEI–low UPF (101.4 mg/dL; $P = .04$), and the high HEI–high UPF (81.1 mg/dL; $P < .001$) categories compared with the reference (115.5 mg/dL). Mean HbA1c was lower in every joint HEI–UPF category compared with the reference, decreasing from 5.49% to 5.31% in the high HEI–high UPF category ($P = .02$). Most categories had lower mean fasting glucose than the reference, decreasing from 106.2 mg/dL in the very low HEI–high UPF category to 96.4 mg/dL in the high HEI–low UPF category ($P = .03$).

Adjusted Differences Within Diet Category

Within each HEI score category, differences in cardiometabolic measures by UPF intake were inconsistent. Among those with very low HEI scores, low UPF intake was associated with lower mean BMI (27.6 kg/m^2 vs 29.6 kg/m^2; $P = .04$), lower prevalence of high waist circumference (42.5% vs 58.3%; $P = .02$), lower prevalence of high HbA1c (19.1% vs 31.9%; $P < .001$), and lower mean fasting glucose (101.2 mg/dL vs 106.2 mg/dL; $P = .004$) compared with the high UPF group. Within the low HEI score category, adults with low UPF consumption had more favorable values across all anthropometric measures, mean HbA1c (5.36% vs 5.45%), prevalence of high HbA1c (17.2% vs 27.8%; $P = .005$), and fasting glucose (101.5 mg/dL vs 105.1 mg/dL; $P = .003$) compared with those with high UPF consumption. There were no differences in anthropometric and cardiometabolic measures by UPF consumption within the moderate HEI score category. In the high HEI category, the low UPF intake group had higher waist circumference (91.3 cm vs 83.8 cm; $P = .01$), prevalence of high waist circumference (33.9% vs 15.1%; $P = .04$), and prevalence of high triglycerides (27.2% vs 1.7%; $P = .006$).

Adjusted Differences in Food Processing Category

When separated by high and low UPF consumption, lower diet quality was associated with less favorable anthropometric and cardiometabolic markers and a higher prevalence of individuals with elevated values in both high and low UPF groups. Within the high UPF group, mean BMI was 29.6 kg/m^2 in the very low HEI category and 23.8 kg/m^2 in the high HEI category ($P < .001$). For those with low UPF consumption, BMI was 27.6 kg/m^2 in the very low HEI category and 25.9 kg/m^2 in the high HEI category ($P = .14$). Lipid profiles showed similar trends. Mean total cholesterol, LDL cholesterol, and triglycerides were higher, and HDL cholesterol was lower in the very low HEI score category compared with the high HEI category within both UPF groups. This finding continued for blood glucose levels. Within the high UPF group, the mean fasting glucose was 106.2 mg/dL for the very low HEI category compared with 98.3 mg/dL for the high HEI category ($P = .03$). Within the low UPF group, the mean fasting glucose was 101.2 mg/dL for the very low HEI category compared with 96.4 mg/dL for the high HEI category ($P = .28$).

DISCUSSION

This nationally representative, descriptive 10-year study found that higher HEI-2020 scores, indicating greater adherence to 2020–2025 Dietary Guidelines for Americans, were associated with better cardiometabolic profiles regardless of UPF intake. These results highlight that overall diet quality remains strongly associated with cardiometabolic health, even in the context of varying UPF consumption.

Previous research has found that higher UPF consumption and lower diet quality are separately associated with poorer diet quality and greater risk of obesity, dyslipidemia, type 2 diabetes, and cardiovascular disease.[2,7,8] However, most existing studies have examined these relationships separately. One prospective cohort study reported that high adherence to the Mediterranean diet combined with low UPF consumption was associated with lower all-cause, cardiovascular, and noncardiovascular, noncancer mortality compared with low adherence and high UPF intake.[29] This analysis extends these findings by assessing cardiometabolic biomarkers across joint HEI scores and UPF consumption in a nationally representative sample. This study finds that diet quality, as measured with the HEI-2020, was more consistently associated with anthropometric and cardiometabolic markers associated with chronic disease than UPF.

These findings may reflect the heterogeneity within the UPF category. UPFs include both nutrient-poor foods like sugar-sweetened beverages and processed meats and nutrient-dense foods, such as whole-grain breads and yogurt.[9] The Nova classification has been important in highlighting the impact of food processing on public health and is the most commonly used definition of UPFs. However, there is ongoing discussion on the best way to define and operationalize UPFs within the US food system because of the different products captured within it.[30,31] Recent prospective cohort studies that have disaggregated UPFs by food group have found that adverse health effects are most consistently associated with a subset of UPFs including sugar-sweetened beverages and red and processed meats.[9,32,33] This analysis did not look at food groups within UPFs, which may be why fewer relationships were observed. In addition, there is currently no agreed-upon threshold that defines high UPF consumption. This analysis identified high UPF consumption as greater than or equal to 40% of total energy intake from UPFs, which is consistent with the top quartile of consumption among NHANES participants.[21,22,34] Future studies should consider higher or lower cut points, as well as further validating methods for estimating usual intake of UPFs.

Strengths and Limitations

Strengths of this study include our use of data from a large, nationally representative sample of US adults spanning recent years. Second, we identified the cut points for HEI categories through multiple sources of health outcome evidence and used validated methods to identify UPFs. Third, we leveraged the rich data sources available from NHANES, validated dietary recalls, physical measurements, and available biomarker data to examine concurrent implications of the HEI score categories and UPF cut points at the individual level.

However, this study is limited by its cross-sectional nature; prospective follow-up is needed to capture changes in clinical outcomes over time. The 24-hour dietary recall is a validated approach but is subject to measurement error and recall bias; however, interviewer-assisted recalls can help reduce error. Diet recalls are not designed to assess food processing level, so applying the Nova classification may involve a degree of misclassification. We were unable to use the NCI HEI–2020 cut points because too few participants had a usual HEI–2020 score of 80 or higher. Excluding participants with one 24-hour recall and the categorization of HEI–2020 scores and UPF intake may have reduced statistical power. While we restricted our study population to people without a chronic disease diagnosis, we were not able to exclude people with undiagnosed or preclinical disease, and this may have attenuated some of the associations, particularly between the high versus low UPF groups.

Public Health Implications

These findings suggest that improving the overall diet quality, as measured by the HEI–2020, should remain a focus of public health efforts to prevent cardiometabolic disease. While reductions in UPFs may support this goal, eating nutrient-dense foods appears to have a stronger association with health markers. Public health recommendations and interventions should continue to promote fruits, vegetables, whole grains, seafood, and plant proteins and recommend limited intake of refined grains and foods high in saturated fat, added sugar, and sodium. Continued research is needed to refine approaches to UPF classification. AJPH

ABOUT THE AUTHORS

Elise Sheinberg, Cindy W. Leung, and Deirdre K. Tobias are with the Department of Nutrition, Harvard T. H. Chan School of Public Health, Boston, MA. Laura A. Schmidt is with the Philip R. Lee Institute for Health Policy Studies and the Department of Humanities and Social Sciences, University of California San Francisco. Jerold R. Mande is with Nourish Science, Boston. Euridice Martinez-Steele is with the Department of Nutrition and Center for Epidemiological Studies in Health and Nutrition, University of São Paulo, Brazil.

CORRESPONDENCE

Correspondence should be sent to Elise Sheinberg, Department of Nutrition, 665 Huntington Ave, Building 2, Boston, MA 02115 (e-mail: esheinberg@g.harvard.edu). Reprints can be ordered at https://www.ajph.org by clicking the "Reprints" link.

PUBLICATION INFORMATION

Full Citation: Sheinberg E, Schmidt LA, Mande JR, Martinez-Steele E, Tobias DK, Leung CW. The intersection of diet quality and ultraprocessed food intake: using evidence-based categories to characterize differences in cardiometabolic profiles. *Am J Public Health*. 2026;116(7): 993–1003.

Acceptance Date: February 12, 2026.

DOI: https://doi.org/10.2105/AJPH.2026.308494

ORCID iDs:

Elise Sheinberg https://orcid.org/0000-0002-5744-6324

Laura A. Schmidt https://orcid.org/0000-0003-4346-7260

Jerold R. Mande https://orcid.org/0009-0006-5208-9854

Euridice Martinez-Steele https://orcid.org/0000-0002-2907-3153

Deirdre K. Tobias https://orcid.org/0000-0003-0020-9552

Cindy W. Leung https://orcid.org/0000-0001-6718-3487

CONTRIBUTORS

C. W. Leung, L. A. Schmidt, J. R. Mande, and D. K. Tobias designed the research. E. Martinez-Steele provided essential materials. C. W. Leung analyzed the data. E. Sheinberg and C. W. Leung wrote the article. E. Sheinberg had primary responsibility for the final content. All authors read and approved the final article.

ACKNOWLEDGMENTS

The linkage of the Nova Classification System for industrial food processing with National Health and Nutrition Examination Survey dietary data are supported by the Center for Epidemiological Studies in Health and Nutrition, University of São Paulo, São Paulo, Brazil, and the National Cancer Institute, Bethesda, MD.

CONFLICTS OF INTEREST

The authors have no conflicts of interest to report.

HUMAN PARTICIPANT PROTECTION

No protocol approval was necessary because this work did not involve human participants.

REFERENCES

1. Micha R, Peñalvo JL, Cudhea F, Imamura F, Rehm CD, Mozaffarian D. Association between dietary factors and mortality from heart disease, stroke, and type 2 diabetes in the United States. *JAMA.* 2017;317(9):912–924. https://doi.org/10.1001/jama.2017.0947
2. Morze J, Danielewicz A, Hoffmann G, Schwingshackl L. Diet quality as assessed by the Healthy Eating Index, Alternate Healthy Eating Index, Dietary Approaches to Stop Hypertension Score, and health outcomes: a second update of a systematic review and meta-analysis of cohort studies. *J Acad Nutr Diet.* 2020;120(12):1998–2031.e15. https://doi.org/10.1016/j.jand.2020.08.076
3. Xu Z, Steffen LM, Selvin E, Rebholz CM. Diet quality, change in diet quality and risk of incident CVD and diabetes. *Public Health Nutr.* 2020;23(2):329–338. https://doi.org/10.1017/S1368980019 00212X
4. US Department of Agriculture, US Department of Health and Human Services. *Dietary Guidelines for Americans, 2020–2025.* Available at: https://www.dietaryguidelines.gov. Accessed August 15, 2025.
5. Monteiro CA, Cannon G, Levy RB, et al. Ultra-processed foods: what they are and how to identify them. *Public Health Nutr.* 2019;22(5):936–941. https://doi.org/10.1017/S13689800 18003762
6. Williams AM, Couch CA, Emmerich SD, Ogburn DF. Ultra-processed food consumption in youth and adults: United States, August 2021–August 2023. *NCHS Data Brief.* 2025;(536). https://doi.org/10.15620/cdc/174612
7. Lane MM, Davis JA, Beattie S, et al. Ultraprocessed food and chronic noncommunicable diseases: a systematic review and meta-analysis of 43 observational studies. *Obes Rev.* 2021;22(3):e13146. https://doi.org/10.1111/obr.13146
8. Vadiveloo MK, Gardner CD, Bleich SN, American Heart Association Council on Lifestyle and Cardiometabolic Health; Council on Cardiovascular and Stroke Nursing; Council on Clinical Cardiology; Council on Genomic and Precision Medicine; and Stroke Council, et al. Ultraprocessed foods and their association with cardiometabolic health: evidence, gaps, and opportunities: a science advisory from the American Heart Association. *Circulation.* 2025;152(12):e245–e263. https://doi.org/10.1161/CIR.0000000000001365
9. Mendoza K, Smith-Warner SA, Rossato SL, et al. Ultra-processed foods and cardiovascular disease: analysis of three large US prospective cohorts and a systematic review and meta-analysis of prospective cohort studies. *Lancet Reg Health Am.* 2024;37:100859. https://doi.org/10.1016/j.lana.2024.100859
10. Valicente VM, Peng CH, Pacheco KN, et al. Ultraprocessed foods and obesity risk: a critical review of reported mechanisms. *Adv Nutr.* 2023;14(4):718–738. https://doi.org/10.1016/j.advnut.2023.04.006
11. Lane MM, Gamage E, Du S, et al. Ultra-processed food exposure and adverse health outcomes: umbrella review of epidemiological meta-analyses. *BMJ.* 2024;384:e077310. https://doi.org/10.1136/bmj-2023-077310
12. Blanton CA, Moshfegh AJ, Baer DJ, Kretsch MJ. The USDA Automated Multiple-Pass Method accurately estimates group total energy and nutrient intake. *J Nutr.* 2006;136(10):2594–2599. https://doi.org/10.1093/jn/136.10.2594
13. Ahluwalia N, Dwyer J, Terry A, Moshfegh A, Johnson C. Update on NHANES dietary data: focus on collection, release, analytical considerations, and uses to inform public policy. *Adv Nutr.* 2016;7(1):121–134. https://doi.org/10.3945/an.115.009258
14. National Cancer Institute. Usual dietary intakes: details of the method. Available at: https://epi.grants.cancer.gov/diet/usualintakes/details.html. Accessed December 19, 2023.
15. Krebs-Smith SM, Pannucci TE, Subar AF, et al. Update of the Healthy Eating Index: HEI-2015. *J Acad Nutr Diet.* 2018;118(9):1591–1602. https://doi.org/10.1016/j.jand.2018.05.021
16. Hu EA, Steffen LM, Coresh J, Appel LJ, Rebholz CM. Adherence to the Healthy Eating Index–2015 and other dietary patterns may reduce risk of cardiovascular disease, cardiovascular mortality, and all-cause mortality. *J Nutr.* 2020;150(2):312–321. https://doi.org/10.1093/jn/nxz218
17. Steele EM, O'Connor LE, Juul F, et al. Identifying and estimating ultraprocessed food intake in the US NHANES according to the Nova classification system of food processing. *J Nutr.* 2023;153(1):225–241. https://doi.org/10.1016/j.tjnut.2022.09.001
18. National Cancer Institute. Linking ASA24 and NHANES data with the Nova classification system for industrial food processing. Available at: https://epi.grants.cancer.gov/nova. Accessed September 12, 2025.
19. Wolfson JA, Tucker AC, Leung CW, Rebholz CM, Garcia-Larsen V, Martinez-Steele E. Trends in adults' intake of un-processed/minimally processed, and ultra-processed foods at home and away from home in the United States from 2003–2018. *J Nutr.* 2025;155(1):280–292. https://doi.org/10.1016/j.tjnut.2024.10.048
20. National Cancer Institute. Usual dietary intakes: SAS macros for analysis of a single dietary component. Available at: https://epi.grants.cancer.gov/diet/usualintakes/macros_single.html. Accessed February 9, 2026.
21. Zhang Z, Jackson SL, Martinez E, Gillespie C, Yang Q. Association between ultraprocessed food intake and cardiovascular health in US adults: a cross-sectional analysis of the NHANES 2011–2016. *Am J Clin Nutr.* 2021;113(2):428–436. https://doi.org/10.1093/ajcn/nqaa276
22. Liu J, Steele EM, Li Y, et al. Consumption of ultra-processed foods and diet quality Among US children and adults. *Am J Prev Med.* 2022;62(2):252–264. https://doi.org/10.1016/j.amepre.2021.08.014
23. Juul F, Parekh N, Martinez-Steele E, Monteiro CA, Chang VW. Ultra-processed food consumption among US adults from 2001 to 2018. *Am J Clin Nutr.* 2022;115(1):211–221. https://doi.org/10.1093/ajcn/nqab305
24. Centers for Disease Control and Prevention. *National Health and Examination Survey Anthropometry Procedures Manual.* 2017. Available at: https://wwwn.cdc.gov/nchs/data/nhanes/public/2017/manuals/2017_Anthropometry_Procedures_Manual.pdf. Accessed June 7, 2024.
25. National Institutes of Health, National Heart, Lung, and Blood Institute. Clinical guidelines on the identification, evaluation, and treatment of overweight and obesity in adults: the evidence report. *Obes Res.* 1998;6(suppl 2):S51–S210. https://doi.org/10.1002/j.1550-8528.1998.tb00690.x
26. Grundy SM, Stone NJ, Bailey AL, et al. 2018 AHA/ACC/AACVPR/AAPA/ABC/ACPM/ADA/AGS/APhA/ASPC/NLA/PCNA Guideline on the Management of Blood Cholesterol: A Report of the American College of Cardiology/American Heart Association Task Force on Clinical Practice Guidelines. *Circulation.* 2019;139(25):e1082–e1143. https://doi.org/10.1161/CIR.0000000000000625
27. Miller M, Stone NJ, Ballantyne C, et al. Triglycerides and cardiovascular disease. *Circulation.* 2011;123(20):2292–2333. https://doi.org/10.1161/CIR.0b013e3182160726
28. American Diabetes Association. *Standards of Care in Diabetes—2023 Abridged for Primary Care Providers. Clin Diabetes.* 2022;41(1):4–31. https://doi.org/10.2337/cd23-as01
29. Liu J, Micha R, Li Y, Mozaffarian D. Trends in food sources and diet quality among US children and adults, 2003–2018. *JAMA Netw Open.* 2021;4(4):e215262. https://doi.org/10.1001/jamanetworkopen.2021.5262
30. Bonaccio M, Di Castelnuovo A, Costanzo S, Moli-sani Study Investigators, et al. Combination of a traditional Mediterranean diet with ultra-processed food consumption in relation to all-cause and cause-specific mortality: prospective findings from the Moli-sani Study. *Clin Nutr.* 2025;50:83–91. https://doi.org/10.1016/j.clnu.2025.04.024
31. Popkin BM, Miles DR, Taillie LS, Dunford EK. A policy approach to identifying food and beverage products that are ultra-processed and high in added salt, sugar and saturated fat in the United States: a cross-sectional analysis of packaged foods. *Lancet Reg Health Am.* 2024;32:100713. https://doi.org/10.1016/j.lana.2024.100713
32. Moran AJ, Khandpur N, Roberto CA. Identifying ultra-processed foods for policy. *Nat Med.* 2026:32(2):410–413. https://doi.org/10.1038/s41591-025-04108-5
33. Chen Z, Khandpur N, Desjardins C, et al. Ultra-processed food consumption and risk of type 2 diabetes: three large prospective US cohort studies. *Diabetes Care.* 2023;46(7):1335–1344. https://doi.org/10.2337/dc22-1993
34. Fang Z, Rossato SL, Hang D, et al. Association of ultra-processed food consumption with all cause and cause specific mortality: population based cohort study. *BMJ.* 2024;385:e078476. https://doi.org/10.1136/bmj-2023-078476

Changes in Neighborhood Foodscapes From 2003 to 2023 by Area Rurality in the United States

Daniel Wiese, PhD, Marissa M. Shams-White, PhD, Zhiyuan Zheng, PhD, Kevin A. Henry, PhD, Marjorie L. McCullough, PhD, and Farhad Islami, MD, PhD

See also Ultraprocessed Food, pp. 898–1029.

AJPH July 2026, Vol. 116, No. 7

Objectives. To evaluate the change in the US foodscape from 2003 to 2023 overall and by area rurality, considering various modes of transportation.

Methods. We conducted this study using longitudinal data on all licensed food retailers, geocoded to census-tract level, and examined changes in the foodscape by estimating the percentages of tracts defined as food deserts (no grocery stores) and food swamps (mostly restaurants or fast-food locations).

Results. We found a considerable increase in the percentage of food swamps and no substantial progress in reducing food deserts. For example, using distance-based foodscape measure (one half of a mile from tract borders), between 2003 and 2023, the percentage of tracts categorized as food swamps increased from 80.2% to 88.5%, while the percentage of food deserts decreased minimally from 6.1% to 5.5%. Across all years, the percentage of food deserts was substantially higher in rural areas, and when people used public transit as a mode of transportation.

Conclusions. The findings underscore the need for improving accessibility to healthy foods across the United States, particularly in rural areas.

Public Health Implications. Expanding public–private partnerships to establish healthy food retailers in food deserts may improve the foodscape quality. (*Am J Public Health*. 2026;116(7):1004–1014. https://doi.org/10.2105/AJPH.2026.308495)

Unhealthy diet has been associated with adverse health outcomes, including excess body weight, diabetes, heart disease, and cancer.[1–5] Although dietary choices may vary by individuals' preferences and food culture, the affordability and availability of foods are important factors contributing to those choices.[6–8] Area-level food environment, also referred to as retail foodscape, often acts as a proxy measure for geographic accessibility to healthy grocery food retailers. Therefore, studies on the retail foodscape often differentiate between food deserts—areas with no access to grocery retailers within a defined distance or travel time—and food swamps—areas with a substantially high number of restaurants and fast-food locations and only a limited number of grocery retailers.

Previous research generally indicates that dietary behaviors are associated with a neighborhood's foodscape. In the United States, for example, the odds of consuming fast food near home increased by 11% to 61%, depending on the model adjustments, for every standard deviation increase in the fast-food density in the neighborhood.[9] By contrast, in another study, fresh produce consumption increased with each additional supermarket in the neighborhood.[10] Several studies have found an association between residing in food deserts or food swamps and adverse health outcomes, including higher body mass index,[11] cardiovascular health risk,[4] obesity,[12] and diabetes-related hospitalization rates in the population.[13]

Given the rising burden of diet-related chronic diseases in the United States, it is essential to track changes in the neighborhood retail foodscape over time. So far, only 1 study has examined these changes to identify geographic and racial disparities in exposure to unfavorable food environment (i.e., neighborhoods with low concentrations of grocery stores) in the United States.[14] However, no studies have examined changes in food deserts and food swamps over time across rural and urban areas and by persistent poverty status. Additionally, it remains unknown how different modes of transportation may influence geographic accessibility to healthy food stores, or if the COVID-19 pandemic coincided with any substantial changes in the neighborhood retail foodscape.

In this study, we examined changes in the US retail foodscape from 2003 to 2023, which includes the COVID-19 era. We also assessed trends in food deserts and food swamps by area rurality, persistent poverty status, and state, and compared accessibility by using distance-, automobile-, and public transit–based measures.

METHODS

We obtained annual data on all licensed businesses in the United States between 2003 and 2023 from DataAxle.[15] Following earlier recommendations for business data refinement,[16] we first selected all relevant business types using the North American Industry Classification System (NAICS) and Standard Industrial Classification (SIC) codes (Table 1) and business names. Next, records for each business were linked across all years based on full street address and geographic coordinates and geocoded to census tract level using the 2010 geometry. For each year, we calculated the number of healthy and unhealthy food retailers in each tract (Table 1). We then reconstructed the tract-level modified Retail Food Environment Index (mRFEI),[17] which estimates the proportion of healthy food retailers from total food retailers in a given geographic area,[18,19] by using the following equation:

$$\text{mRFEI} = 100 \times \frac{\text{Healthy Food Retailers}}{\left\{\begin{array}{l}\text{Healthy Food Retailers} \\ + \text{Unhealthy Food Retailers}\end{array}\right\}} \quad (1)$$

In this study, we define accessibility as geographic access—the ease of reaching food retailers on the basis of proximity or travel time. We used 3 different methods: first, the traditional half-mile buffer zone around the tract boundary (distance-based mRFEI); second, 20-minute drive time zones from the population-weighted tract centroid by personal automobile (20-minute drive time corresponds to approximately 6–10 miles travel distance in urban areas and up to 20 miles travel distance in rural areas); third, 20-minute ride zones by public transit (including bus, local and regional rail, and ferries) using the TravelTime tool.[20,21] A 20-minute threshold was selected on the basis of empirical evidence indicating that after accounting for regional variation and urban–rural context, over 80% of the US population can access a supermarket within approximately 19.6 minutes (considered optimal access).[22]

We then evaluated the US retail foodscape by estimating the percentages of tracts defined as food deserts (no healthy food retailers; mRFEI = 0), food swamps (mostly restaurants or fast-food locations; mRFEI < 33.3), and tracts with a good food environment (mRFEI ≥ 33.3), and the number of people living in food deserts and food swamps overall, by area rurality (based on the Urban Rural Indicator Codes, where rural census tracts are defined as those with an urban population of < 50%),[23] persistent poverty status (defined as a census tract with a poverty rate ≥ 20.0% in 4 consecutive measurement periods between 1990 and 2019),[24] and by state. Population data were derived from the American Community Survey's 5-year estimates for 2015 to 2019 (for tract level) and 2019 to 2023 (for state level). We selected these mRFEI thresholds in accordance with an earlier study.[25] We also examined the association between changes in the percentage of food swamps and food deserts by calculating the swamp-to-desert ratio (overall, by area rurality, and by state), and we mapped changes in the number of healthy and unhealthy food retailers and in the proportion of food deserts and food swamps by state (including the District of Columbia) for the contiguous United States. We conducted data preprocessing using Python (Python Software Foundation, Wilmington, DE); data analysis and visualization were executed using R statistical software (R Foundation for Statistical Computing, Vienna, Austria).

RESULTS

The total number of food retailers in the United States steadily increased by 62.6%—from 756 668 in 2003 to 1 208 797 in 2020—but then decreased from 2020, coinciding with the start of the COVID-19 pandemic in the United States, by 11.6% to 1 067 984 in 2023 (Table 1). Similarly, the number of unhealthy and healthy food retailers rose from 2003 to 2020 by 66.0% (from 623 738 to 1 035 370) and 30.4% (from 132 930 to 173 280), respectively. Between 2020 and 2023, however, the number of both unhealthy and healthy food retailers decreased by 11.2% (to 919 199) and 14.1% (to 148 785), respectively. As a result, the overall increase in numbers from 2003 to 2023

TABLE 1— Changes in the Number of Food Retailers in the United States Between 2003 and 2023

Retail Category	Standard Industrial Classification Code	2003, No.	2020, No.	2023, No.	Change 2003–2020, %	Change 2020–2023, %	Change 2003–2023, %
All retailers combined		756 668	1 208 797	1 067 984	62.6	−11.6	41.1
Unhealthy food retailers							
Total		623 738	1 035 370	919 199	66.0	−11.2	47.4
Bakery/coffee/tea shop	546101, 546105, 546107, 546108, 546109, 549915, 549938	26 157	42 468	37 796	62.4	−11.0	44.5
Convenience store (including gas station shops, dollar stores)	541103, 541104, 549999	98 473	137 258	120 119	39.4	−12.5	22.0
Dairy produce retailer (including ice-cream shops)	545101, 545102, 545103	3 874	10 214	8 241	163.7	−19.3	112.7
Full-service restaurant	581208	404 417	708 003	624 408	75.1	−11.8	54.4
Limited-service restaurant	581201, 581202, 581203, 581204, 581205, 581206, 581209, 581211, 581213, 581214, 581215, 581217, 581218, 581219, 581221, 581222, 581224, 581227, 581228, 581229, 581236, 581237, 581246, 581248, 581240, 581241, 581244, 581249, 581250, 581251, 581252, 581254, 581255	90 817	137 427	128 635	51.3	−6.4	41.6
Healthy food retailers							
Total		132 930	173 280	148 785	30.4	−14.1	11.9
Department store/club store (carrying fresh produce)	531102, 531110	2 060	7 250	7 119	251.9	−1.8	245.6
Ethnic grocery store	541106, 541107, 541108, 549912, 549916, 549917, 549918, 549919, 549923, 549926, 549927, 549930, 549937, 549945	2 119	2 204	1 932	4.0	−12.3	−8.8
Fruit and vegetable market	543101, 543102, 543103, 543104, 543105, 543106	10 021	14 061	11 369	40.3	−19.1	13.5
Grocery store/supermarket	541101, 541105, 541109, 549928	104 044	131 213	112 729	26.1	−14.1	8.3
Meat/fish market	542101, 542104, 542105, 542106, 542107, 542108, 542109, 542110, 542111, 542113, 542114, 542116, 542118, 542117	14 686	18 552	15 636	26.3	−15.7	6.5

Note. Although full-service restaurants are categorized as "unhealthy," several may offer healthy meals. This categorization was adopted from the initial modified Retail Food Environment Index (mRFEI)[17] definition. A more granular categorization of full-service restaurants was not possible because information on food types served was not available.

was substantially greater for unhealthy food retailers (47.4%) than for healthy food retailers (11.9%).

Changes in the Foodscape Nationally

Using distance-based mRFEI (Figure 1), the percentage of food deserts first decreased by 1.9 percentage points between 2003 and 2020 (from 6.1% to 4.2%), but then increased to 5.5% in 2023. The percentage of food swamps increased between 2003 and 2020 by 9.6 percentage points (from 80.2% to 89.8%) but decreased to 88.5% in 2023. By contrast, the percentage of tracts with a good food environment decreased by 7.7 percentage points (from 13.7% to 6.0%) between 2003 and 2020 and remained at this level through 2023.

Using the drive time–based mRFEI (Appendix Figure A, available as a supplement to the online version of this article at http://www.ajph.org), the percentage of food deserts was stable at 2.0% between 2003 and 2020 and increased minimally by 0.1 percentage point by 2023. The percentage of food swamps rose by 2 percentage points between 2003 and 2020 (from 94.8% to 96.8%) but then decreased by 0.1 percentage point by 2023. The percentage of tracts with a good food environment decreased by 2.0 percentage points (from 3.2% to 1.2%) between 2003 and 2020 and remained unchanged thereafter.

When using the public transit-based mRFEI (Appendix Figure A), the percentage of food deserts decreased by 2.0 percentage points, from 53.1% to 51.1%, between 2003 and 2020, but increased to 52.7% in 2023. The percentage of food swamps increased by 6.9 percentage points between 2003 and 2020, from 33.3% to 40.2%, but decreased to 38.7% in 2023. The percentage of tracts with a good food environment decreased by 5.0 percentage points,

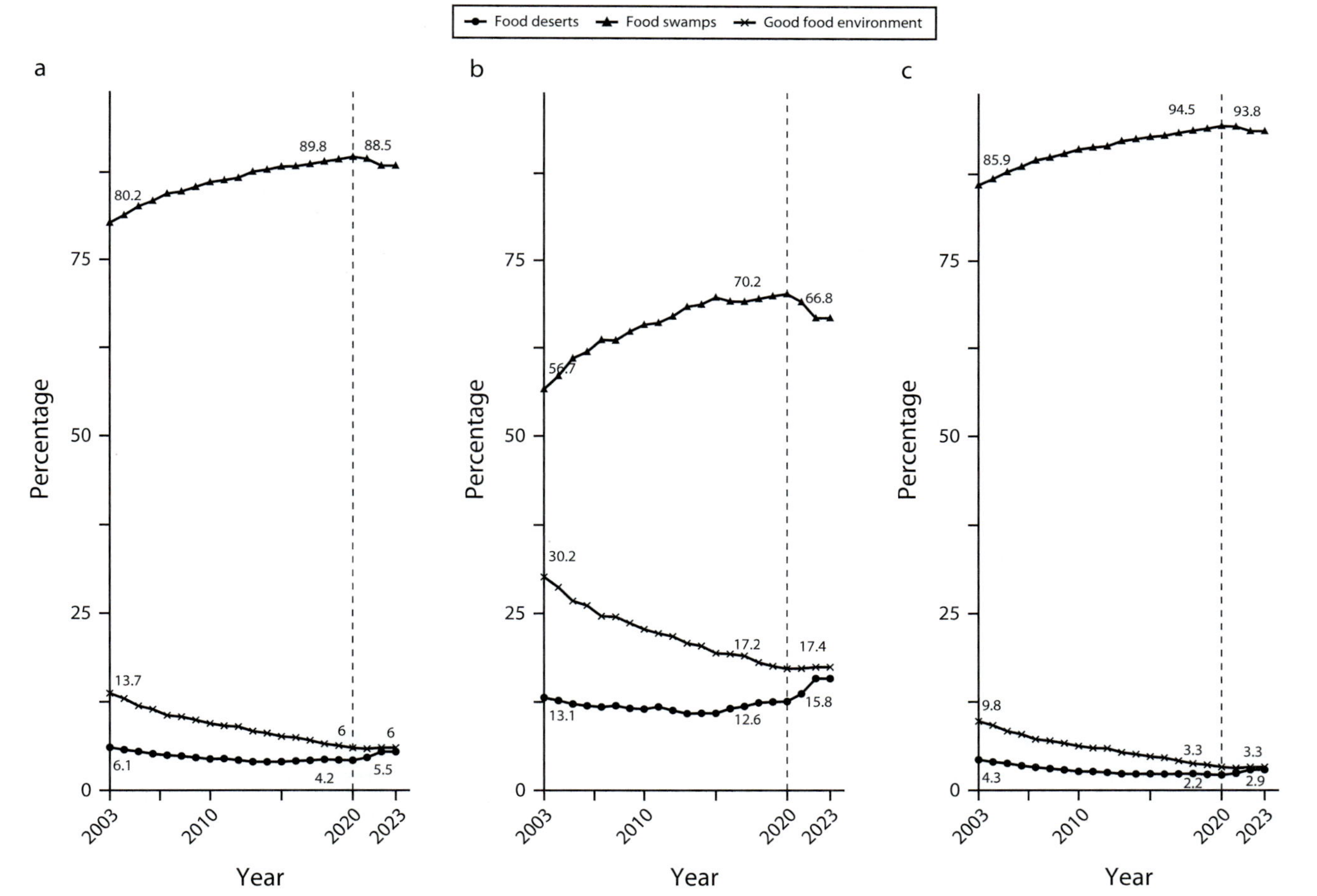

FIGURE 1— Change in the US Foodscape From Overall, (b) Rural Areas, and (c) Urban Areas Using Distance-Based mRFEI Measure: 2003–2023

Note. mRFEI = modified Retail Food Environment Index. Dashed line indicates the beginning of the COVID-19 pandemic (2020).

from 13.7% to 8.7%, during 2003 to 2020, and decreased further to 8.6% in 2023.

Stratified by rurality status (Figure 1, Appendix Figure A), the overall patterns were generally similar and reflected the nationwide trajectories. Regardless of the mode of transportation, in both rural and urban areas there was a minimal decrease or no change in the percentage of food deserts between 2003 and 2020, but an increase from 2020 to 2023. By contrast, the percentage of food swamps increased substantially between 2003 and 2020, then decreased slightly by 2023. The percentage of tracts with a good food environment either consistently decreased over time or remained consistently low, depending on the mode of transportation. However, in rural areas, the percentage of food deserts was substantially higher than in urban areas, whereas the percentage of food swamps was generally lower. In 2023, for example, the percentage of food swamps in rural and urban areas was 66.8% and 93.8% and the percentage of food deserts was 15.8% and 2.9%, respectively. The percentage of food deserts was lower in both rural (10.2%) and urban (0.2%) areas when we used automobile-based mRFEI, but it was substantially higher when we used public transit–based mRFEI (93.8% and 42.8%, respectively). Regardless of the mRFEI measure used, we found that a decrease in the percentage of food deserts was generally associated with an increase in the percentage of food swamps, as indicated by the swamp-to-desert ratio (Appendix Figure B). This relationship was more pronounced in urban than rural areas.

In 2023, the number of people residing in food deserts ranged from 4.9 million (1.5% of the total US population) using drive time–based mRFEI to 14 million (4.4%) using distance-based mRFEI to 178 million (55.3%) using public transit–based mRFEI (Appendix Table A). In rural areas, the total population residing in food deserts ranged from 4.5 million (8.1% of the total rural population) using drive time–based mRFEI to 7.1 million (2.2%) using distance-based mRFEI to 51.6 million (93.9%) using public transit–based mRFEI. Food swamp residents included over 290 million people, or more than 90% of the total US population, using distance-based or drive time–based mRFEI, and approximately 116 million (36%) using public transit–based mRFEI. (Appendix Table A).

Changes in the Foodscape by Poverty Status

Among 68 106 (94.4%) census tracts with available poverty data, 8244 tracts (11.4%) were categorized as persistent poverty areas (> 30 million residents). Regardless of the mRFEI measure used, the overall patterns in both persistent poverty tracts and nonpersistent poverty tracts reflected the nationwide trajectories (Appendix Figure C). However, selection of the mode of transportation substantially influenced the number of food deserts, especially in persistent poverty areas. For example, using distance-based or drive time–based mRFEI, 1.9% of tracts with persistent poverty were categorized as food deserts in 2003 and 2023. When we used public transit–based mRFEI, this percentage was 22.0% in 2003 and increased to 23.3% by 2023. The total population residing in food deserts and food swamps in persistent poverty areas in 2023 varied by the mRFEI measure used (Appendix Table A). The estimated numbers of people living in food deserts were approximately 476 000 (distance-based mRFEI), 0.5 million (drive time–based mRFEI), and 7.4 million (public transit–based mRFEI). The numbers of people living in food swamps were 26 million (distance-based mRFEI), 29 million (drive time–based mRFEI), and 18 million (public transit–based mRFEI).

Changes in the Foodscape by State

Despite some variation in foodscape changes between states (Figure 2, Appendix Figure D), most state-specific trajectories reflected nationwide patterns (i.e., a minimal decrease to a slight increase in food deserts and a substantial increase in food swamps). Between 2003 and 2023, the percentage of food deserts decreased in 26, 14, and 25 states using distance-based (Figure 2a), drive time–based, or public transit–based mRFEI, respectively (Appendix Figure D). The percentage of food swamps increased in 48, 38, and 47 states using distance-based (Figure 2b), drive time–based, or public transit–based mRFEI, respectively (Appendix Figure D). In the majority of states, the foodscape patterns during the COVID-19 period were similar to the national patterns. From 2020 to 2023, regardless of the mRFEI measure used, the percentage of food deserts generally increased, whereas the percentage of food swamps decreased (Appendix Tables B–D).

Geographically, by 2023, regardless of the mRFEI measure used, states with the highest percentage of food deserts were predominantly located in the North and Great Plains regions, whereas those with the lowest percentage were concentrated in the mid-Atlantic region and along the West Coast (Figure 3, Appendix Figure E). States with a lower percentage of food deserts often had the highest percentage of food swamps. In 2023, approximately 14.1 million people (4.4% of the total population) in the United States resided in

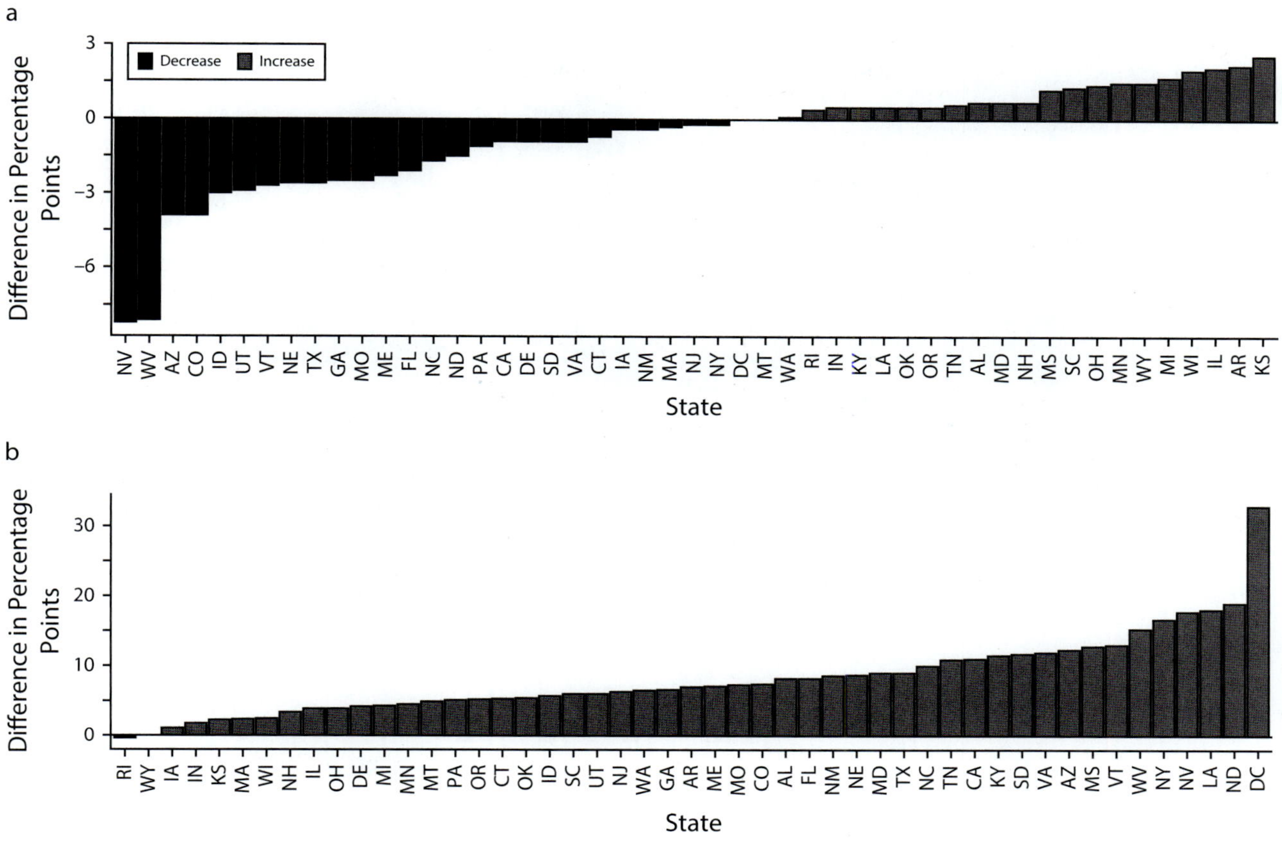

FIGURE 2— State-Specific Change in the Proportion of (a) Food Deserts and (b) Food Swamps Using Distance-Based mRFEI: United States, 2003–2023

Note. mRFEI = modified Retail Food Environment Index.

food deserts and 292.1 million (90.7%) resided in food swamps (Appendix Table A). Across states (Appendix Tables B–D), Texas had the largest population living in food deserts (> 1 million; 3.6% of the state population). The largest populations living in food swamps were found in California (36 million; 91.2% of the state population) and in Texas (26.7 million; 94.6%).

DISCUSSION

Our findings indicate little progress in reducing the number of food deserts and a substantial increase in the number of food swamps in the United States in the past 2 decades, resulting in at least 4.9 million people living in food deserts and up to 314 million people living in food swamps. This trend is largely driven by a substantially greater increase in the number of restaurants and fast-food locations compared with grocery retailers nationwide, which is consistent with earlier findings.[14] The slower growth in the number of grocery retailers may be attributed to the complexities of their business structure, including logistics, supply chains, and financial sustainability,[26] or to challenges finding appropriate property size, especially in urban areas.[19] Similar to previous research, we found that among healthy food retailers, the greatest increase was observed in the number of club stores and department stores,[27] many of which operate as franchises or chains. Although the establishment of such large club "superstores" may allow them to serve a broader customer base and act as anchor locations for several areas, their presence does not necessarily improve the geographic accessibility to healthy foods.[27] These stores are frequently located in commercial districts rather than residential neighborhoods, which may limit their role in alleviating food deserts,[28] especially for individuals with limited access to transportation. Additionally, club stores generally require a membership fee, which may not be affordable to some individuals; therefore, they are not considered a

AJPH July 2026, Vol. 116, No. 7

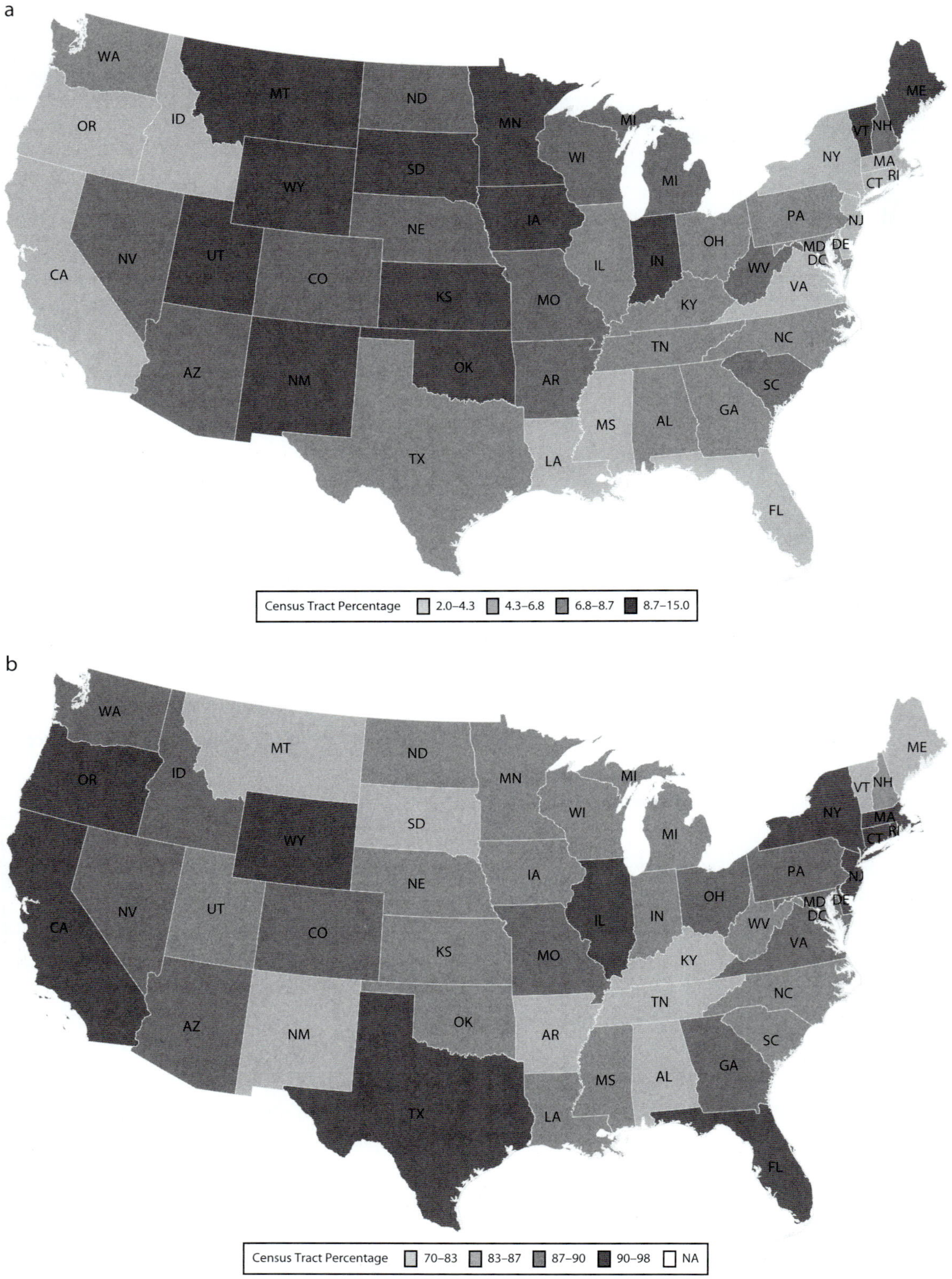

FIGURE 3— Geographic Distribution of (a) Food Deserts and (b) Food Swamps Using Distance-Based mRFEI: United States, 2023

Note. mRFEI = modified Retail Food Environment Index. NA indicates that the percentage of census tracts is 0 (only in the District of Columbia).

potential source for grocery shopping.[27,29] Public–private healthy food financing programs to improve access to grocery retailers have been implemented at the federal and state levels. For example, the Healthy Food Financing Initiative and related programs (including Pennsylvania's Fresh Food Financing Initiative) provide grants and low-interest financing to support the development of healthy grocery retailers in rural and urban underserved areas.[30–32] Such investments could improve healthy food access in food desert settings and may yield measurable benefits for residents.[33] Additionally, local policies to control the growth of unhealthy food retailers have been proposed and implemented across many US jurisdictions, including zoning, land-use restrictions, or partial and temporal bans on the opening of new fast-food retailers.[34] However, their success must be further evaluated because many policies, especially bans, have generally been subject to strong opposition from businesses and other stakeholders.[34] Moreover, although higher taxes on unhealthy foods may not directly change the neighborhood foodscape, it has the potential to reduce unhealthy food consumption.[35]

Although the overall pattern of foodscape changes was similar across urban and rural areas, food deserts were disproportionately concentrated in rural areas regardless of the mRFEI measure used, but especially when we used public transit-based mRFEI because of generally underdeveloped public transit networks in rural areas. This disparity is likely attributable to the larger sizes of census tracts in rural areas, which results in longer travel distances to healthy food retailers.[36] Additionally, rural tracts with small populations may lack the consumer base necessary to sustain large grocery stores, further exacerbating limited food access.[37]

Our findings also highlight that accessibility to healthy food retailers varies by the mode of transportation. When using a private automobile, only a small fraction of the US population lacks access to healthy food retailers. Automobile-based measures, however, assume universal car ownership and may underestimate inequities in food access because many individuals do not have access to a private automobile[36]; approximately 8% of the US population and 19% of individuals with incomes below the federal poverty level do not own a car.[38] Our findings also show that populations living in persistent poverty areas have more limited accessibility to grocery stores when relying on public transit only. Additionally, the majority of census tracts with available public transit connections were categorized as food swamps, confirming previous findings that many public transit users, especially bus riders, have easier access to unhealthy than to healthy food retailers.[39] Prior work also suggests that food shopping may be influenced by the design of the public transit routes and their interaction with access to fast-food retailers and convenience stores.[39] Evidence suggests that transit-focused interventions—such as modifying fixed-route bus service to connect socioeconomically disadvantaged areas to supermarkets[40] or establishing grocery shuttles and "shopper links"[41]—could enhance access to healthy food options for public transit users.

The nationwide foodscape trends were also largely reflected at the state level. In general, by 2023, states with the highest percentages of food deserts were predominantly located in the North and Great Plains regions (including states with the highest number of food deserts nationwide[37]), whereas those with the lowest percentages were concentrated in the mid-Atlantic region and along the West Coast. We also observed that states with a lower percentage of food deserts often had a higher percentage of food swamps. This pattern may be related to population distribution. States with higher population densities and large urban centers tend to have a greater number of food retailers, particularly fast-food restaurants and convenience stores, but also healthy food retailers.[42] Thus, having fewer deserts in a state may not necessarily mean having a healthier food environment. Additionally, a dense network of major arterial roads may contribute to a higher proportion of food swamps, as these areas often attract fast-food establishments serving the bypassing traffic.[43]

The COVID-19 pandemic coincided with substantial changes in the foodscape, as the nationwide lockdown, reduction of dining-in opportunities, and decrease in the number of customers resulted in the closure and bankruptcy of many food retailers. The reduction of healthy food retailers during the pandemic is likely among the reasons for an overall increase in the number of food deserts during the pandemic and postpandemic periods, especially in rural areas, leaving many residents with very limited accessibility to healthy food. By contrast, a substantially larger decrease in the number of unhealthy food retailers resulted in an overall decrease in the number of food swamps. The number of food retailers should be monitored for a longer period, as some businesses continue to recover from the economic impact from the COVID-19 pandemic. Future monitoring should also account for structural changes such as the growth of e-grocery shopping and food delivery platforms,[44] which may reshape access independent of physical retail density. Increasing the advertising of food deliveries (beyond fast-food and restaurant delivery) and the number of grocery retailers participating in food delivery programs may be beneficial for populations with limited geographic accessibility to healthy food and for individuals with limited mobility.

Limitations

This study is the first to examine temporal changes in the US neighborhood-level foodscape, nationally and by area rurality, persistent poverty status, and state, over the past 2 decades, including the COVID-19 pandemic era. However, several limitations related to data and methodology should be acknowledged. First, some businesses might have changed their NAICS or SIC codes over time, potentially leading to misclassification within specific retail subcategories. For example, although the number of ethnic grocery stores appeared to decrease, many were reassigned to other categories, such as fruit and vegetable stores or meat markets. However, these reclassifications did not affect the broader "healthy" or "unhealthy" classification of food retailers. Second, defining the foodscape at the tract level may not fully capture actual food accessibility and availability. Additionally, using the number of food retailers alone does not allow us to evaluate the quality and volume of the supplied foods and may not guarantee a healthy dietary pattern. According to a study on the consumption behavior of approximately 60 000 US households in 2020, 48% of purchased foods in supermarkets are considered unhealthy ultraprocessed foods.[45] Higher taxes or implementing front-of-package warning labels, similar to practices in some other countries, may limit the consumption of these foods.[46,47]

We also did not account for potential changes in access to healthy food retailers among the commuting population. However, a study from Florida reported only minimal changes in accessibility to healthy food retailers when considering commuting patterns as compared with primary residency only.[48] We were also not able to include digital food access (e.g., delivery zones) into our study because of the limited data. Although a recent report by the Brookings Institution states that over 90% of the US population should have access to at least 1 grocery delivery option,[49] actual use of these services depends on various factors, including broadband access or number of consumers in the areas, and thus remains largely unknown.[50] Lastly, there is no universally accepted mRFEI threshold for defining food swamps. Despite this, the substantially greater increase in the number of restaurants and fast-food locations compared with healthy food retailers will result in an increase in the number of food swamps, regardless of the threshold used.

Conclusions

In conclusion, our findings highlight the need to improve access to healthy food retailers across the United States, particularly in rural and socioeconomically disadvantaged areas. Expanding public–private partnerships to establish new healthy food retailers in food deserts, including in sparsely populated areas or areas with lower-income populations, may help increase access to healthy foods. Additionally, further expansion and strategic planning of public transit networks could help reduce accessibility barriers for socioeconomically marginalized populations. AJPH

ABOUT THE AUTHORS

Daniel Wiese, Zhiyuan Zheng, and Farhad Islami are with the Department of Surveillance, Prevention, & Health Services Research, American Cancer Society, Atlanta, GA. At the time of the study, Marissa M. Shams-White and Marjorie L. McCullough were with the Population Science Department, American Cancer Society, Atlanta. Kevin A. Henry is with the Department of Geography, Temple University, Philadelphia, PA.

CORRESPONDENCE

Correspondence should be sent to Daniel Wiese, Department of Surveillance, Prevention, & Health Services Research, American Cancer Society, 270 Peachtree St NW, Suite 1300, Atlanta, GA 30303 (e-mail: daniel.wiese@cancer.org). Reprints can be ordered at https://www.ajph.org by clicking the "Reprints" link.

PUBLICATION INFORMATION

Full Citation: Wiese D, Shams-White MM, Zheng Z, Henry KA, McCullough ML, Islami F. Changes in neighborhood foodscapes from 2003 to 2023 by area rurality in the United States. *Am J Public Health*. 2026;116(7):1004–1014.

Acceptance Date: February 12, 2026

DOI: https://doi.org/10.2105/AJPH.2026.308495

ORCID iDs:

Daniel Wiese https://orcid.org/0000-0002-1603-7583

Marissa M. Shams-White https://orcid.org/0000-0002-7824-4545

Farhad Islami https://orcid.org/0000-0002-7357-5994

CONTRIBUTORS

D. Wiese and F. Islami conceptualized the study and led article development. D. Wiese and K. A. Henry acquired the data and performed data quality assurance. D. Wiese performed statistical analysis and wrote the original draft. All authors interpreted the data, critically revised the article, and reviewed and approved the final version of the article.

ACKNOWLEDGMENTS

We thank Molly Catlin of the Rollins School of Public Health at Emory University for providing assistance with data management and preparation for this project during the internship at the American Cancer Society.

CONFLICTS OF INTEREST

The authors do not have any conflicts of interest to report. D. Wiese, M. M. Shams-White, Z. Zheng, and F. Islami are employed by the American Cancer Society, which receives grants from private and corporate foundations, including foundations associated with companies in the health sector for research outside the submitted work.

HUMAN PARTICIPANT PROTECTION

No protocol approval was needed for this study because no human participants were involved.

REFERENCES

1. Cooksey-Stowers K, Schwartz MB, Brownell KD. Food swamps predict obesity rates better than food deserts in the United States. *Int J Environ Res Public Health.* 2017;14(11):1366. https://doi.org/10.3390/ijerph14111366
2. Rock CL, Thomson C, Gansler T, et al. American Cancer Society guideline for diet and physical activity for cancer prevention. *CA Cancer J Clin.* 2020;70(4):245–271. https://doi.org/10.3322/caac.21591
3. Clinton SK, Giovannucci EL, Hursting SD. The World Cancer Research Fund/American Institute for Cancer Research Third Expert Report on Diet, Nutrition, Physical Activity, and Cancer: impact and future directions. *J Nutr.* 2020;150(4):663–671. https://doi.org/10.1093/jn/nxz268
4. Testa A, Jackson DB, Semenza DC, Vaughn MG. Food deserts and cardiovascular health among young adults. *Public Health Nutr.* 2021;24(1):117–124. https://doi.org/10.1017/S1368980020001536
5. Centers for Disease Control and Prevention. FastStats: leading causes of death. 2021. Available at: https://www.cdc.gov/nchs/fastats/leading-causes-of-death.htm. Accessed April 2026.
6. Diez-Roux AV, Nieto FJ, Caulfield L, Tyroler HA, Watson RL, Szklo M. Neighbourhood differences in diet: the Atherosclerosis Risk in Communities (ARIC) Study. *J Epidemiol Community Health.* 1999;53(1):55–63. https://doi.org/10.1136/jech.53.1.55
7. Chen PJ, Antonelli M. Conceptual models of food choice: influential factors related to foods, individual differences, and society. *Foods.* 2020;9(12). https://doi.org/10.3390/foods9121898
8. McCullough ML, Chantaprasopsuk S, Islami F, et al. Association of socioeconomic and geographic factors with diet quality in US adults. *JAMA Netw Open.* 2022;5(6):e2216406. https://doi.org/10.1001/jamanetworkopen.2022.16406
9. Moore LV, Diez Roux AV, Nettleton JA, Jacobs DR, Franco M. Fast-food consumption, diet quality, and neighborhood exposure to fast food: The Multi-Ethnic Study of Atherosclerosis. *Am J Epidemiol.* 2009;170(1):29–36. https://doi.org/10.1093/aje/kwp090
10. Morland K, Wing S, Roux AD. The contextual effect of the local food environment on residents' diets: The Atherosclerosis Risk in Communities Study. *Am J Public Health.* 2002;92(11):1761–1767. https://doi.org/10.2105/ajph.92.11.1761
11. Woodruff RC, Haardörfer R, Raskind IG, Hermstad A, Kegler MC. Comparing food desert residents with non-food desert residents on grocery shopping behaviours, diet and BMI: results from a propensity score analysis. *Public Health Nutr.* 2020;23(5):806–811. https://doi.org/10.1017/S136898001900363X
12. Chen D, Jaenicke EC, Volpe RJ. Food environments and obesity: household diet expenditure versus food deserts. *Am J Public Health.* 2016;106(5):881–888. https://doi.org/10.2105/AJPH.2016.303048
13. Phillips AZ, Rodriguez HP. US county "food swamp" severity and hospitalization rates among adults with diabetes: a nonlinear relationship. *Soc Sci Med.* 2020;249:112858. https://doi.org/10.1016/j.socscimed.2020.112858
14. Jiang Q, Ghosh D, Steinbach S, Cooksey Stowers K. A longitudinal assessment of racial and ethnic inequities in food environment exposure and retail market concentration. *Public Health Nutr.* 2023;26(9):1850–1861. https://doi.org/10.1017/S1368980023001179
15. DataAxle. Consumer data. 2024. Available at: https://www.data-axle.com/our-data/consumer-data. Accessed October 2024.
16. Hirsch JA, Moore KA, Cahill J, et al. Business data categorization and refinement for application in longitudinal neighborhood health research: a methodology. *J Urban Health.* 2021;98(2):271–284. https://doi.org/10.1007/s11524-020-00482-2
17. Center for Disease Control and Prevention. Census tract level state maps of the modified Retail Food Environment Index (mRFEI). 2011. Available at: https://www.cdc.gov/obesity/downloads/census-tract-level-state-maps-mrfei_TAG508.pdf. Accessed April 2026.
18. Kraft AN, Thatcher EJ, Zenk SN. Neighborhood food environment and health outcomes in US low-socioeconomic status, racial/ethnic minority, and rural populations: a systematic review. *J Health Care Poor Underserved.* 2020;31(3):1078–1114. https://doi.org/10.1353/hpu.2020.0083
19. Walker RE, Keane CR, Burke JG. Disparities and access to healthy food in the United States: a review of food deserts literature. *Health Place.* 2010;16(5):876–884. https://doi.org/10.1016/j.healthplace.2010.04.013
20. Ryan GE, Tierney N, Golding N, Weiss DJ. traveltime: an R package to calculate travel time across a landscape from user-specified locations. *Gates Open Res.* 2025;9:50. https://doi.org/10.12688/gatesopenres.16356.1
21. TravelTime. traveltimeR: interface to "Travel Time" API (R package) version 1.3.1. Comprehensive R Archive Network. 2025. Available at: https://cran.r-project.org/web/packages/traveltimeR/index.html. Accessed April 2026.
22. Mathis WS, Kahn PA, Tang S, Berenbrok LA, Hernandez I. Empirically-derived, locally responsive travel time thresholds for optimal geographic supermarket access using national commuting data. *J Transp Geogr.* 2024;118:103945. https://doi.org/10.1016/j.jtrangeo.2024.103945
23. Surveillance Epidemiology, and End Results Program. Census tract attributes. 2024. Available at: https://seer.cancer.gov/seerstat/variables/countyattribs/census-tract-attribs.html. Accessed September 2025.
24. US Dept of Agriculture. Poverty area measures—documentation. 2025. Available at: https://www.ers.usda.gov/data-products/poverty-area-measures/documentation. Accessed February 2026.
25. Baxter C, Park YM. Food swamp versus food desert: analysis of geographic disparities in obesity and diabetes in North Carolina using GIS and spatial regression. *Prof Geogr.* 2024;76(4):409–424. https://doi.org/10.1080/00330124.2024.2306642
26. Ver Ploeg M, Breneman V, Farrigan T, et al. Access to affordable and nutritious food: measuring and understanding food deserts and their consequences: report to Congress. US Dept of Agriculture. 2009. Available at: https://ers.usda.gov/sites/default/files/_laserfiche/publications/42711/12716_ap036_1_.pdf?v=36657. Accessed April 2026.
27. Leibtag ES. Where you shop matters: store formats drive variation in retail food prices. In: Amber waves: the economics of food, farming, natural resources, and rural America. AgEcon Search Waite Library, Dept. of Applied Economics, University of Minnesota, St. Paul. 2005:13–18. Available at: https://ageconsearch.umn.edu/record/127354/files/FeatureWhereYouShopNovember2005.pdf. Accessed April 2026.
28. Larsen K, Gilliland J. A farmers' market in a food desert: evaluating impacts on the price and availability of healthy food. *Health Place.* 2009;15(4):1158–1162. https://doi.org/10.1016/j.healthplace.2009.06.007
29. Ver Ploeg M, Breneman V, Dutko P, et al. Access to affordable and nutritious food: updated estimates of distance to supermarkets using 2010 data. 2012. Available at: https://www.ers.usda.gov/sites/default/files/_laserfiche/publications/45032/33845_err143.pdf?v=23542. Accessed April 2026.
30. US Dept of Agriculture Reinvestment Fund. About the Healthy Food Financing Initiative. 2026. Available at: https://www.investinginfood.com/about-hffi. Accessed February 2026.
31. Pennsylvania Dept of Agriculture. Apply for the PA Fresh Food Financing Initiative. 2026. Available at: https://www.pa.gov/services/pda/apply-for-the-pa-fresh-food-financing-initiative. Accessed February 2026.
32. US Dept of Agriculture. Healthy Food Financing Initiative. 2026. Available at: https://www.rd.usda.gov/about-rd/initiatives/healthy-food-financing-initiative. Accessed February 2026.
33. Richardson AS, Ghosh-Dastidar M, Beckman R, et al. Can the introduction of a full-service supermarket in a food desert improve residents' economic status and health? *Ann Epidemiol.* 2017;27(12):771–776. https://doi.org/10.1016/j.annepidem.2017.10.011
34. Nixon L, Mejia P, Dorfman L, et al. Fast-food fights: news coverage of local efforts to improve food environments through land-use regulations, 2001–2013 [erratum in: *Am J Public Health.* 2015;105(4):e10]. *Am J Public Health.* 2015;105(3):490–496. https://doi.org/10.2105/AJPH.2014.302368
35. Zhang D, Giabbanelli PJ, Arah OA, Zimmerman FJ. Impact of different policies on unhealthy dietary behaviors in an urban adult population: an agent-based simulation model. *Am J Public Health.* 2014;104(7):1217–1222. https://doi.org/10.2105/AJPH.2014.301934
36. Dutko P, Ver Ploeg M, Farrigan T. Characteristics and influential factors of food deserts. US Dept of Agriculture. 2012. Available at: https://ers.usda.gov/sites/default/files/_laserfiche/publications/45014/30940_err140.pdf. Accessed April 2026.
37. Morton LW, Blanchard TC. Starved for access: life in rural America's food deserts. *Rural Realities.* 2007;1(4):1–10.
38. National Equality Atlas. Car access: everyone needs reliable transportation access and in most American communities that means a car. 2022. Available at: https://nationalequityatlas.org/indicators/Car_access. Accessed February 2026.
39. Abdul Razak S, Atoloye AT, Antrum CJ, et al. Food swamps and transportation access: intersecting

structural determinants of food shopping and access in marginalized urban communities. *Int J Environ Res Public Health.* 2025;22(10):1481. https://doi.org/10.3390/ijerph22101481

40. Sisk A, Rappazzo K, Luben T, Fefferman N. Connecting people to food: a network approach to alleviating food deserts. *J Transp Health.* 2023;31:1–12. https://doi.org/10.1016/j.jth.2023.101627
41. National Aging and Disability Transportation Center. Best practices: access to healthy food. 2021. Available at: https://www.nadtc.org/wp-content/uploads/USAging-NADTC-Access-to-Healthy-Food-508.pdf. Accessed April 2026.
42. James P, Arcaya MC, Parker DM, Tucker-Seeley RD, Subramanian SV. Do minority and poor neighborhoods have higher access to fast-food restaurants in the United States? *Health Place.* 2014;29:10–17. https://doi.org/10.1016/j.healthplace.2014.04.011
43. Hurvitz PM, Moudon AV, Rehm CD, Streichert LC, Drewnowski A. Arterial roads and area socioeconomic status are predictors of fast food restaurant density in King County, WA. *Int J Behav Nutr Phys Act.* 2009;6(1):46. https://doi.org/10.1186/1479-5868-6-46
44. Capital One Shopping Research. Online grocery shopping statistics (2025): sales + growth rate. 2025. Available at: https://capitaloneshopping.com/research/online-grocery-shopping-statistics/?utm_source=chatgpt.com. Accessed February 2026.
45. Dunford EK, Miles DR, Popkin BM. Exploring disparities in the proportion of ultra-processed foods and beverages purchased in grocery stores by US households in 2020. *Public Health Nutr.* 2025;28(1):e85. https://doi.org/10.1017/S1368980025000606
46. Crosbie E, Gomes FS, Olvera J, Rincón-Gallardo Patiño S, Hoeper S, Carriedo A. A policy study on front-of-pack nutrition labeling in the Americas: emerging developments and outcomes. *Lancet Reg Health Am.* 2023;18:100400.
47. *Preventing Childhood Obesity: The Impact of Food Warning Labels.* Los Angeles, CA: UCLA Latino Policy and Politics Institute; 2023.
48. Glover B, Mao L, Hu Y, Zhang J. Enhancing the Retail Food Environment Index (RFEI) with neighborhood commuting patterns: a hybrid human–environment measure. *Int J Environ Res Public Health.* 2022;19(17):10798. https://doi.org/10.3390/ijerph191710798
49. George C, Tomer A. Delivering to deserts: New data reveals the geography of digital access to food in the US. Brookings. 2022. Available at: https://www.brookings.edu/articles/delivering-to-deserts-new-data-reveals-the-geography-of-digital-access-to-food-in-the-us. Accessed April 2026.
50. Haider Z, Hu Y, Charkhgard H, Himmelgreen D, Kwon C. Creating grocery delivery hubs for food deserts at local convenience stores via spatial and temporal consolidation. *Socioecon Plan Sci.* 2022;82:101301. https://doi.org/10.1016/j.seps.2022.101301

Ultraprocessed Food Versus Diet Quality in Relation to Cardiometabolic Health and All-Cause Mortality: NHANES 1999–2018

Juna Hatta-Langedyk, Lu Wang, PhD, Bingbing Fan, PhD, Peilin Shi, PhD, and Dariush Mozaffarian, MD, DrPH

See also Ultraprocessed Food, pp. 898–1029.

Objectives. To examine associations of ultraprocessed foods (UPFs, defined by Nova) with cardiometabolic risk factors, prevalent conditions, and mortality, before and after comprehensively adjusting for nutritional quality.

Methods. We analyzed data from 47 999 adults in the National Health and Nutrition Examination Survey (NHANES) 1999–2018. Survey-weighted, multivariable adjusted linear or logistic regression evaluated cross-sectional associations with risk factors and disease prevalence, and Cox models evaluated prospective associations with all-cause mortality. Models were compared before and after adjustment for each individual's Food Compass Score (i.FCS) to test independence from nutritional quality.

Results. Every 10% of energy supplied from UPFs was associated with higher body mass index, HbA1c, diastolic blood pressure, total-to-high-density lipoprotein cholesterol (HDL-C); lower HDL-C and low-density lipoprotein cholesterol (LDL-C); greater prevalence of metabolic syndrome (odds ratio [OR] = 1.07; 95% confidence interval [CI] = 1.05, 1.09), diabetes (OR = 1.03; 95% CI = 1.00, 1.07), and cancer (OR = 1.05; 95% CI = 1.02, 1.08); and higher risk of all-cause mortality (hazard ratio = 1.04; 95% CI = 1.02, 1.07). When we adjusted for i.FCS, associations were only partly attenuated, remaining significant. By comparison, adjustment for saturated fat, added sugar, or sodium had little effect. Findings were consistent in population subgroups, except for stronger associations among lower-income adults.

Conclusions. UPF consumption is associated with adverse risk factors, disease conditions, and all-cause mortality, only partly explained by nutritional quality. (*Am J Public Health*. 2026;116(7):1015–1024. https://doi.org/10.2105/AJPH.2026.308499)

AJPH July 2026, Vol. 116, No. 7

Ultraprocessed foods (UPFs) are characterized by industrial processes and additives uncommon in home cooking that alter shelf life, flavor, texture, fat content, or production costs.[1] The potential health risks of UPFs are drawing significant public and policy attention, based on growing evidence from observational studies and randomized controlled trials linking UPF consumption with adverse health outcomes.[2–6] With UPFs supplying approximately 53% of adults' and 62% of children's energy,[7] understanding health effects is critical.

Controversy exists over the independent relevance of ultraprocessing per se.[8] Observed harms may be attributable to poor nutritional profiles, notably saturated fat, sodium, and sugar, rather than processing itself. If so, renewed focus would be needed on such nutrients, and the concept of UPFs may be a distraction from effective clinical, public health, and policy efforts targeting nutrient goals. Conversely, other features of UPFs—such as loss of natural cell structure, reduced polyphenols and other bioactives, presence of industrial additives, and packaging contaminants[2]—could also produce harms not captured by traditional nutrient-focused metrics or policies.[2]

The nutritional profiles of UPFs are considered part of the mechanisms of harm, but whether processing itself has long-term harms, independent of major nutrients, remains unclear. Two randomized controlled trials found that UPFs increase short-term calorie consumption independent of major nutrient characteristics.[3,7] Understanding whether UPFs are linked to harms beyond nutritional characteristics is critical for informing research, clinical, and policy efforts to improve healthful eating and address diet-related diseases.[9]

We investigated the relationship of UPFs with cardiometabolic risk factors, prevalent disease conditions, and all-cause mortality in the National Health and Nutrition Examination Survey (NHANES), a nationally representative survey of US adults. We evaluated these associations with and without adjusting for diverse aspects of nutritional quality, comprehensively measured by a validated nutrient profiling score. We also explored UPF subtypes—sugar-sweetened beverages (SSBs), processed meats, and other UPFs—and population subgroups. We hypothesized that adjustment for nutrient quality would attenuate but not eliminate associations between UPFs and adverse outcomes.

METHODS

We analyzed 47 999 adults aged 20 to 85 years from 10 cycles of NHANES (1999–2000 to 2017–2018), a nationally representative survey of the noninstitutionalized US population.[10] The sample included all participants with 1 or more dietary recall, with no additional exclusion criteria. We evaluated all-cause and cause-specific mortality via National Death Index linkage through 2018 (81 participants excluded for missing National Death Index data).[11] We examined UPF associations with cardiometabolic risk factors and disease conditions cross-sectionally and, with mortality, prospectively.

Ultraprocessed Foods and Nutrient Quality

NHANES interviewers conducted dietary recalls using the Automated Multiple Pass Method. One 24-hour dietary recall was available for participants in the 1999–2002 cycles, and 2 were available for most participants from 2003 onward, which were averaged. Two investigators independently classified foods using the Nova system: unprocessed or minimally processed (group 1), culinary ingredients (group 2), processed foods (group 3), and UPFs (group 4).[12] Foods were defined as UPFs if they were industrial formulations using ingredients uncommon in home cooking (e.g., flavorings, colorings, emulsifiers, and other additives) or undergoing multiple processing stages. We also separated SSBs and ultraprocessed meats, which include preservatives other than sodium (e.g., nitrites) and are linked with adverse health outcomes.

We assessed nutritional quality using Food Compass 2.0, a comprehensive food rating system validated against healthy diet patterns, including the Healthy Eating Index, and health outcomes.[13] This system evaluates a broader range of nutritional attributes than most nutrient profiling systems and is energy-weighted, providing a standardized measure of food healthfulness. The algorithm scores foods and beverages from 1 (least healthy) to 100 (most healthy) based on 54 attributes across 9 domains (Table 1). To isolate nutritional quality independent of UPFs, we modified the Food Compass Score to remove Nova classification and artificial additives from the

TABLE 1— Food Compass 2.0 Attributes

Nutrient Ratios	Unsaturated-to-Saturated Fat Ratio, Fiber-to-Carbohydrate Ratio, Potassium-to-Sodium Ratio
Vitamins (top 5)	Vitamin A, thiamin (B1), riboflavin (B2), niacin (B3), vitamin B6, folate (B9), cobalamin (B12), vitamin C, vitamin D, vitamin E, vitamin K, choline
Minerals (top 5)	Calcium, phosphorus, magnesium, iron, zinc, copper, selenium, sodium, potassium, iodine
Food-based ingredients	Fruits, vegetables (nonstarchy), beans and legumes, whole grains, nuts and seeds, seafood, yogurt, plant oils, refined carbohydrates, red or processed meat
Additives[a]	Added sugar, nitrites, artificial sweeteners, flavors, or colors, partially hydrogenated oils, interesterified or hydrogenated oils, high fructose corn syrup, monosodium glutamate (MSG)
Processing[b]	Nova classification, fermentation, frying
Specific lipids (top 3) (0.5 weight)	α-Linolenic acid, eicosapentaenoic acid (EPA) and docosahexaenoic acid (DHA), medium-chain fatty acids, dietary cholesterol, trans fats
Fiber and protein (0.5 weight)	Total fiber, total protein
Phytochemicals (0.5 weight)	Total flavonoids, total carotenoids

[a]The additives domain was modified in this analysis to remove artificial additives including artificial sweeteners, flavors, or colors, partially hydrogenated oils, interesterified or hydrogenated oils, high fructose corn syrup, and monosodium glutamate (MSG).
[b]The processing domain was modified in this analysis to remove Nova classification.

processing domain. An individual-level Food Compass Score (i.FCS) was calculated from calorie-weighted scores of all foods and beverages consumed.[13]

Outcomes

Risk factors included body mass index (BMI; kg/m^2); systolic and diastolic blood pressure (BP; mm Hg); high-density lipoprotein cholesterol (HDL-C; mg/dL), low-density lipoprotein cholesterol (LDL-C; mg/dL), triglycerides (mg/dL), total-to-high-density lipoprotein cholesterol (HDL-C) ratio; and hemoglobin A1c (HbA1c; %) and fasting plasma glucose (mg/dL).[10] Prevalent disease conditions included the following: metabolic syndrome (≥ 3 criteria: waist circumference ≥ 88 cm [women] or 102 cm [men], triglycerides ≥ 150 mg/dL or on lipid-lowering medication, HDL-C < 50 mg/dL [women] or < 40 mg/dL [men] or on lipid-lowering medication, BP ≥ 130 mmHg systolic or ≥ 85 mmHg diastolic or on antihypertensive medication, and fasting plasma glucose ≥ 100 mg/dL or on diabetes medication)[14]; diabetes (HbA1c > 6.5%, fasting plasma glucose > 126 mg/dL, or diabetes medication)[15]; cardiovascular disease (CVD; self-reported coronary heart disease, heart failure, stroke, myocardial infarction, angina or use of angina, hypertension or lipid-lowering medication); cancer (self-reported); lung disease (self-reported history of emphysema, bronchitis, asthma, chronic obstructive pulmonary disease); optimal cardiometabolic health (defined by adiposity: (BMI < 25 kg/m^2 and waist circumference (WC) ≤ 88 cm [women]/ WC ≤ 102 cm [men]); blood glucose (fasting plasma glucose < 100 mg/dL and HbA1c < 5.7% without diabetes medication); blood lipids (total-to-HDL-C ratio < 3.5:1 without lipid-lowering medication); blood pressure (systolic BP < 120 mmHg, diastolic BP < 80 mmHg without antihypertensive medication); and history of CVD (no self-reported coronary heart disease, heart failure, myocardial infarction, stroke, or angina).[16] We assessed missing outcomes using Predictive Means Matching based on available predictors.[17,18]

Covariates

We assessed major demographic characteristics and lifestyle factors by standard NHANES methods, including age, gender, race/ethnicity, education, household income, smoking, alcohol use, and physical activity as Metabolic Equivalent of Task (MET)-hours per week.[10]

Statistical Analysis

We calculated descriptive statistics across quintiles of percentage of total energy (%E) consumed from UPFs, incorporating NHANES survey weight to generate nationally representative estimates.[19] In analyses of relationships with clinical risk factors, prevalent health conditions, and mortality, UPF consumption was evaluated per 10%E, and i.FCS was evaluated per standard deviation (SD; approximately 10 units). Survey-weighted linear regression with robust standard errors assessed associations of UPFs and i.FCS with continuous risk factors, and survey-weighted logistic regression with robust standard errors evaluated associations with prevalent health conditions. Cox proportional hazards assessed associations of UPFs and i.FCS with all-cause and cause-specific mortality, with study time as the time scale and time at risk calculated from the date of each participant's baseline dietary assessment until death or end of follow-up on December 31, 2019. We tested the proportional hazards assumption using Schoenfield residuals, and it was not violated.

We adjusted all models for age (years, years squared), gender, race and ethnicity (non-Hispanic White, non-Hispanic Black, Mexican American, Asian/other), education (< high school graduate, high school graduate, some college education [or associate degree], college graduate or more), household income (based on poverty-to-income ratio, continuous), smoking status (never, former, current), alcohol use (%E from alcohol), total physical activity (MET-hours per week), and prevalent diabetes (given evidence for reverse causation in sugar intake in this group). To assess effects independent of nutritional quality, we evaluated all risk estimates for UPFs with and without adjustment for i.FCS, calculating for each outcome the percent change and absolute change in the β coefficient for UPFs mediated through nutritional quality.[20] Additional models separately adjusted for added sugar (%E), saturated fat (%E), and sodium intake (mg/day).

In secondary analyses, we explored subcategories of UPF in relation to clinical risk factors, prevalent health conditions, and mortality risk, including SSBs, processed meats, and other UPFs (per 10%E), and population subgroups in relation to mortality risk, including by age (< 65, ≥ 65 years), gender, race (Asian/ other race, non-Hispanic Black, other Hispanic, Mexican American, non-Hispanic White), education (≤ high school, > high school), and income (at the median, lower [poverty-to-income ratio ≤ 2.15], higher [poverty-to-income ratio > 2.15]). To assess statistical significance of differences by subgroup, multiplicative interaction terms were added to each model to compute *P* values for interaction. We evaluated trends in consumption of these UPF subgroups over time across the survey cycles.

RESULTS

Among the included 47 999 US adults, those with higher UPF consumption were more likely to be younger, non-Hispanic White or Black, and a current smoker, and to have lower education and income, higher overall energy intake, and higher physical activity (Table 2).

Ultraprocessed Foods and Risk Factors

Higher UPF consumption was associated with major cardiometabolic risk factors, including (per 10%E) higher BMI (0.30 kg/m^2; 95% confidence interval [CI] = 0.26, 0.35), HbA1c (0.01%; 95% CI = 0.00, 0.01), diastolic BP (0.13 mmHg; 95% CI = 0.04, 0.22), and total-to-HDL-C ratio (0.02 units; 95% CI = 0.01, 0.03) and lower HDL-C (−0.53 mg/dL; 95% CI = −0.63, −0.42; Table 3). UPF consumption was not significantly associated with systolic BP, triglycerides, LDL-C, or fasting plasma glucose. When we evaluated prevalent diseases, UPF consumption was further associated with higher prevalence of metabolic syndrome (odds ratio [OR] = 1.07; 95% CI = 1.05, 1.09), diabetes (1.03; 95% CI = 1.00, 1.07), CVD (1.05; 95% CI = 1.02, 1.08), lung disease (1.07; 95% CI = 1.05, 1.09), and lower prevalence of optimal cardiometabolic health (0.93; 95% CI = 0.90, 0.96).

After further adjustment for i.FCS, many of these associations of UPFs were partly attenuated but remained significant (Table 3). For example, the association of UPFs with higher BMI was attenuated by 16.7%, diastolic BP by 84.6%, and HDL-C by 81.1%. Associations of UPFs with higher total-to-HDL-C ratio were actually reversed (−0.02 units; 95% CI = −0.03, −0.01), whereas an inverse association with LDL-C became apparent (−1.04 mg/dL; 95% CI = −1.40, −0.68). When we evaluated prevalent diseases, associations of UPFs with metabolic syndrome were attenuated by 27.9%, CVD by 39.4%, and lower optimal cardiometabolic health by 43.7%, whereas the association with diabetes was strengthened by 65.1%. No appreciable changes were observed for cancer or lung disease. Findings were similar in posthoc sensitivity analyses excluding individuals with prevalent diabetes (Table A, available as a supplement to the online version of this article at http://www.ajph.org).

Ultraprocessed Foods and Mortality

During 20.8 years of follow-up, 7481 deaths occurred, including 2619 from cardiometabolic disease and 1691 from cancer. Each 10% greater UPF consumption was prospectively associated with a 4% higher risk of all-cause mortality (hazard ratio [HR] = 1.04; 95% CI = 1.02, 1.07; Table 4). After adjustment for i.FCS, the relationship of UPF consumption with total mortality was attenuated by 24.6% but remained significant (1.03; 95% CI = 1.00, 1.05). Cause-specific associations were directionally similar but not statistically significant.

Saturated Fat, Added Sugar, and Sodium

In analyses evaluating saturated fat, added sugar, and sodium as potential mediators of the associations between UPFs and each outcome, little consistent attenuation was observed (Table B). Adjustment for added sugar (%E) attenuated UPF associations with diastolic BP, HDL-C, CVD, cancer, and lung disease; strengthened associations with BMI, systolic BP, triglycerides, LDL-C, fasting plasma glucose, and diabetes; and reversed associations with the total-to-HDL ratio. Adjustment for saturated fat attenuated UPF associations with BMI, systolic BP, diastolic BP, fasting plasma glucose, and diabetes; and strengthened associations with LDL-C and HDL-C. Generally, most associations remained statistically significant even following attenuation. Adjustment for sodium (mg/day) attenuated UPF associations with systolic BP, LDL-C, and fasting plasma glucose. UPF associations with all-cause mortality were only slightly attenuated after adjusting for added sugar, were unchanged after adjusting for saturated fat, and were slightly strengthened after adjusting for sodium.

Ultraprocessed Food Subgroups

SSB consumption (per 10%) positively associated with BMI (0.34 kg/m^2; 95% CI = 0.22, 0.46), systolic BP (0.35 mmHg; 95% CI = 0.12, 0.59), diastolic BP (0.40 mmHg; 95% CI = 0.21, 0.60), LDL-C (1.05 mg/dL; 95% CI = 0.34, 1.76), and the total-to-HDL-C ratio (0.14 units; 95% CI = 0.12, 0.16), and inversely with HDL-C (−1.79 mg/dL; 95% CI = −2.01, −1.58; Table C). SSB consumption also was associated with higher prevalence of metabolic syndrome (OR = 1.14; 95% CI = 1.10, 1.19), CVD (1.13; 95% CI = 1.06, 1.20), cancer (1.10; 95% CI = 1.04, 1.17), and lung disease (1.10; 95% CI = 1.07, 1.16), and

TABLE 2— Characteristics of 47 999 US Adults Aged 20 Years and Older According to Quintiles of Ultraprocessed Food (UPF) Consumption: National Health and Nutrition Examination Survey (NHANES), 1999–2018

	Unweighted No. (Weighted %)[a] or Mean ±SD				
	Quintile 1[b] (n = 9600)	Quintile 2[b] (n = 9600)	Quintile 3[b] (n = 9600)	Quintile 4[b] (n = 9600)	Quintile 5[b] (n = 9599)
Age group, y					
20–34	2006 (23.8)	2179 (24.6)	2290 (25.2)	2566 (27.7)	3438 (37.0)
35–49	2360 (27.9)	2345 (28.4)	2415 (28.6)	2380 (28.2)	2457 (27.8)
50–64	2618 (28.4)	2448 (26.2)	2339 (26.1)	2305 (25.1)	1998 (22.3)
≥ 65	2616 (20.0)	2628 (20.8)	2556 (20.1)	2349 (19.0)	1706 (12.9)
Gender					
Male	4710 (49.2)	4542 (46.7)	4594 (47.8)	4662 (48.2)	4521 (47.0)
Female	4890 (50.8)	5058 (53.3)	5006 (52.2)	4938 (51.8)	5078 (53.0)
Race/ethnicity					
Asian/other	1740 (14.8)	798 (6.4)	586 (5.1)	510 (4.5)	486 (4.5)
Non-Hispanic Black	1619 (10.0)	1742 (9.4)	1938 (10.4)	2116 (11.3)	2547 (14.0)
Mexican American	1792 (8.3)	2028 (9.7)	1895 (9.1)	1592 (7.9)	1112 (6.2)
Other Hispanics	1316 (9.5)	889 (6.1)	693 (4.9)	555 (4.0)	455 (3.2)
Non-Hispanic White	3133 (57.4)	4143 (68.5)	4488 (70.4)	4827 (72.4)	4999 (72.1)
Education level					
< HS graduate	3045 (19.7)	2621 (16.6)	2520 (16.4)	2379 (16.2)	2204 (16.5)
HS graduate	1782 (19.5)	2009 (20.9)	2241 (23.7)	2377 (25.4)	2729 (29.6)
Some college	2235 (26.4)	2622 (30.9)	2706 (30.3)	2933 (32.5)	3161 (34.7)
≥ College graduate	2538 (34.5)	2348 (31.6)	2133 (29.6)	1911 (25.8)	1505 (19.3)
Ratio of family income to poverty[c]					
< 1.30	3124 (23.0)	2683 (19.1)	2792 (20.2)	2834 (20.9)	3301 (26.5)
1.30–2.49	2898 (27.2)	3095 (28.1)	3080 (28.5)	3103 (28.7)	3208 (31.1)
≥ 2.50	3578 (49.7)	3822 (52.8)	3728 (51.3)	3663 (50.4)	3090 (42.4)
Smoking status					
Never	5549 (55.5)	5442 (55.4)	5239 (54.5)	5000 (52.3)	4837 (51.0)
Former	2404 (25.9)	2486 (25.9)	2568 (26.9)	2482 (25.4)	2099 (21.4)
Current	1647 (18.6)	1672 (18.7)	1793 (18.6)	2118 (22.3)	2663 (27.6)
Total energy intake, kcal/d	1966.2 ±801.6	2065.1 ±791.5	2093.8 ±784.1	2158.1 ±807.5	2140.2 ±815.6
Alcohol intake, %E	4.6 ±8.2	3.3 ±6.1	2.6 ±5.6	2.1 ±5.0	1.6 ±5.0
Physical activity, MET-hours/week	60.5 ±97.3	60.8 ±100.4	61.2 ±103.2	63.5 ±104.3	67.9 ±110.9

Note. HS = high school; MET = metabolic equivalent of task; %E = percentage of total energy intake.

[a]Data are presented as unweighted no. (NHANES survey weighted %) for categorical variables and mean ±SD for continuous variables. All estimates were calculated using NHANES dietary sample weights to be representative of the noninstitutionalized US adult population aged 20 years and older from 1999 to 2018.

[b]Quintiles of UPF consumption were defined based on the percentage of total daily energy (%E) from UPFs. The ranges for each quintile were as follows: quintile 1 = 0–37.3%E; quintile 2 = 37.3–48.6%E; quintile 3 = 48.6–57.9%E; quintile 4 = 57.9–68.5%E; quintile 5 = 68.5–100%E.

[c]Represents the ratio of family income to the federal poverty threshold (according to US Census), adjusting for household size.

TABLE 3— Association of Ultraprocessed Food (UPF) Consumption With Risk Factors and Disease Outcomes Among 47 999 Adults: National Health and Nutrition Examination Survey (NHANES), 1999–2018

	Multivariable-Adjusted Association of UPF, per 10%E (95% CI)[a]	Association of UPF After Further Adjustment for i.FCS (95% CI)[b]	% Change in the Association[c]	Absolute Unit Change in the Association[c]
Cardiometabolic risk factors (difference)				
BMI, kg/m^2	0.30 (0.26, 0.35)	0.25 (0.20, 0.31)	−16.7	−0.05
Systolic BP, mmHg	0.09 (−0.02, 0.20)	−0.05 (−0.17, 0.07)	−155.6	−0.14
Diastolic BP, mmHg	0.13 (0.04, 0.22)	0.02 (−0.08, 0.12)	−84.6	−0.11
Triglycerides, mg/dL	−0.19 (−1.10, 0.72)	−0.71 (−1.71, 0.28)	+237.7	−0.52
LDL-C, mg/dL	−0.20 (−0.53, 0.12)	−1.04 (−1.40, −0.68)	+420.0	−0.84
HDL-C, mg/dL	−0.53 (−0.63, −0.42)	−0.10 (−0.22, 0.02)	−81.1	+0.43
Total-to-HDL-C ratio, 1 unit	0.02 (0.01, 0.03)	−0.02 (−0.03, −0.01)	−200.0	−0.04
HbA1c, %	0.01 (0.00, 0.01)	0.01 (0.00, 0.01)	0.0	0.00
Fasting plasma glucose, mg/dL	0.16 (−0.01, 0.33)	0.14 (−0.05, 0.33)	−12.5	−0.02
Prevalent conditions (odds ratio)				
Metabolic syndrome	1.07 (1.05, 1.09)	1.05 (1.03, 1.07)	−27.9	N/A
Diabetes	1.03 (1.00, 1.07)	1.05 (1.01, 1.09)	+65.1	N/A
Cardiovascular disease	1.05 (1.02, 1.08)	1.03 (1.00, 1.06)	−39.4	N/A
Cancer	1.05 (1.02, 1.08)	1.05 (1.01, 1.08)	0.0	N/A
Lung disease	1.07 (1.05, 1.09)	1.07 (1.04, 1.09)	0.0	N/A
Optimal cardiometabolic health	0.93 (0.90, 0.96)	0.96 (0.93, 1.00)	−43.7	N/A

Note. BMI = body mass index; BP = blood pressure; CI = confidence interval; HbA1c = hemoglobin A1c; HDL-C = high-density lipoprotein cholesterol; i.FCS = individual Food Compass Score; LDL-C = low-density lipoprotein cholesterol; N/A = not applicable; %E = percentage of total energy intake.

[a]Based on multivariable-adjusted linear (or logistic regression models, using NHANES dietary sample weights to provide effect estimates (or odds ratios) for a nationally representative noninstitutionalized US population. All models were adjusted for age (years), gender, race/ethnicity (Asian/other race, non-Hispanic Black, other Hispanic, Mexican American, non-Hispanic White), education level (< high school graduate, high school graduate, some college or associates degree, ≥ college graduate), income (poverty: income ratio), smoking status (nonsmoker, former smoker, current smoker), total physical activity (Metabolic Equivalent of Task [MET]-hours/week), alcohol use (%energy), and self-reported diabetes (yes, no; except for analyses of diabetes as an outcome).

[b]Including additional adjustment for i.FCS as a continuous variable.

[c]Percent change calculated from the β coefficients (from linear regression or the natural log of odds ratio from logistic regression) using the formula $(\beta_{after} - \beta_{before})/\beta_{before}$. Absolute unit change for continuous risk factors calculated by subtracting these coefficients.

lower prevalence of optimal cardiometabolic health (0.86; 95% CI = 0.71, 0.92). After adjustment for i.FCS, these associations were attenuated by 20.6% for BMI, 68.6% for systolic BP, 45% for diastolic BP, 38% for HDL-C, 50% for total-to-HDL-C ratio, 20.4% for metabolic syndrome, 22% for cardiovascular disease, 0% for lung disease, and 44.7% for optimal cardiometabolic health. Associations of SSBs with LDL-C were reversed after adjusting for i.FCS.

Processed meat consumption (per 10%) was positively associated with BMI (0.82 kg/m^2; 95% CI = 0.37, 1.00), systolic BP (0.60 mmHg; 95% CI = 0.22, 0.98), diastolic BP (0.47 mmHg; 95% CI = 0.20, 0.75), fasting plasma glucose (0.55 mg/dL; 95% CI = 0.01, 1.09), metabolic syndrome (1.17; 95% CI = 1.11, 1.23), and diabetes (1.14; 95% CI = 1.04, 1.25), and inversely associated with optimal cardiometabolic health (0.81; 95% CI = 0.71, 0.92; Table C). Adjusting for i.FCS attenuated these associations by 6.1% for BMI, 25% for systolic BP, 23.4% for diastolic BP, 5.5% for fasting plasma glucose, 11% for metabolic syndrome, and 17.3% for optimal cardiometabolic health. Associations with diabetes were unchanged after adjusting for i.FCS.

Other UPF consumption (per 10%) was positively associated with BMI (0.24 kg/m^2; 95% CI = 0.19, 0.29), HbA1c (0.01%; 95% CI = 0.00, 0.02), metabolic

TABLE 4— Association of Ultraprocessed Food (UPF) Consumption With Mortality Among 47 918 Adults: National Health and Nutrition Examination Survey (NHANES), 1999–2018

Outcomes	Multivariable-Adjusted Association of UPF per 10%E,[a] HR (95% CI)[b]	Association of UPF After Further Adjustment for i.FCS,[c] HR (95% CI)[b]	% Change in the Association (β Coefficient)[d]
All-cause mortality (n = 7481 events)	1.04 (1.02, 1.07)	1.03 (1.00, 1.05)	−24.6
Cardiometabolic mortality (n = 2619 events)	1.03 (0.99, 1.07)	1.02 (0.98, 1.06)	−33.0
Cancer mortality (n = 1691 events)	1.03 (0.98, 1.07)	1.00 (0.96, 1.05)	−100.0

Note. i.FCS = individual Food Compass Score; %E = percentage of total energy intake.

[a]All models were adjusted for age (years), age squared (years), gender, race/ethnicity (Asian/other race, non-Hispanic Black, other Hispanic, Mexican American, non-Hispanic White), education level (< high school graduate, high school graduate, some college or associates degree, ≥ college graduate), income (poverty: income ratio), smoking status (nonsmoker, former smoker, current smoker), total physical activity (Metabolic Equivalent of Task [MET]-hours/week), alcohol use (%energy), and self-reported diabetes (yes, no; except for analyses of diabetes as an outcome).

[b]HRs (hazard ratios) and 95% CIs (confidence intervals) were estimated by using multivariable Cox proportional hazards models. NHANES dietary sample weights were incorporated in the models to provide hazard ratios for a nationally representative noninstitutionalized US population.

[c]Including additional adjustment for i.FCS as a continuous variable.

[d]Percent change calculated from the β coefficients (from the natural log of hazard ratio from Cox proportional hazards models) using the formula $(\beta_{after}-\beta_{before})/\beta_{before}$.

syndrome (1.05; 95% CI = 1.03, 1.07), CVD (1.04; 95% CI = 1.01, 1.07), cancer (1.05; 95% CI = 1.01, 1.08), and lung disease (1.06; 95% CI = 1.04, 1.09), and inversely associated with LDL-C (−0.55 mmHg; 95% CI = −0.90, 0.20), HDL-C (−0.28 mmHg; 95% CI = −0.39, 0.17) and optimal cardiometabolic health (0.96; 95% CI = 0.92, 0.99). These associations were only partly attenuated after adjusting for i.FCS, including 12.5% attenuation for BMI and 92.9% attenuation for HDL-C. Associations were strengthened by 109.1% for LDL-C and 200% for the total-to-HDL-C ratio, and unchanged for HbA1c after adjusting for i.FCS (Table C).

In prospective assessment of mortality, other UPFs (1.03; 95% CI = 1.01, 1.06) and SSBs (1.16; 95% CI = 1.09, 1.23) each were positively associated with all-cause mortality; Table C). SSBs also were positively associated with cardiometabolic disease-specific (1.11; 95% CI = 1.02, 1.21) and cancer-specific (1.18; 95% CI = 1.06, 1.30) mortality. Processed meats were not significantly associated with all-cause or cause-specific mortality. Adjusting for i.FCS only partly attenuated associations for other UPFs and SSBs with all-cause mortality, with 33% and 17.7% attenuations, respectively. SSB association was attenuated by 8.7% for cardiometabolic-disease specific mortality and 15.6% for cancer-specific mortality after adjusting for i.FCS.

When we evaluated trends in UPF subgroups over time, consumption of ultraprocessed sweet snacks and sweets, savory snacks, ready-to-eat or ready-to-heat mixed dishes, animal-based products, whole-grain foods, and dairy foods increased, whereas ultraprocessed SSBs, refined grain foods, vegetables and beans, fats and oils, condiments, and sauces decreased; Figure A).

Population Subgroups

The relationships of UPFs with all-cause mortality, and the partial attenuation after adjustment for i.FCS, were similar in all population groups except by household income (*P* interaction = .005; Figure B). A positive association between UPFs and mortality was observed among lower-income adults (1.07; 95% CI = 1.04, 1.11), but not higher-income adults (1.02; 95% CI = 0.98, 1.05), and little attenuation occurred among lower income adults after adjustment for i.FCS (13.9%).

DISCUSSION

UPF consumption was associated with adverse cardiometabolic risk profiles, greater chronic disease prevalence, and higher all-cause mortality. After adjustment for the nutritional quality (i.FCS), many associations were attenuated, but generally only partly, suggesting that common nutritional metrics explain only part of the observed harms. Adjustment for saturated fat, added sugar, and sodium had little effect, suggesting these are not key mediators. SSBs, processed meats, and other UPFs associated with cardiometabolic risk factors and conditions; SSBs and other UPFs were also associated with all-cause mortality. Findings were generally consistent across most demographic subgroups, except income: associations of UPFs with mortality were stronger, and largely unaffected by adjustment for nutritional quality, among lower-income adults.

The adverse health effects of UPFs may operate through multiple mechanisms. Evidence from observational, animal, in vitro, and human studies have raised concerns about the adverse features of UPFs, including harmful nutrients like starch, sugar, and salt; loss of fiber, polyphenols, and other bioactives; loss of natural food structure, speeding digestion in the stomach and small intestine and reducing nourishment to the gut microbiome; the harms of certain additives like specific sweeteners, flavorings, colorants, emulsifiers, or preservatives; introduction of toxins like furans, heterocyclic amines, polycyclic aromatic hydrocarbons, or acrylamide; and packaging contaminants such as phthalates, bisphenols, mineral oils, or microplastics.[2,7] Combinations of relevant pathways can vary across UPF products, but the Nova classification suggests that processing confers risk beyond nutrients.

Our new findings support this concept. Food Compass includes types of fat, carbohydrate and added sugar, fiber, protein, vitamins, minerals, sodium, omega 3's and other trace lipids, and even certain bioactives such as carotenoids and polyphenols. Food Compass also incorporates food-based ingredients (e.g., quantities of fruits, vegetables, nuts, fish) and other aspects of processing that do not qualify as UPFs (e.g., fermentation). Adjustment for these features only partly attenuated most of the observed associations. Our results are consistent with short-term randomized controlled trials demonstrating that UPF diets increase energy intake and body weight compared with unprocessed diets, despite being matched for macronutrients, fiber, sugar, and sodium.[3]

At least 20 US states have passed or proposed bills addressing different aspects of UPFs, using varying definitions, from bans or warning labels on certain additives to restrictions on UPFs in school meals. Laws or bills in Alabama, Arizona, Arkansas, Connecticut, Florida, Kentucky, Louisiana, Maryland, Missouri, New Jersey, North Carolina, South Carolina, Texas, and West Virginia focus on a small number of specific food or color additives, which may fail to capture most UPFs. Other states, such as Pennsylvania and Massachusetts, have proposed—but not yet passed—broader definitions consistent with Nova: industrial formulations containing cosmetic, functional, or technical additives uncommon in home kitchens. In October 2025, California passed a definition of UPFs with 2 required criteria: (1) the presence of industrial ingredients with cosmetic, technical, or functional effects,[21] similar to criteria in Pennsylvania[22] and Massachusetts,[23] and (2) a requirement for minimum levels of sodium, added sugar, or saturated fat. The latter criterion creates a loophole, excluding many current and future UPF formulations that meet the thresholds for the 3 targeted nutrients but still have adverse characteristics. Our findings that saturated fat, added sugar, and sodium generally have little influence on the associations of UPFs with adverse health outcomes suggest that policies defining and addressing UPFs should not include these nutrients as additional criteria.

No current states have included nitrite preservatives, widely used in processed meats, as part of the UPF definition. We found that processed meat consumption was associated with greater BMI, higher BP and glucose levels, metabolic syndrome, and diabetes, and less optimal cardiometabolic health, but not with all-cause mortality.

The current administration recently released the MAHA Strategy to address chronic disease in youths, which included several plans related to UPFs.[24] This included plans to develop a federal definition of UPFs, enabling coherent standards across labeling, marketing, procurement, and research. In July 2025, the Food and Drug Administration (FDA) and Department of Agriculture jointly released a public Request for Information on this topic. In addition, the strategy includes plans to reform the FDA's "Generally Recognized as Safe" pathway, which allows industrial ingredients to enter the food supply through self-affirmed safety determinations by manufacturers.[25] Our new findings support the need to consider UPFs separately from conventional nutritional criteria. The recently published 2025 Dietary Guidelines for Americans has also included recommendations discouraging consumption of highly processed foods.

Our observation that associations with mortality were strongest among lower-income adults was not expected and requires further evaluation in other studies. UPFs exhibit considerable heterogeneity, and it is plausible that lower-income Americans consume UPFs with more adverse features than higher-income Americans do because of challenges around cost, access, knowledge, time to shop and cook, health and nutrition literacy, and more.[26]

Our findings in a nationally representative US population align with findings from large-scale prospective cohorts in other populations (NutriNet-Santé, Moli-Sani, Seguimiento Universidad de Navarra [SUN], Framingham, National Institutes of Health–AARP).[5,27–29] Across multiple large cohorts, associations between high UPF intake and increased risks for all-cause mortality, CVD, and type-2 diabetes largely persisted after adjusting for the overall nutritional quality (e.g., via Programme National Nutrition Santé—Guidelines Score, Healthy Eating Index–2015, Modified Food Standard Agency–Nutrient Profiling System, or Mediterranean diet adherence) or selected nutrients or indices such as energy density, carbohydrates, protein, total fat, fiber, saturated fat, and sodium. For example, although these adjustments sometimes attenuated the risk estimates (e.g., SUN type 2 diabetes HR from 1.65 to 1.50; NutriNet-Santé CVD HR from 1.13 to 1.11), the associations were not eliminated, and in several cases were not materially altered (e.g., Moli-Sani mortality HR from 1.19 to 1.20; Framingham mortality remains HR = 1.09).[5,27–29] Our new findings build upon these limited prior results by using a comprehensive validated nutritional profiling score in a large, nationally representative population, evaluating risk factors, prevalent disease, and all-cause mortality.

Strengths and Limitations

The large study population of nearly 50 000 adults provided statistical power to test associations. The use of 24-hour recalls provided product-specific assessment of UPFs and nutritional quality compared with food frequency questionnaires, which only assess broad food categories. NHANES includes a range of well-measured sociodemographic, dietary, lifestyle, and outcome data, reducing measurement error and increasing the ability to adjust for confounding factors.

Although repeated 24-hour recalls are a gold standard approach for assessing population dietary consumption, individuals' intakes may be partly misclassified because of diet variation over time, which would attenuate associations. Processed foods may be more commonly misreported in dietary recalls than minimally processed foods.[13] Associations with risk factors and prevalent diseases were cross-sectional, subject to reverse causation; however, the findings were broadly consistent in prospective analyses of all-cause mortality. These findings are observational, and residual confounding cannot be excluded.

Public Health Implications

UPFs constitute a substantial portion of the American diet, accounting for more than 50% of adult and about 60% of child caloric intake.[7] The observed associations, such as a 0.3-unit difference in BMI and 4% higher risk of all-cause mortality, therefore translate into meaningful estimated public health burdens when considered at the population level. These findings emphasize the value of incorporating more unprocessed and minimally processed foods into the diet and limiting UPF intake. Efforts to improve overall nutritional quality among both individuals and communities, including reducing UPFs, can contribute to chronic disease prevention and help alleviate health care costs. Addressing structural and policy-related barriers to accessing healthier foods remains critical for promoting equitable dietary improvements across populations. AJPH

ABOUT THE AUTHORS

Juna Hatta-Langedyk, Lu Wang, Bingbing Fan, Peilin Shi, and Dariush Mozaffarian are with the Friedman School of Nutrition Science and Policy, Tufts University, Boston, MA. Juna Hatta-Langedyk is also with the Department of Biology, Tufts University, Medford, MA. Dariush Mozaffarian is also with the Division of Cardiology, Tufts Medical Center, Boston, MA.

CORRESPONDENCE

Correspondence should be sent to Juna Hatta-Langedyk (e-mail: juna.hatta_langedyk@tufts.edu). Reprints can be ordered at https://www.ajph.org by clicking the "Reprints" link.

PUBLICATION INFORMATION

Full Citation: Hatta-Langedyk J, Wang L, Fan B, Shi P, Mozaffarian D. Ultraprocessed food versus diet quality in relation to cardiometabolic health and all-cause mortality: NHANES 1999–2018. *Am J Public Health*. 2026;116(7):1015–1024.

Acceptance Date: February 13, 2026.

DOI: https://doi.org/10.2105/AJPH.2026.308499

ORCID iDs:

Juna Hatta-Langedyk https://orcid.org/0009-0006-9330-6077

Dariush Mozaffarian https://orcid.org/0000-0001-7958-9492

CONTRIBUTORS

D. Mozaffarian conceptualized and supervised the study. J. Hatta-Langedyk did the statistical analyses and wrote the first draft of the manuscript. L. Wang, B. Fan, and J. Hatta-Langedyk interpreted the data. L. Wang and P. Shi acquired the data. L. Wang and D. Mozaffarian critically reviewed the manuscript for intellectual content. J. Hatta-Langedyk, L. Wang, and D. Mozaffarian drafted the manuscript.

ACKNOWLEDGMENTS

This study was supported by funding from the National Institutes of Health (R01HL115189; principal investigator: D. Mozaffarian). L. Wang was supported by American Diabetes Association's Pathway to Stop Diabetes Award (1-24-INI-04). J. Hatta-Langedyk was supported by the Laidlaw Foundation's Laidlaw Scholars Program.

CONFLICTS OF INTEREST

D. Mozaffarian reports service on scientific advisory boards for Beren Therapeutics, Brightseed, Calibrate, Elysium Health, Filtricine, HumanCo, Instacart Health, January Inc, WndrHLTH; scientific consulting for Amazon Health; equity in Calibrate and HumanCo; and chapter royalties from UpToDate. All other authors declare no conflict of interests.

HUMAN PARTICIPANT PROTECTION

The Tufts University institutional review board exempted this investigation from human participant review because it was based on nationally representative, de-identified data sets.

REFERENCES

1. Monteiro CA, Cannon G, Levy RB, et al. Ultra-processed foods: what they are and how to identify them. *Public Health Nutr.* 2019;22(5):936–1023. https://doi.org/10.1017/S1368980018003762

2. Touvier M, da Costa Louzada ML, Mozaffarian D, Baker P, Juul F, Srour B. Ultra-processed foods and cardiometabolic health: public health policies to reduce consumption cannot wait. *BMJ.* 2023;383:e075294. https://doi.org/10.1136/bmj-2023-075294

3. Hall KD, Ayuketah A, Brychta R, et al. Ultra-processed diets cause excess calorie intake and weight gain: an inpatient randomized controlled trial of ad libitum food intake. *Cell Metab.* 2019; 30(1):67–77.e63. https://doi.org/10.1016/j.cmet.2019.05.008

4. Wang L, Du M, Wang K, et al. Association of ultra-processed food consumption with colorectal cancer risk among men and women: results from three prospective US cohort studies. *BMJ.* 2022;378:e068921. https://doi.org/10.1136/bmj-2021-068921

5. Bonaccio M, Di Castelnuovo A, Ruggiero E, et al. Joint association of food nutritional profile by Nutri-Score front-of-pack label and ultra-processed food intake with mortality: Moli-Sani Prospective Cohort Study. *BMJ.* 2022;378:e070688. https://doi.org/10.1136/bmj-2022-070688

6. Wang L, Steele EM, Du M, et al. Association between ultraprocessed food consumption and mortality among US adults: Prospective Cohort Study of the National Health and Nutrition Examination Survey, 2003–2008. *J Acad Nutr Diet.* 2025;125(7):875–887.e7. https://doi.org/10.1016/j.jand.2024.11.014

7. Hamano S, Sawada M, Aihara M, et al. Ultra-processed foods cause weight gain and increased energy intake associated with reduced chewing frequency: a randomized, open-label, crossover study. *Diabetes Obes Metab.* 2024; 26(11):5431–5443. https://doi.org/10.1111/dom.15922

8. Scientific Advisory Committee on Nutrition. Processed foods and health: rapid evidence update. GOV.UK. 2025. Available at: https://www.gov.uk/government/publications/processed-foods-and-health-sacns-rapid-evidence-update. Accessed October 11, 2025.

9. Dietary Guidelines Advisory Committee. *Scientific Report of the 2025 Dietary Guidelines Advisory Committee: Advisory Report to the Secretary of Health and Human Services and Secretary of Agriculture.* Washington, DC: US Dept of Agriculture; 2024.

10. Zipf G, Chiappa M, Porter KS, et al. National Health and Nutrition Examination Survey: plan and operations, 1999–2010. *Vital Health Stat 1.* 2013;1(56):1–37.

11. *The Linkage of National Center for Health Statistics Survey Data to the National Death Index–2019 Linked Mortality File (LMF): Linkage Methodology and Analytic Considerations, June 2022.* Hyattsville, MD: National Center for Health Statistics; 2022.

12. Williams AM, Couch CA, Emmerich SD, Ogburn DF. Ultra-processed food consumption in youth and adults: United States, August 2021–August 2023. *NCHS Data Brief.* 2025;536(536):1–11. https://doi.org/10.15620/cdc/174612

13. Barrett EM, Shi P, Blumberg JB, O'Hearn M, Micha R, Mozaffarian D. Food Compass 2.0 is an improved nutrient profiling system to characterize healthfulness of foods and beverages. *Nat Food.* 2024;5(11):911–915. https://doi.org/10.1038/s43016-024-01053-3

14. Grundy SM, Cleeman JI, Daniels SR, et al. Diagnosis and management of the metabolic syndrome: an American Heart Association/National Heart, Lung, and Blood Institute scientific statement. *Circulation.* 2005;112(17):2735–2752. https://doi.org/10.1161/circulationaha.105.169404

15. American Diabetes Association. 2. Classification and Diagnosis of Diabetes: Standards of Care in Diabetes—2024. *Diabetes Care.* 2024;47(suppl 1): S20–S42. https://doi.org/10.2337/dc24-S002

16. Lloyd-Jones DM, Hong Y, Labarthe D, et al. Defining and setting national goals for cardiovascular health promotion and disease reduction: the American Heart Association's strategic impact goal through 2020 and beyond. *Circulation.* 2010;121(4):586–613. https://doi.org/10.1161/circulationaha.109.192703

17. Rubin DB. Statistical matching using file concatenation with adjusted weights and multiple imputations. *J Bus Econ Stat.* 1986;4(1):87–94. https://doi.org/10.1080/07350015.1986.10509497

18. Little RJA. Missing-data adjustments in large surveys. *J Bus Econ Stat.* 1988;6(3):287–296. https://doi.org/10.1080/07350015.1988.10509663

19. Chen TC, Clark J, Riddles MK, Mohadjer LK, Fakhouri THI. National Health and Nutrition Examination Survey, 2015 – 2018: sample design and estimation procedures. *Vital Health Stat 2.* 2020;2(184):1–35.

20. Nevo D, Liao X, Spiegelman D. Estimation and inference for the mediation proportion. *Int J Biostat.* 2017;13(2). https://doi.org/10.1515/ijb-2017-0006

21. California State Legislature. AB 1264 (2025). Available at: https://leginfo.legislature.ca.gov/faces/billNavClient.xhtml?bill_id=202520260AB1264. Accessed October 20, 2025.

22. Pennsylvania General Assembly. House Bill 1132 (2025–2026 legislative session). Available at: https://www.palegis.us/legislation/bills/2025/hb1132. Accessed October 20, 2025.

23. Massachusetts General Court. Bill H.4562 (2025–2026 legislative session). Available at: https://malegislature.gov/Bills/194/H4562. Accessed October 20, 2025.

24. *Make Our Children Healthy Again Strategy Report.* Washington, DC: MAHA Commission; 2025.

25. Pomeranz JL, Broad Leib EM, Mozaffarian D. Regulation of added substances in the food supply by the Food and Drug Administration Human Foods Program. *Am J Public Health.* 2024;114(10): 1061–1070. https://doi.org/10.2105/AJPH.2024.307755

26. Craig HC, Sharib JR, Ridberg R, et al. Development and validation of a brief Nutrition Security Screener (NSS) for clinical and public health settings. *Am J Clin Nutr.* 2025;122(6):1689–1700. https://doi.org/10.1016/j.ajcnut.2025.08.017

27. Schnabel L, Kesse-Guyot E, Alles B, et al. Association between ultraprocessed food consumption and risk of mortality among middle-aged adults in France. *JAMA Intern Med.* 2019;179(4):490–498. https://doi.org/10.1001/jamainternmed.2018.7289

28. Juul F, Vaidean G, Lin Y, Deierlein AL, Parekh N. Ultra-processed foods and incident cardiovascular disease in the Framingham Offspring Study. *J Am Coll Cardiol.* 2021;77(12):1520–1531. https://doi.org/10.1016/j.jacc.2021.01.047

29. Llavero-Valero M, Escalada-San Martín J, Martínez-González MA, Basterra-Gortari FJ, de la Fuente-Arrillaga C, Bes-Rastrollo M. Ultra-processed foods and type-2 diabetes risk in the SUN project: a prospective cohort study. *Clin Nutr.* 2021;40(5): 2817–2824. https://doi.org/10.1016/j.clnu.2021.03.039

Operationally Defining and Targeting Ultraprocessed Foods: Insights From US Policy Proposals

Aline D'Angelo Campos, PhD, MPP, James W. Krieger, MD, MPH, Carmen E. Prestemon, BSPH, Bridget A. Hollingsworth, MPH, RD, and Lindsey Smith Taillie, PhD, MPH

See also Ultraprocessed Food, pp. 898–1029.

Objectives. To examine operational ultraprocessed food (UPF) definitions and policy scope in existing US policy proposals.

Methods. We conducted a search for federal and state policy proposals targeting UPFs through December 2025.

Results. We identified 43 proposals targeting UPFs between 2021 and 2025. Most (93%) hailed from states. About a third (35%) defined UPFs by listing narrow sets of specific food additives. Some provided definitions more closely related to Nova's: 9% referenced classes of additives considered "cosmetic" by Nova, whereas 21% directly referenced or paraphrased Nova but lacked comprehensive lists of targeted ingredients. A final third (35%) did not provide any definition. Most targeted foods served or sold in schools (58%). Others proposed UPF warning labels (12%) and marketing restrictions (5%).

Conclusions. Proposals mostly targeted school foods and frequently defined UPFs using narrow lists of additives that lack evidence as reliable UPF indicators.

Public Health Implications. Informing policymakers about existing and emerging operational UPF definitions consistent with science-based approaches is urgent. (*Am J Public Health*. 2026;116(7): 1025–1029. https://doi.org/10.2105/AJPH.2026.308464)

AJPH July 2026, Vol. 116, No. 7

NOVA, a system that classifies foods based on processing level, defines ultraprocessed foods (UPFs) as formulations of edible ingredients rarely used in home kitchens, containing little to no whole foods, and assembled using intense industrial processing.[1] Since Nova's introduction in 2009, a substantial evidence base has linked UPFs to ill health,[1,2] sparking interest in regulating them.

Presently, no consensus exists on how best to define UPFs for policy purposes. To maximize health benefits, operational UPF definitions should reliably identify products classified as UPFs by Nova, the framework underlying the overwhelming majority of the evidence linking UPFs to health harms.[3] Critically, Nova was developed for research purposes, and translating it into policy contexts, which requires criteria that are both precise and easy for nonexperts to apply, can be challenging. However, Nova's use of ingredients as proxy indicators ("markers") of processing level[4]—developed because manufacturers are not required to disclose food processing methods—could, as previously demonstrated,[5] feasibly be adapted to policy contexts in the United States, where ingredient disclosure is mandatory.

The United States has recently seen an unprecedented spike in the number of policy proposals targeting UPFs, leading the Food and Drug Administration (FDA) to announce plans to develop a federal UPF definition.[6] To inform this and other efforts, we reviewed policy proposals introduced through 2025 to assess how they defined UPFs and their scope.

METHODS

In December 2025, we conducted a search in Nexis Uni, a comprehensive database for federal and state legal instruments. We searched for policy proposals that mentioned UPFs through the terms ultraprocess* or ultraprocess*. The search was restricted to the United States; no date limits were applied.

One researcher screened all results obtained under "statutes and legislation" or "administrative codes and regulations" to determine eligibility (Figure A, available as a supplement to the online version of this article at http://www.ajph.org). Eligible proposals were those explicitly showing intent to target UPFs (i.e., clearly identifying UPFs as the target and proposing actions to address them). Only the most recent version of each proposal was included. For comprehensiveness, we included companion bills (i.e., matching bills introduced to different legislative chambers) and identical bills introduced in different years separately. We then examined eligible proposals in full and coded key information (i.e., jurisdiction, timeline, status, UPF definition, and policy scope).

RESULTS

We identified 54 proposals mentioning UPFs. Of these, 43 (36 bills, 6 resolutions, 1 executive order) met our inclusion criteria (Figure A). Eight proposals (19%) dated from 2021 to 2024, and the remaining 35 (81%) were introduced in 2025. As of December 2025, 10 (23%) had been enacted or adopted. Proposals hailed from the US Congress and the states of Alabama, Arizona, Arkansas, California, Florida, Hawaii, Indiana, Kentucky, Louisiana, Massachusetts, Missouri, New Jersey, North Carolina, Pennsylvania, South Carolina, Tennessee, and Texas (online Table A).

Operational Ultraprocessed Food Definitions

As shown in Table 1, about a third of proposals (n = 15; 35%) defined UPFs based on the presence of specific food additives—most commonly Blue 1, Blue 2, Green 3, Red 3, Red 40, titanium dioxide, Yellow 5, Yellow 6, potassium bromate, brominated vegetable oil, and propylparaben. One proposal additionally included azodicarbonamide and butylated hydroxyanisole, and another included aspartame. The latter also included certain seed oils, which are not UPF markers.[4]

Fewer proposals used criteria more closely related to Nova's. Three (7%) defined UPFs based on the presence of any additive from entire classes whose function is considered "cosmetic" by Nova (e.g., emulsifiers, colors, flavors).[4] One (2%) specified both nutrient content (i.e., high added sugar, saturated fat, sodium) and cosmetic additive classes. One (2%) directly referenced Nova without providing its own definition, and 8 (15%) used language closely aligned with Nova's (i.e., industrial processing, lack of whole foods, nonculinary ingredients) but only provided examples of marker ingredients rather than comprehensive lists.

Lastly, 15 proposals (35%) targeted UPFs without providing or referring to any definition.

Policy Scope

Although all policy proposals included in this review stated the intent to target UPFs, not all their proposed actions applied uniformly across all UPFs as defined in their text. Notably, some included actions targeting only a subset of UPFs based on specific criteria (e.g., UPFs "of concern" or "foods with certain ultraprocessed ingredients").

Schools were the most common target: 18 proposals (42%) banned and 7 (16%) limited UPFs or a subset of UPFs in schools. Five (12%) commissioned studies on UPFs to guide school food policy. Only 3 (7%) allocated funds for staff training and equipment to remove UPFs from schools, and 1 (2%) called for federal financial support for this purpose (Table A).

Four proposals (9%) introduced mandatory warning labels on UPFs or a subset of UPFs, and 2 (5%) introduced UPF marketing restrictions. Two (5%) stated support for UPF exclusions from the Supplemental Nutrition Assistance Program, 2 (5%) for reducing UPFs in prisons and hospitals, and 1 (2%) for redirecting agricultural subsidies from UPF inputs (Table B).

DISCUSSION

This review found that most US policy proposals targeting and defining UPFs to date focus on the presence of 10 to 13 specific food additives, substantially departing from Nova's approach. The reliability of this narrow set of additives as UPF indicators is unknown and very likely low, considering that Nova uses over 3000 ingredients as UPF markers.[5] For reference, although previous studies found that over 70% of products in the US market qualify as UPFs based on Nova,[7] only 19% contain dyes, which constitute most of the ingredients in the narrow definitions identified.[8] Moreover, 2 of the listed additives (i.e., Red 3 and brominated vegetable oil) are being phased out of the US market per FDA decision, limiting their future usefulness as UPF indicators.[9]

Policies using UPF definitions that largely depart from Nova's cannot be considered evidence-based, and it is unclear what health benefits could result from them. Although some evidence suggests that the additives targeted by the narrow UPF definitions identified in this review may individually

AJPH July 2026, Vol. 116, No. 7

TABLE 1— Operational Definitions of Ultraprocessed Foods (UPFs) in Policy Proposals

Definition Specification	Legal Instruments	No. (%)	Notes
Based on Specific Additives/Ingredients[a]			
Foods containing 1 or more of the following additives: • Colors: Blue 1, Blue 2, Green 3, Red 3, Red 40, titanium dioxide, Yellow 5, Yellow 6 • Dough conditioners: potassium bromate • Emulsifiers: brominated vegetable oil • Preservatives: propylparaben	AL HB 580 (2025), AZ HB 2213 (2025), AZ HB 2164 (2025),[b] FL SB 1826 (2025), KY HB 439 (2025), MO SB 1290 (2026), MO SB 802 (2025), NC HB 874 (2025), NJ SB 4560 (2025), SC SB 589 (2025), SC HB 4339 (2025), TX HB 3292 (2025)	12 (28)	N/A
Foods containing 1 or more of the following additives: • Colors: Blue 1, Blue 2, Green 3, Red 3, Red 40, titanium dioxide, Yellow 5, Yellow 6 • Dough conditioners: potassium bromate • Preservatives: propylparaben	AR HB 1962 (2025)	1 (2)	N/A
Foods containing 1 or more of the following additives: • Colors: Blue 1, Blue 2, Green 3, Red 3, Red 40, titanium dioxide, Yellow 5, Yellow 6 • Dough conditioners: potassium bromate, azodicarbonamide • Emulsifiers: brominated vegetable oil • Preservatives: propylparaben, butylated hydroxyanisole	MO HB 1412 (2025)	1 (2)	N/A
Foods containing 1 or more of the following additives/ingredients: • Colors: Blue 1, Blue 2, Green 3, Red 3, Red 40, titanium dioxide, Yellow 5, Yellow 6 • Dough conditioners: potassium bromate • Emulsifiers: brominated vegetable oil • Preservatives: propylparaben • Sweeteners: aspartame • Oils: cottonseed oil, grapeseed oil, safflower oil	LA SB 117 (2025)	1 (2)	The original version of LA SB 117 simply defined UPFs based on the presence of the additives/ingredients listed, whereas the most recent version changed its language to "foods with certain ultraprocessed ingredients." The additives listed are UPF markers per Nova, but the seed oils listed are not.
Based on Classes of Additives With "Cosmetic" Functions (per Nova)			
Foods containing 1 or more additive in the following classes: surface-active agents, stabilizers and thickeners, propellants, aerating agents, color and coloring adjuncts, emulsifiers and emulsifier salts, flavoring agents and adjuvants, flavor enhancers, surface-finishing agents, nonnutritive sweeteners	HR 10199 (2024), S 4195 (2024), PA HB 1132 (2025)	3 (7)	N/A
Foods (a) high in saturated fat, sodium, and added sugars, and containing nonnutritive sweeteners, and (b) containing 1 or more additives in the following classes: surface-active agents, stabilizers and thickeners, propellants, aerating agents, color and coloring adjuncts, emulsifiers and emulsifier salts, flavoring agents and adjuvants, flavor enhancers, surface-finishing agents	CA AB 1264 (2025)[b]	1 (2)	CA AB 1264 additionally targets specific food colors (i.e., Blue 1, Blue 2, Green 3, Red 40, Yellow 5, Yellow 6), but does not include these in its definition of UPF.
Paraphrasing Nova			
Mentioning industrial processing, absence of whole-food ingredients, presence of ingredients never or rarely used in kitchens, and presence of additives to make the final product palatable, appealing, or preservable	CA EO1 (2025),[b] MA HB 4562 (2025), MA HB 539 (2025), MA S 401 (2025), MA SB 308 (2023), MA HB 451 (2023), MA HB 564 (2021), MA SB 363 (2021)	8 (19)	Definitions provide *examples* of UPFs, of ingredients never or rarely used in kitchens, and of additives to make the final product palatable, appealing, or preservable; but do not provide a *comprehensive* list of the types of substances that would identify UPFs.
Directly Referencing Nova			
Foods described in group 4 of the Nova classification system	HR 2530 (2025)	1 (2)	N/A

Continued

TABLE 1— Continued

Definition Specification	Legal Instruments	No. (%)	Notes
No Definition			
N/A	CA SB 121 (2025), CA AB 121 (2025),[b] CA SB 147 (2025),[b] HI SCR 101 (2025), HI SR 82 (2025), IN SCR 22 (2025), LA HR 3 (2025),[b] LA HR 4 (2025),[b] MA HB 4040 (2023),[b] MA HB 3901 (2023), TN HJR 69 (2025),[b] TX HB 4210 (2025), TX SB 1645 (2025), TX SB 25 (2025),[b] TX HB 25 (2025)	15 (35)	TX SB 25 and TX HB 25 explicitly target UPFs (without providing a definition) when establishing an advisory committee to examine evidence and provide education on the health effects of UPFs. Later, these bills list 44–52 ingredients for warning labels, but do not tie such ingredients to a UPF definition. Most of the ingredients listed are UPF markers, but not all.

Note. N/A = not applicable. The total sample size was n = 43.
[a]Ingredient categories are provided only for clarity; the proposals themselves did not distinguish ingredients by type or function.
[b]Enacted (bills) or adopted (resolutions and executive orders) as of December 2025.

pose health concerns,[10] which likely provided the rationale for their inclusion, such additives are neither the sole nor the main drivers of the link between UPFs and ill health. Because of its broadness, Nova's UPF category captures products that affect health through several synergistic mechanisms: hyper-palatability and digestibility, sensory appeal, unbalanced nutrient content, presence of contaminants from processing and contact materials, and microbiome disruptions.[11,12] The narrow UPF definitions identified are unlikely to adequately target most of these mechanisms.

Lack of clarity and objectivity were also common issues identified. Some proposals ambiguously targeted ingredients without explicitly linking them to a UPF definition, despite previously stating the intent to target UPFs. Some targeted ingredients that are not considered UPF markers by Nova, such as seed oils and agrochemicals. Others used Nova-like criteria but did not comprehensively list targeted ingredients, limiting their policy readiness.

Lastly, schools were the primary policy target identified, perhaps because food dyes predominantly pose concerns for youths.[10] Although schools may be a useful initial target, UPFs are linked to ill health across age groups,[2] making population-wide interventions also necessary.

PUBLIC HEALTH IMPLICATIONS

There is an urgent need to inform policymakers about existing[5] and emerging approaches that could better approximate scientific UPF identification methods in policy contexts. Clearly communicating the goal of ingredients-based criteria (i.e., reliably identifying UPFs rather than eliminating the source of their harm) is critical. Additionally, policies should aim for more comprehensive scope to meaningfully reduce the health risks posed by UPFs. AJPH

ABOUT THE AUTHORS

Aline D'Angelo Campos, Lindsey Smith Taillie, Carmen E. Prestemon, and Bridget A. Hollingsworth are with the Carolina Population Center, University of North Carolina at Chapel Hill. Lindsey Smith Taillie and Carmen E. Prestemon are also with the Department of Nutrition, Gillings School of Global Public Health, University of North Carolina at Chapel Hill. James W. Krieger is with the Department of Health Systems and Population Health, School of Public Health, University of Washington, Seattle, and with Healthy Food America, Seattle.

CORRESPONDENCE

Correspondence should be sent to Aline D'Angelo Campos, 123 W Franklin St, Chapel Hill, NC 27516 (e-mail: adangelo-campos@unc.edu). Reprints can be ordered at https://www.ajph.org by clicking the "Reprints" link.

PUBLICATION INFORMATION

Full Citation: D'Angelo Campos A, Krieger JW, Prestemon CE, Hollingsworth BA, Taillie LS. Operationally defining and targeting ultraprocessed foods: insights from US policy proposals. *Am J Public Health*. 2026;116(7):1025–1029.

Acceptance Date: February 2, 2026.

DOI: https://doi.org/10.2105/AJPH.2026.308464

ORCID iDs:
Aline D'Angelo Campos https://orcid.org/0000-0001-7382-5976

Carmen E. Prestemon https://orcid.org/0000-0002-5978-8061

CONTRIBUTORS

A. D'Angelo Campos led the search and data analysis and drafted the article. A. D'Angelo Campos, L. S. Taillie, and J. W. Krieger designed the study. B. A. Hollingsworth and C. E. Prestemon assisted with data analysis. All authors contributed to the writing and editing of the article.

ACKNOWLEDGMENTS

This work was supported by Healthy Eating Research.

CONFLICTS OF INTEREST

The authors declare no conflicts of interest.

HUMAN PARTICIPANT PROTECTION

This study did not require institutional review board approval because it only used data from publicly available legal documents.

REFERENCES

1. Monteiro CA, Louzada ML, Steele-Martinez E, et al. Ultra-processed foods and human health: the main thesis and the evidence. *Lancet.* 2025; 406(10520):2667–2684. https://doi.org/10.1016/S0140-6736(25)01565-X
2. Lane MM, Gamage E, Du S, et al. Ultra-processed food exposure and adverse health outcomes: umbrella review of epidemiological meta-analyses. *BMJ.* 2024;384:e077310. https://doi.org/10.1136/bmj-2023-077310
3. Medin AC, Gulowsen SR, Groufh-Jacobsen S, Berget I, Grini IS, Varela P. Definitions of ultra-processed foods beyond Nova: a systematic review and evaluation. *Food Nutr Res.* Published online June 16, 2025:69. https://doi.org/10.29219/fnr.v69.12217
4. Martinez-Steele E, Khandpur N, Batis C, et al. Best practices for applying the Nova food classification system. *Nat Food.* 2023;4(6):445–448. https://doi.org/10.1038/s43016-023-00779-w
5. Popkin BM, Miles DR, Taillie LS, Dunford EK. A policy approach to identifying food and beverage products that are ultra-processed and high in added salt, sugar and saturated fat in the United States: a cross-sectional analysis of packaged foods. *Lancet Reg Health Am.* 2024;32:100713. https://doi.org/10.1016/j.lana.2024.100713
6. US Food and Drug Administration. Ultra-processed foods. July 24, 2025. Available at: https://www.fda.gov/food/nutrition-food-labeling-and-critical-foods/ultra-processed-foods. Accessed August 19, 2025.
7. Baldridge AS, Huffman MD, Taylor F, et al. The healthfulness of the US packaged food and beverage supply: a cross-sectional study. *Nutrients.* 2019;11(8):1704. https://doi.org/10.3390/nu11081704
8. Dunford EK, Galligan TM, Taillie LS, Musicus AA. All the colors of the rainbow: synthetic dyes in US packaged foods and beverages in 2020. *J Acad Nutr Diet.* 2025;125(9):1207–1217.e9. https://doi.org/10.1016/j.jand.2025.05.007
9. US Food and Drug Administration. List of select chemicals in the food supply under FDA review. August 21, 2025. Available at: https://www.fda.gov/food/food-chemical-safety/list-select-chemicals-food-supply-under-fda-review. Accessed December 23, 2025.
10. Schab DW, Trinh NHT. Do artificial food colors promote hyperactivity in children with hyperactive syndromes? A meta-analysis of double-blind placebo-controlled trials. *J Dev Behav Pediatr.* 2004;25(6):423–434. https://doi.org/10.1097/00004703-200412000-00007
11. Srour B, Kordahi MC, Bonazzi E, Deschasaux-Tanguy M, Touvier M, Chassaing B. Ultra-processed foods and human health: from epidemiological evidence to mechanistic insights. *Lancet Gastroenterol Hepatol.* 2022;7(12):1128–1140. https://doi.org/10.1016/S2468-1253(22)00169-8
12. Touvier M, da Costa Louzada ML, Mozaffarian D, Baker P, Juul F, Srour B. Ultra-processed foods and cardiometabolic health: public health policies to reduce consumption cannot wait. *BMJ.* 2023;383:e075294. https://doi.org/10.1136/bmj-2023-075294

Protecting US Children From Lead Exposures: Applications of a Data-Mapping Blueprint for Focusing High-Impact Interventions

Valerie Zartarian, PhD, MS, Alan Walts, JD, Carol Ann Gross-Davis, PhD, MS, Antonios Poulakos, BA, Kathy Triantafillou, BS ChE, Kristi Rea Simoneau, MA, Nicholas Spalt, MS, Chloe Durand, BA, Shayna Sellars, MEEd, Maxwell Kromer, BS, Alexa Burnett, MPH, BS, Rashad Taylor, MPH, Colleen Neely, MPA, Thomas Speth, PhD, Nichole Kulikowski, BA, Veronica Helms Garrison, DrPH, MPH, Peter Han, PhD, Rogelio Tornero-Velez, PhD, MSPH, and Lindsay Wichers Stanek, PhD, MSPH

AJPH July 2026, Vol. 116, No. 7

Objectives. To describe a data-mapping blueprint for identifying US locations at high risk for childhood lead exposure and to apply this approach to inform targeted public health interventions.

Methods. We developed a stepwise, flexible blueprint integrating environmental and housing data, blood lead level data, and geospatial mapping to identify potential lead exposure hotspots, characterize contributing sources, and guide intervention prioritization. We applied the blueprint in multiple federal and state case studies through interagency collaboration.

Results. Application of the blueprint identified high-risk locations for childhood lead exposure and informed targeted actions across diverse contexts. In data-rich settings, integration of blood lead level and environmental data enabled identification of exposure hotspots and prioritization of outreach, enforcement, and remediation. In data-limited settings, lead exposure indices and environmental indicators supported targeted surveillance and resource allocation. Across applications, the blueprint facilitated coordination among agencies, improved lead-based paint and infrastructure intervention targeting, and supported expansion of screening and prevention efforts.

Conclusions. A coordinated, data-driven mapping approach can improve identification of lead exposure hotspots and support prioritization of impactful interventions.

Public Health Implications. Broader implementation of the blueprint, along with enhanced data integration and interagency collaboration, may strengthen efforts to reduce childhood lead exposures and improve public health outcomes. (*Am J Public Health*. 2026;116(7):1030–1037. https://doi.org/10.2105/AJPH.2026.308440)

Lead has historically been used in a variety of commodities and is found in air, water, soil, paint, dust, food, consumer products, and other sources. There is no known safe level of lead in children's blood, and many lead sources aggregate across exposure pathways. Lead exposure is particularly harmful to children younger than 6 years, among whom it can lead to permanent neurological damage, among other harms.[1] The United States has made great progress in reducing lead exposures in recent decades. National data show significant declines in children's blood lead levels (BLLs).[2–5] However, reducing exposure remains a critical public health challenge.[6,7] Figure A (available as a supplement to the online version of this article at http://www.ajph.org) illustrates reductions in BLLs from national- and state-collected data as well as the power of hotspot mapping to identify progress and locations needing more attention. Pinpointing high lead exposure risk locations can inform primary and secondary prevention efforts, including lead hazard control, inspection, and enforcement targeting, outreach, and education.

Mapping lead exposures has been a federal priority.[6,7] The Federal Action Plan to Reduce Childhood Lead Exposures and Associated Health Impacts includes an action to "generate data, maps, and mapping tools to identify high exposure . . . locations . . . to prioritize efforts for reducing children's blood lead levels."[7] Together with the US Department of Housing and Urban Development (HUD), the US Department of Health and Human Services, and other federal and state partners, the US Environmental Protection Agency (EPA) is addressing this need by advancing a US interagency partnership to protect public health by applying a recently developed lead blueprint.[8] The blueprint provides a systematic science-based approach for targeting primary and secondary lead prevention actions in communities. It supports the use of data and science in prioritizing federal, state, and local resources to reduce children's lead exposures across the nation. Central to the blueprint is the mapping approach using indices and models based on publicly available old housing and other data, as described in Zartarian et al.[9]

We build on previous work to provide examples of how federal and state agencies are using the published analytic lead-mapping methods and blueprint steps to inform government decision-making and public health practice.

METHODS

The blueprint originated in a 2019 EPA lead-mapping coordination workshop and was introduced as a data integration roadmap for whole-of-government exposure prevention efforts.[9] The methodology steps include partner engagement and problem formulation, selection and compilation of data, identification and verification (i.e., ground truthing) of potential high-risk locations, determination of the primary lead sources in those locations, mitigation and prevention actions, and impact assessment of actions taken (Figure 1). Depending on data availability and analytical context, following all steps sequentially may not always be feasible or necessary (as illustrated by, e.g., the dashed line from steps 1 to 5 in Figure 1). Partner collaborations throughout the project are critical. Supplement A (available as a supplement to the online version of this article at http://www.ajph.org) provides details of each step; Supplement B (available as a supplement to the online version of this article at http://www.ajph.org) provides a standard operating procedure (SOP) for the peer-reviewed, published mapping methodology,[10] including options to scale the national analysis method to regional, state, or local geographies of choice; and Supplements C–F (available as a supplement to the online version of this article at http://www.ajph.org) provide detailed science in action examples.

The examples in the Results section reflect interagency government collaborations. Initial demonstration projects in Michigan and West Virginia were based on a set of informal EPA selection criteria (Supplement A). The blueprint is not prescriptive but fosters a consistent, evidence-based approach among federal, state, and local entities working to address lead. This builds collective capacity to collaborate in improving children's health outcomes in places where the evidence shows such action is most needed. The approach uses state-of-science geospatial mapping, modeling, and data analysis methods through collaborative engagement, including the use of local information. Its development, evolution, and applications reflect input from various workshops, conferences, advisory committees, and discussions with federal, state, and local agencies and nongovernmental organizations.

Step 1 of the blueprint is to identify and engage partners to join in collaborative scoping discussions. Discussions formulate general and specific questions of interest, focused on decisions that can be informed by lead data mapping. Examples include (1) Where are the most affected communities that might be eligible for federal or state lead grants or mitigation programs and resources for lead source reduction, surveillance, and outreach efforts? and (2) Where could resources and actions be focused in a more coordinated way, and what are the impacts of actions taken for lead-based paint programs (LBPs), such as outreach and investigations; for prioritizing lead service line replacements and technical assistance; and for increasing environmental monitoring and blood lead testing surveillance?

Step 2 is to select and compile BLL data, exposure indices based on publicly available housing data, environmental lead data indicators of BLLs, and data on other lead sources that can contribute to exposures (e.g., take-home exposures and consumer products). Zartarian et al.[9,10] provide details of these data categories and sources of information (e.g., composite lead exposure indices [Figure B, available as a supplement to the online version of this article at http://www.ajph.org]; EPA's Lead Occurrence and Source Tool [POST][11]). POST brings together national environmental data sets related to lead in numerous layers in the ArcGIS GeoPlatform (Esri, Redlands, CA)

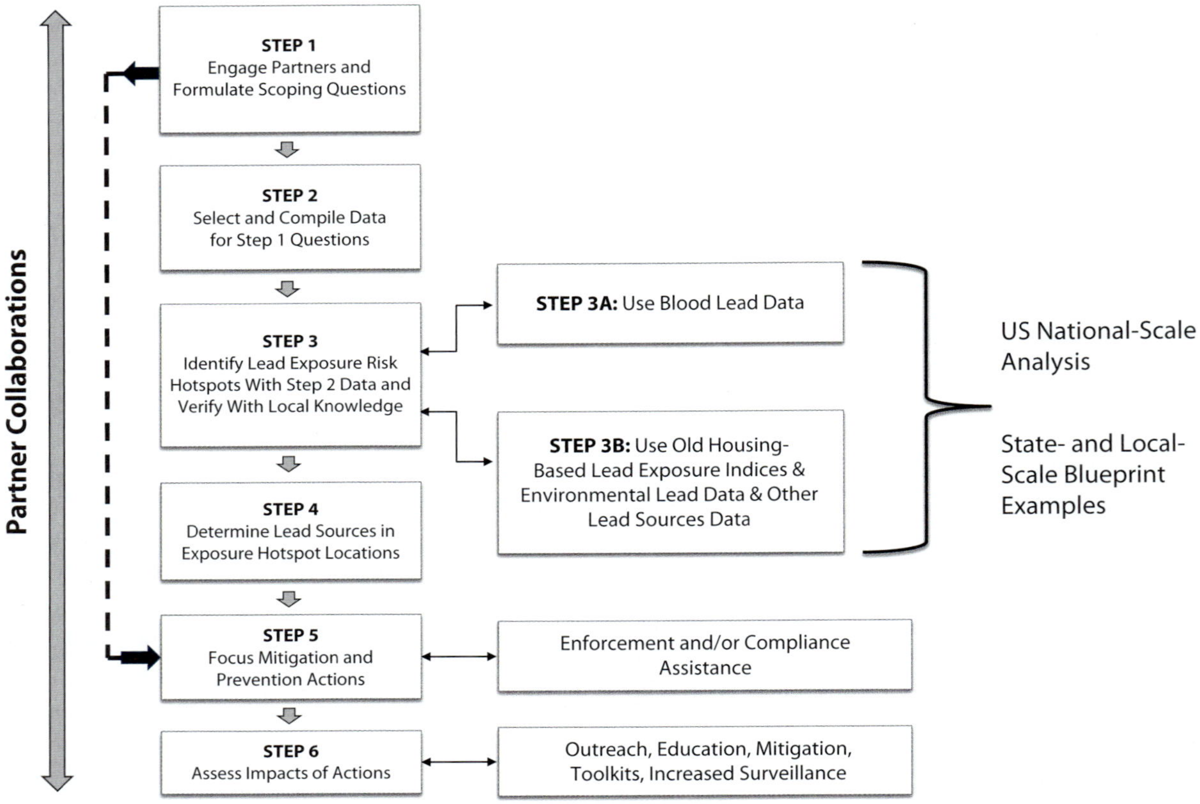

FIGURE 1— **Blueprint to Identify and Address High Lead Exposure Risk Locations**

to facilitate data analysis and visualization.

Step 3 is to use maps and data analyses from step 2 and the peer-reviewed, published results and methods in Zartarian et al.[10] to identify lead exposure hotspots and to ground truth, or verify, this information with local expertise (e.g., health department reports, data). Step 3A uses BLL data where available. Step 3B uses other exposure data (old housing-based lead exposure indices, environmental lead sources and concentrations data, other lead sources data, e.g., consumer products)—either alone or in conjunction with BLL data. We emphasize that even if no BLL data are available or step 3A is not used, step 3B can inform primary lead exposure prevention efforts.[12]

Step 4 is to determine lead sources contributing to identified potential exposure hotspots (e.g., source apportionment analyses to determine relative contributions of sources to BLL[12]). Approaches include visual inspection and analysis of mapped lead sources and BLL data, modeling and data analyses, and local information and expertise. Supplement A provides references with examples, and challenges are noted in the Discussion.

Step 5 is to focus resources and prioritize actions to address key lead sources in identified exposure hotspots. Examples include delivering compliance assistance, monitoring and assurance, risk communication, outreach and education, and technical assistance.

Step 6 is to assess (i.e., evaluate and monitor) the impacts of lead actions taken, such as reducing children's BLL,[5,13,14] increasing blood lead testing rates in high lead exposure risk locations, and observing improvements in children's health in the community (i.e., absence of illness and conditions associated with lead exposure or increased well-being).

RESULTS

In this section, we provide case study examples of applying the blueprint with the published mapping research to inform decisions that address lead. The examples illustrate lessons learned to help other entities interested in applying the blueprint.

Data-Rich State Example

Michigan has many robust blood lead–screening programs.[5,15] Children enrolled in Michigan Medicaid programs must be tested for lead by age 3 years, and testing is also required for Michigan children enrolled in the Women, Infants, and Children program (Michigan Compiled Law 333.5474). In 2023, more than 126 000 children were tested, corresponding to almost 20% of children younger than 6 years, with a similar number tested in other years.[16] The Michigan blueprint example stemmed from Xue et al.,[5] which was a collaboration among EPA Region 5, Office of Research and Development, Office of Enforcement and Compliance Assurance and state, local, and federal partners. For step 1, the EPA formed a workgroup with the Michigan Department of Health and Human Services; Environment, Great Lakes, and Energy; and HUD. Maps were used to define scoping questions and focus actions to address multiple lead sources contributing to higher BLLs among children.

In step 2, published maps[5] were examined that displayed the predictive capability of higher BLLs among children based on old housing-based indices and other data described in Zartarian et al.[9] Based on the outcomes of workgroup discussions, outlier census tracts (i.e., those with higher BLLs that were not identified by the analysis) became the focus to evaluate potential lead sources beyond old housing. In addition, EPA Region 5 evaluated multiple environmental indicators of potential lead exposure using POST to facilitate informed decision-making across regional lead programs (Figure C, available as a supplement to the online version of this article at http://www.ajph.org).

For step 3, 3 pilot locations with high risks of children's BLLs above action levels were selected for scoping and screening: Jackson, Adrian, and Grand Rapids. For step 4, EPA Region 5 used POST to examine lead exposure factors and presented its analysis to other internal programs to facilitate informed decision-making. Other analyses were conducted for potential exposure sources in these areas, including internal EPA data on lead service line replacements and purchased data from Dunn and Bradstreet containing information on potential lead sources (e.g., airports, shooting ranges, and inactive mines). For step 5, EPA Region 5 completed considerable outreach work, focusing on education and risk communication, including multiple sessions of the Agency for Toxic Substances and Disease Registry's soilSHOP program and a community lead awareness session. EPA Region 5 also provided recommendations on locations to receive renovation, repair, and painting certification classes for contractors.

In addition, the Michigan Department of Health and Human Services cited Xue et al.[5] and continued investigations of the EPA–Michigan workgroup as justification for the validity and efficacy of using blood lead data to identify and prioritize communities and resources for prevention and intervention activities.

Data-Limited State Example

West Virginia has historically low blood lead testing rates. EPA Region 3 partnered with the West Virginia Department of Health and HUD on joint, community-focused planning to apply the science with environmental and public health agency programs: compliance assistance, monitoring, and assurance; risk communication; outreach and education; and technical assistance. The overall goal was to collaborate on a public health practice informed by science to support West Virginia and federal lead strategies and to provide lessons learned that may be helpful for other similarly situated states.

For step 1, the team met to collaboratively brainstorm and formulate questions of interest: where to focus blood lead surveillance in areas with potentially high exposures; how to use maps to guide funds allocation for lead service line replacement, testing, and outreach; and where to focus other lead outreach and public health awareness (e.g., for lead in drinking water, paint, and soil).

For steps 2 and 3, the approach was to use and enhance existing lead exposure indices and published lead exposure mapping results to inform focused efforts in the absence of complete BLL data. Figure D (available as a supplement to the online version of this article at http://www.ajph.org) highlights potential lead exposure risk locations identified by old housing-based indices and by 2023 percentages of children (aged ≤ 6 years) tested from the West Virginia Department of Health. Environmental lead data from POST and public Web sites (e.g., mining data) were mapped. For step 4, maps were generated showing environmental lead source data (e.g., lead waste and cleanup, air lead concentrations, lead in drinking water and coal mines) that can inform locations for BLL surveillance (Figure E, available as a supplement to the online version of this article at http://www.ajph.org).

For step 5, multiple outreach strategies were implemented to increase BLL surveillance in locations identified using the published mapping approach,[10] scaled to West Virginia. These included engagement with primary care physicians through the EPA Region 3 Pediatric Environmental Health Specialty Unit at Villanova University and collaboration with 3 West Virginia Special Supplemental Nutrition Program for Women,

Infants, and Children centers in 3 counties to provide on-site blood lead testing. Additionally, EPA Region 3 led the development of the EPA's *Local Lead Action Plan Guide* to provide information resources, science translation, and best practices to inform lead reduction actions that will be used in West Virginia.

For step 6, the West Virginia case study highlights where novel approaches are being implemented to increase blood lead testing. This effort will provide a more focused and deliberate strategy to increase childhood screening and to evaluate the effectiveness of the outreach efforts.

Lead-Based Paint Example

National-scale EPA and HUD lead-based paint coordination. To strengthen data-driven decision-making nationally and support a whole-of-government approach, EPA regions have been encouraged to use the published lead exposure mapping data[10] with other criteria to support collaboration across LBP outreach and enforcement activities under the Toxics Substances Control Act Lead Renovation, Repair, and Painting Program.

For step 1, coordination between outreach activities, such as EPA Community Lead Awareness Sessions,[17] and compliance assurance activities, such as inspection targeting, supports common program objectives of reducing lead exposure in communities. This blueprint framework can help regional EPA outreach and enforcement programs select high-priority areas for their initiatives. Multiple EPA regions have voluntarily started using the mapping data as part of steps 2 and 3 to support coordinated action. Such collaboration demonstrates how other regional, lead-based paint outreach and enforcement programs could benefit from incorporating the data into their own strategic efforts.

For step 4, Figure F (available as a supplement to the online version of this article at http://www.ajph.org) highlights locations of EPA lead-based paint community awareness, inspection, and enforcement activities conducted during fiscal year 2023. Of these locations, 84% are in communities (defined using the Census 2023 Places file[18]), with at least 1 high-potential lead exposure hotspot census tract, based on Zartarian et al.[10] The purple and red dots highlight the success of lead-based paint efforts, and shaded areas show that there are more census tracts needing attention. The green dots display communities where HUD awarded 2023 healthy homes grants. HUD and the EPA are collaborating to bring published maps together and use the information collectively for advancing interagency LBP coordination efforts for step 5. Future efforts include overlaying these data with other federal data sources and sharing these data with federal partners for improved collaboration and coordination of LBP outreach, enforcement, and grant distribution.

Examples of state-specific applications of the blueprint and maps. The Tennessee Department of Environment and Conservation's LBP used the lead indices maps[10] together with publicly available screening rates for children's blood lead by county (from Tennessee Department of Health's Childhood Lead Poisoning Prevention Program 2023 data) for steps 2 through 4 to help inform LBP outreach and compliance monitoring activities. For step 5, Tennessee's LBP is using the results in Figure F to target outreach and education efforts and to identify parts of the state where workforce development might be needed for LBP training and certifications.

Figure G (available as a supplement to the online version of this article at http://www.ajph.org) shows the Maine map being used to focus EPA Region 1's cross-office initiative work including LBPs and other media. The gray areas represent the combination of all 5 lead indices in Zartarian et al.,[10] and the black represent the intersection (using both statistical methods in that article), which identifies concentrations of old housing in Portland, Lewiston, and rural areas.

Supplement F provides another example of how the blueprint is being applied for lead in drinking water at the national scale.

DISCUSSION

The legacy issue of lead exposure is a persistent public health "wicked problem"[20,21] (a complex problem that defies a solution) in the United States and globally.[22] The ubiquitous presence of lead in the environment is the consequence of a multifaceted system with many interacting elements. To address this serious challenge, these key overarching questions need to be answered at local, national, and global scales: Where are remaining lead exposure hotspots? What is the relative contribution of different lead sources to exposures and BLLs? How should resources and actions be focused and prioritized to prevent, reduce, and eliminate lead exposures? What are the impacts of actions taken?

The blueprint presented in this article represents the evolution of research to public health practice to help address these questions through federal, state, and local collaborations. It includes examples of projects informed by applying peer-reviewed, published science and local expertise to deliver compliance assistance, monitoring, and assurance; outreach and education; and technical assistance in areas identified by exposure maps. The blueprint is not intended to be "the" solution but rather to capture the complexity of the problem and provide a framework for interventions that will make strides toward reducing the problem.

Interagency collaborations are vital in obtaining, interpreting, and communicating available data and results. The examples present national and state-specific success stories operationalizing a deliberative approach to reduce lead exposures across the nation and improve children's health. The supplemental mapping SOP based on the EPA's published national-scale methodology can be scaled to identify exposure risk hotspots in specific states and locations. This supports capacity building with entities trying to address similar questions for prioritizing resources and program attention.

The steps of this lead-specific blueprint are similar to those in other environmental health practices, such as Health Impact Assessment. Significant progress has been made to identify and address remaining lead exposure hotspots in the United States, and there are still data gaps and coordination needs,[8] particularly for steps 4 and 6. Source apportionment analyses (step 4), to identify the relative contribution of various lead sources to exposures and prioritize lead source reduction actions, require integrated data sets. Some states have mapped lead sources and BLL data together in the same data portals (e.g., the Wisconsin environmental public health tracker,[23] the DataOhio catalog[24]), but typically integrated, multimedia lead data are not available.

Figure 2 illustrates a vision for interagency coordination efforts to identify and address lead exposure locations. The vision is to bring together blood lead data; environmental, drinking water–related, and other lead sources data; and lead exposure indices to enhance the identification of potential exposure locations and relative source contribution for prioritizing actions. Such a vision would benefit from machine learning and artificial intelligence approaches. Step 6 of the blueprint,

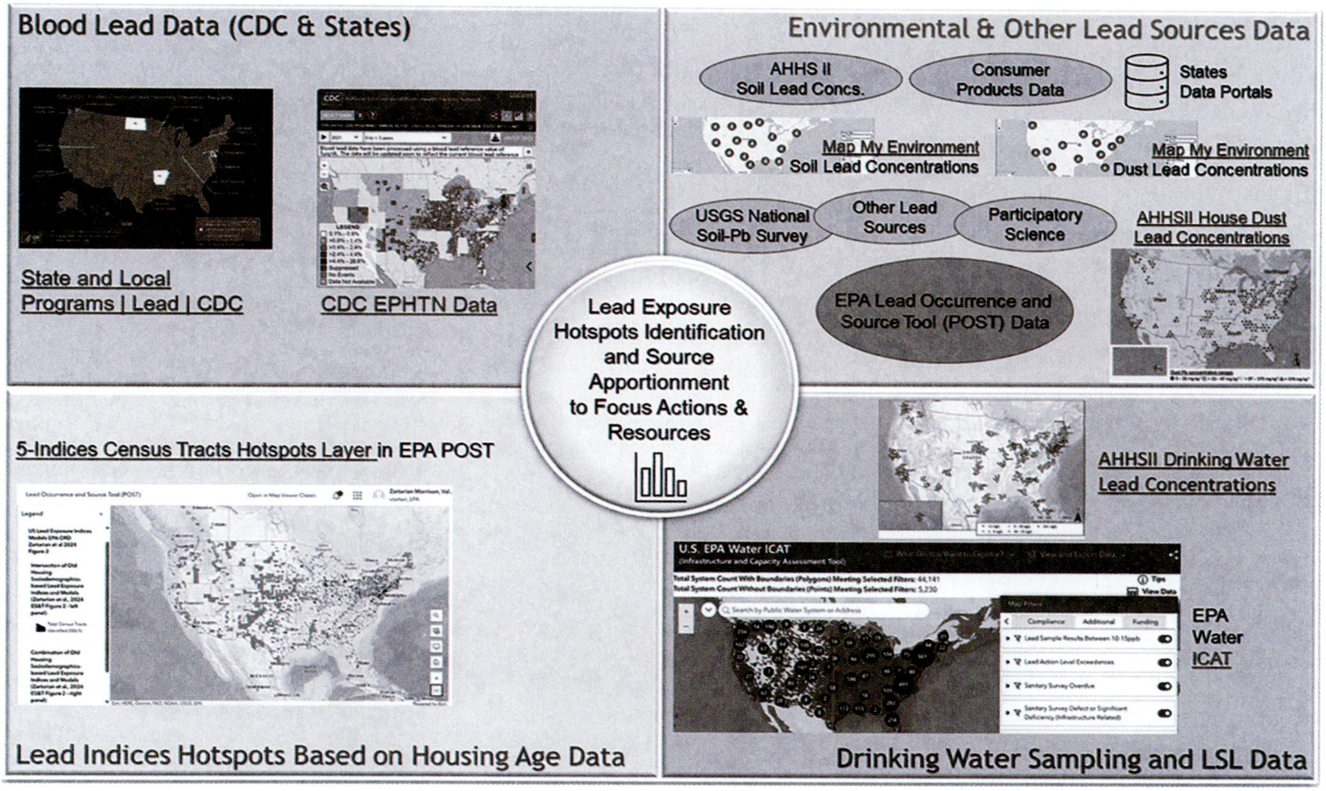

FIGURE 2— **Vision for Data Integration and Mapping Coordination for Interagency Efforts to Identify and Address Lead Exposure Locations**

Note. AHHS = American Healthy Homes Survey; CDC = Centers for Disease Control and Prevention; EPHTN = Environmental Public Health Tracking Network; LSL = lead service lines; POST = lead occurrence and source tool; Water ICAT = water infrastructure and capacity assessment tool.

to assess impacts of step 5 actions, can involve monitoring BLL decreases after lead intervention actions are implemented or improving lead testing rates. Data from the Centers for Disease Control and Prevention's Childhood Blood Lead Surveillance System[25,26] in 2021 indicated that testing rates for children younger than 3 years ranged from 3% to 45% in 25 states, with different lead testing policies.

Another area to explore under step 5 is public health improvements compared with cost and resource requirements for specific actions. Next steps toward the vision and enhancing the blueprint for greater impact include further interagency coordinated and data sharing,[27] broader communication of the mapping SOP, and on-the-ground engagement of many partners beyond government agencies. Additional benefits to the collaborative blueprint approach are efficiencies gained and strategic use of resources.

PUBLIC HEALTH IMPLICATIONS

The work presented supports federal agencies' commitments to work collectively to reduce childhood BLLs from multiple environmental and other sources in the United States, for example, by using available data-mapping tools to increase blood lead screening where exposures are high. Lead-mapping science has increased capacity to help agencies prioritize risk reduction actions and optimize resource allocations, as shown by examples of successful blueprint applications. Lessons learned from implementing the blueprint and hotspots mapping SOP through public health practice will help operationalize a powerful community of practice to optimize health interventions at national, state, local, and household scales. AJPH

ABOUT THE AUTHORS

Valerie Zartarian was with the Environmental Protection Agency (EPA) Office of Research and Development (ORD), Boston, MA. Alan Walts and Alexa Burnett were with EPA Region 5, Chicago, IL. Carol Ann Gross-Davis was with EPA Region 3, Philadelphia, PA. Antonios Poulakos is with LinTech Global, Inc. under contract to EPA Region 1, Boston, MA. Kathy Triantafillou is with EPA Region 5, Chicago, IL. Kristi Rea Simoneau is with EPA Region 1, Boston, MA. Nicholas Spalt and Maxwell Kromer are with EPA Office of Enforcement and Compliance Assurance (OECA), Washington, DC. Chloe Durand and Shayna Sellars are with EPA Office of Chemical Safety and Pollution Prevention (OCSPP), Washington, DC. Rashad Taylor was with EPA Office of Children's Health Protection, Washington, DC. Colleen Neely is with EPA Office of Water, Washington, DC. Thomas Speth was with EPA ORD, Cincinnati, OH. Nichole Kulikowski was with EPA ORD, Washington, DC. Veronica Helms Garrison and Peter Han are with the Department of Housing and Urban Development, Washington, DC. Rogelio Tornero-Velez and Lindsay Wichers Stanek were with EPA ORD in Research Triangle Park, NC.

CORRESPONDENCE

Correspondence should be sent to Lindsay Wichers Stanek, MSPH, PhD, US EPA Office of the Administrator, Office of Applied Science and Environmental Solutions, 109 T.W. Alexander Dr, Research Triangle Park, NC 27709 (e-mail: stanek.lindsay@epa.gov). Reprints can be ordered at https://www.ajph.org by clicking the "Reprints" link.

PUBLICATION INFORMATION

Full Citation: Zartarian V, Walts A, Gross-Davis CA, et al. Protecting US children from lead exposures: applications of a data-mapping blueprint for focusing high-impact interventions. *Am J Public Health*. 2026;116(7):1030–1037.

Acceptance date: December 17, 2025.

DOI: https://doi.org/10.2105/AJPH.2026.308440

ORCID iDs:
Alan Walts https://orcid.org/0000-0001-5953-104X

Nicholas Spalt https://orcid.org/0009-0008-2980-5458

Shayna Sellars https://orcid.org/0009-0006-0858-5738

Maxwell Kromer https://orcid.org/0009-0003-2540-532X

Alexa Burnett https://orcid.org/0009-0004-1223-1452

Rashad Taylor https://orcid.org/0009-0009-1048-5295

Colleen Neely https://orcid.org/0009-0006-6128-0677

Thomas Speth https://orcid.org/0000-0002-6640-2737

Lindsay Wichers Stanek https://orcid.org/0000-0002-9921-7458

CONTRIBUTORS

V. Zartarian developed the idea for the article, led conceptual design of the blueprint, coordinated the project, and had primary responsibility for writing and revising the article and files for critical intellectual content. A. Walts envisioned the Michigan example and built out the blueprint concept. A. Walts, C. A. Gross-Davis, and L. Wichers Stanek edited the work product for critical intellectual content. A. Walts, K. Triantafillou, K Rea Simoneau, N. Spalt, and L. Wichers Stanek contributed to conceptual design of the blueprint. C. A. Gross-Davis envisioned the West Virginia example and built out the blueprint concept. C. A. Gross-Davis, N. Poulakos, K. Triantafillou, C. Durand, S. Sellars, M. Kromer, A. Burnett, R. Taylor, C. Neely, T. Speth, V. Helms Garrison, P. Han, R. Tornero-Velez, and L. Wichers Stanek interpreted the data. C. A. Gross-Davis, C. Durand, S. Sellars, M. Kromer, A. Burnett, R. Taylor, C. Neely, T. Speth, and V. Helms Garrison developed the study objectives. C. A. Gross-Davis and L. Wichers Stanek acquired the data. A. Poulakos generated the tables and had primary responsibility for supplemental standard operating procedure material. A. Poulakos and N. Spalt generated the maps. K. Triantafillou developed the Michigan study objectives. K Triantafillou and A Burnett performed community outreach. K. Rea Simoneau created the Environmental Protection Agency (EPA) Region 1 examples. N. Spalt coordinated the data. C. Durand, S. Sellars, and M. Kromer created the national lead-based paint example. A. Burnett led creation of the Michigan example. R. Taylor created the Tennessee lead-based paint example and tested the standard operating procedure. C. Neely and T. Speth created the drinking water example. N. Kulikowski developed and applied the modeling specific to Michigan and was responsible for supplemental standard operating procedure material. V. Helms Garrison and P. Han created the national lead-based paint example and refined research ideas. R. Tornero-Velez developed and applied modeling and analyzed the data specific to the blueprint. All authors provided approval for the final version of the article to be published.

ACKNOWLEDGMENTS

The data mapping and analyses described in this article was funded in part by the EPA (Office of Research and Development [ORD] Sustainable and Healthy Communities Research Program) under the Environmental Compliance History Online (ECHO)–Multi Region Information Technology (IT) Services Support Contract and the EPA Region 1 IT Services Support Task Order, specifically, LinTech Global, Inc.'s ECHO contract (GS-35F-0343W/68HE0319F0020) with EPA Regions 1, 2, and 3. The Tennessee example was supported by an appointment to the EPA Research Participation Program administered by the Oak Ridge Institute for Science and Education (ORISE) through an interagency agreement between the US Department of Energy (DOE) and the EPA. ORISE is managed by Oak Ridge Associated Universities under the DOE (contract DE-SC0014664).

Michigan Department of Health and Human Services (MDHHS) provided blood lead data used in this article (Data Use Agreement 201909-157). Ohio data in Figure A maps were provided by the Ohio Department of Health (ODH) through the Ohio Public Health Information Warehouse.

We appreciate technical reviewers Grace Robiou and Wayne Cascio and managers from our agencies who supported this article and related research. We also broadly acknowledge individuals from the following organization for their contributions: from EPA Regional Offices, ORD; Office of Water; Office of the Administrator; Office of Chemical Safety and Pollution Prevention; Centers for Disease Control and Prevention's Agency for Toxic Substances and Disease Registry; MDHHS; West Virginia Department of Health; ODH; Tennessee Department of Health; EPA Regional Science Liaisons, standard operating procedure testers from EPA Regions 1, 4, 5, 7, 8; ORD lead data-mapping and analysis team, managers, and support staff; coauthors and collaborators of lead-mapping articles in epa.gov/lead/mapping; EPA Lead Strategy Team and Lead Coordinating Committee; Lead Subcommittee of the President's Task Force and interagency mapping working group; and other federal, state, and local collaborators on blueprint examples. We are thankful to state and local agencies who provided data sources.

Note. This work has been reviewed by the EPA and the US Department of Housing and Urban Development (HUD), and approved for publication. The views and opinions expressed in this article are those of the authors and do not necessarily reflect the views or policies of the EPA, Department of Housing and Urban Development, DOE, Oak Ridge Associated Universities' ORISE, or federal, state, or local partners. Any mention of trade names, products, or services does not imply an endorsement by the US government or individual agencies. The coauthors and their agencies do not endorse any commercial products, services, or enterprises. In addition, the contractor's role did not include establishing agency policy.

MDHHS and ODH disclaim responsibility for any analyses, interpretations, or conclusions from the data used in this study. The EPA assumes full responsibility for the analysis and interpretation of the data.

CONFLICTS OF INTEREST

The authors have no conflicts of interest to report.

HUMAN PARTICIPANT PROTECTION

Research included in this analysis was approved under institutional review boards through the University of North Carolina (16-2302), MDHHS (201703-12-EA), and ODH (2019-41).

REFERENCES

1. Centers for Disease Control and Prevention. Lead exposure symptoms and complications. April 10, 2024. Available at: https://www.cdc.gov/lead-prevention/symptoms-complications/index.html. Accessed April 17, 2026.
2. Egan KB, Cornwell CR, Courtney JG, Ettinger AS. Blood lead levels in US children ages 1–11 years, 1976–2016. *Environ Health Perspect.* 2021;129(3):37003. https://doi.org/10.1289/EHP7932
3. Environmental Protection Agency. Biomonitoring—lead. 2023. Available at: https://www.epa.gov/americaschildrenenvironment/biomonitoring-lead. Accessed May 29, 2026.
4. Stanek LW, Xue J, Zartarian VG, et al. Identification of high lead exposure locations in Ohio at the census tract scale using a generalizable geospatial hotspot approach. *J Expo Sci Environ Epidemiol.* 2024;34(4):718–726. https://doi.org/10.1038/s41370-024-00666-x
5. Xue J, Zartarian V, Tornero-Velez R, et al. A generalizable evaluated approach, applying advanced geospatial statistical methods, to identify high lead exposure locations at census tract scale: Michigan case study. *Environ Health Perspect.* 2022;130(7):77004. https://doi.org/10.1289/EHP9705
6. Breysse P. Welcome to the *AJPH* supplement on ubiquitous lead: risks, prevention–mitigation programs, and emerging sources of exposure. *Am J Public Health.* 2022;112(suppl 7):S632–S634. https://doi.org/10.2105/AJPH.2022.306986
7. Presidents' Task Force on Environmental Health Risks and Safety Risks to Children. Federal Action Plan to Reduce Childhood Lead Exposures and Associated Health Impacts. December 2018. Available at: https://ptfcehs.niehs.nih.gov/featured-resources/federal-action-plan-reduce-childhood-lead-exposures-and-associated-health. Accessed April 16, 2026.
8. Environmental Protection Agency. Data mapping to identify high lead exposure risk locations in the US. 2025. Available at: https://www.epa.gov/lead/mapping. Accessed May 29, 2026.
9. Zartarian V, Poulakos A, Helms Garrison V, et al. Lead data mapping to prioritize US locations for whole-of-government exposure prevention efforts: state of the science, federal collaborations, and remaining challenges. *Am J Public Health.* 2022;112(suppl 7):S658–S669. https://doi.org/10.2105/AJPH.2022.307051
10. Zartarian VG, Xue J, Poulakos AG, et al. A US lead exposure hotspots analysis. *Environ Sci Technol.* 2024;58(7):3311–3321. https://doi.org/10.1021/acs.est.3c07881
11. Environmental Protection Agency. Lead occurrence and source tool (POST). 2024. Available at: https://epa.maps.arcgis.com/home/item.html?id=89142e6a55d14248a021594553d67bbd. Accessed March 14, 2025.
12. Centers for Disease Control and Prevention. Preventing childhood lead poisoning. June 12, 2024. Available at: https://www.cdc.gov/lead-prevention/prevention/index.html. Accessed May 29, 2026.
13. Klemick H, Mason H, Sullivan K. Superfund cleanups and children's lead exposure. *J Environ Econ Manage.* 2020;100:102289. https://doi.org/10.1016/j.jeem.2019.102289
14. Ye D, Brown JS, Umbach DM, et al. Estimating the effects of soil remediation on children's blood lead near a former lead smelter in Omaha, Nebraska, USA. *Environ Health Perspect.* 2022;130(3):037008. https://doi.org/10.1289/ehp8657
15. Roberts EM, Madrigal D, Valle J, King G, Kite L. Assessing child lead poisoning case ascertainment in the US, 1999–2010. *Pediatrics.* 2017;139(5):10. https://doi.org/10.1542/peds.2016-4266
16. Michigan Health & Human Services. MiTracking. 2026. Available at: https://mitracking.state.mi.us. Accessed May 29, 2026.
17. Environmental Protection Agency. Community lead awareness sessions. May 5, 2026. Available at: https://www.epa.gov/lead/community-lead-awareness-sessions. Accessed May 29, 2026.
18. US Census Bureau. Cartographic boundary files. April 10, 2025. Available at: https://www.census.gov/geographies/mapping-files/time-series/geo/cartographic-boundary.html. Accessed March 17, 2025.
19. Garrison VEH, Ashley PJ. Identifying jurisdictions at risk of containing housing units with deteriorated paint: results and targeting implications for the US Department of Housing and Urban Development. *J Public Health Manag Pract.* 2021;27(6):546–557. https://doi.org/10.1097/PHH.0000000000001191
20. Burke TA, Cascio WE, Costa DL, et al. Rethinking environmental protection: meeting the challenges of a changing world. *Environ Health Perspect.* 2017;125(3):A43–A49. https://doi.org/10.1289/EHP1465
21. Caron RM, Serrell N. Community ecology and capacity: keys to progressing the environmental communication of wicked problems. *Appl Environ Educ Commun.* 2009;8(3–4):195–203. https://doi.org/10.1080/15330150903269464
22. Larsen B, Sánchez-Triana E. Global health burden and cost of lead exposure in children and adults: a health impact and economic modelling analysis. *Lancet Planet Health.* 2023;7(10):e831–e840. https://doi.org/10.1016/S2542-5196(23)00166-3
23. Wisconsin Department of Health Services. Environmental health data dashboards. February 24, 2026. Available at: https://www.dhs.wisconsin.gov/epht/data.htm. Accessed May 29, 2026.
24. State of Ohio. DataOhio. Available at: https://data.ohio.gov/wps/portal/gov/data/view. Accessed May 29, 2026.
25. Centers for Disease Control and Prevention. Childhood blood lead surveillance: national data. September 23, 2025. Available at: https://www.cdc.gov/lead-prevention/php/data/national-surveillance-data.html. Accessed May 29, 2026.
26. Centers for Disease Control and Prevention. National environmental public health tracking network. January 20, 2026. Available at: https://ephtracking.cdc.gov/. Accessed May 29, 2026.
27. Environmental Protection Agency. EPA, HUD and HHS announce interagency commitments to more robust collaboration on addressing risks of exposures to lead. February 26, 2024. Available at: https://www.epa.gov/newsreleases/epa-hud-and-hhs-announce-interagency-commitments-more-robust-collaboration-addressing. Accessed April 16, 2026.

Access to Abortion for US Military Service Members in 2024 After the *Dobbs v Jackson* Supreme Court Decision

Caila Brander, MSc, Kate Grindlay, MSPH, Caitlin Russell, PhD, MBE, MSHP, Elisa Cardnell, MA, and Caitlin Gerdts, PhD, MHS

US military service members have long faced challenges accessing reproductive health care, especially abortion. The 2022 *Dobbs v Jackson Women's Health Organization* (*Dobbs*) Supreme Court decision and subsequent state-level abortion policy restrictions have exacerbated barriers to care for many communities, especially those with marginalized identities.

To assess the impact of *Dobbs* on abortion access for US active-duty service members, we launched a qualitative study among active-duty service members who experienced pregnancy and considered or obtained abortion care after the *Dobbs* decision. Recruitment was challenging, and we completed only 3 interviews. The complexity of accessing abortion care for active-duty military service members has intensified, with long-standing barriers related to insurance, mobility, finances, and confidentiality compounded by post-*Dobbs* abortion restrictions in states where many service members are stationed and by the failure of policies to provide support.

We drew on the existing literature and illustrative quotations from interview participants to explore the impacts of *Dobbs* on this population and reflected on the need to address barriers to abortion access for active-duty service members—a critical issue for military readiness as well as the health and well-being of service members. (*Am J Public Health*. 2026;116(7):1038–1043. https://doi.org/10.2105/AJPH.2026.308431)

AJPH July 2026, Vol. 116, No. 7

More than 225 000 active-duty female service members serve in the US military, the majority of whom are of reproductive age.[1] Despite constituting approximately one fifth (and growing) of the active-duty force, female service members consistently experience challenges to accessing reproductive health services. Active-duty service members who seek to terminate their pregnancies face a unique and complex web of constraints. *Dobbs v Jackson Women's Health Organization* (*Dobbs*; 597 US 215 [2022]), the Supreme Court decision that overturned federal protections for abortion, raised concerns at the Department of Defense (DOD) about military readiness, as barriers to abortion care that preexisted the *Dobbs* decision were likely to worsen as a result.[2]

METHODS

Recognizing the impact of the *Dobbs* decision on this population, we designed a qualitative study to explore experiences of active-duty service members who experienced a pregnancy and considered or obtained abortion care after *Dobbs*. The interview guide explored pregnancy decision-making and, for those who sought abortion, constraints and facilitators to care. Anticipating recruitment challenges owing to the actual and perceived consequences of discussing abortion care in the military,[3] our study team consisted of researchers and organizations with experience on the topic and trusted ties to service members. We relied on convenience sampling to recruit participants through study flyers distributed at abortion clinics, word of mouth through military advocacy groups, online via Reddit posts and advertisements on Meta platforms, and through snowball sampling among participants. We conducted interviews over the encrypted messaging service Signal, and participants provided verbal consent before their interview began.

Over the course of 6 months (June–November 2024), our team was successful in recruiting only 3 participants into our study. The literature has documented recruitment challenges (e.g., heightened state surveillance, increasing fears of criminalization) among populations who face unique barriers to abortion access.[3] However, the specific circumstances and experiences of active-duty service members who considered or sought abortion after the *Dobbs* decision remain undocumented and may have contributed to fears about participating in our study. In this essay, we drew on both the published literature and a selection of illustrative quotations (selected for relevance to the themes addressed in this essay) from our 3 study participants to describe what abortion access for service members was like before the *Dobbs* decision, and we reflect on implications of the *Dobbs* decision and subsequent state and federal policy changes for the current state of abortion access among service members.

RESULTS

It is difficult to determine how many service members access abortion each year. Yet, we know access to contraception in the US military is fraught with challenges,[4] and, simultaneously, studies have documented a higher prevalence of unintended pregnancy among active-duty service members than among the general US population (5.6%–5.9% vs 3.6% of girls and women aged 15–44 years in 2018–2019).[5,6]

Unintended pregnancy was more prevalent among service members who were younger, had a high school degree or less, and were married or cohabitating.[5] Although annual abortion incidence in the military is not reliably measured, 1 study estimated that of the 11 000 to 11 900 unintended pregnancies among active-duty service members each year, roughly 2573 to 4136 end in abortion.[7]

Why Service Members Seek Abortion

Service members seek abortion for many of the same reasons that have been documented among civilians, including financial insecurity, feeling it is not the right time in their life to have a child, or feeling their family is already complete.[8,9] As a study participant serving in the Army in a state with an abortion ban with limited exceptions said, "I had a plan and being pregnant just wasn't in the plan."

There are also reasons specific to military service that may contribute to abortion decision-making among active-duty service members, such as the mental and physical demands of the job, wanting to remain in training or on a deployment, and challenging work schedules that may not accommodate raising a baby. Fear of termination of duty, being reprimanded, and negative impacts on promotions and career growth during pregnancy or parenting can also affect pregnancy decision-making.[8,9] A study participant serving in the Army in a state with gestational limits on abortion reported, "I was nervous because I thought that I was going to get a dishonorable discharge [for] being pregnant." This participant was unsure how pregnancy would affect her current assignment:

> I didn't know if [the pregnancy] would affect my role . . . being as though I'm dealing with, you know, infantry weapons and things of that nature. So, it was kind of like, "What do I do? What do I do?"

Importantly, more than 1 in 10 female service members report experiencing sexual assault in their military careers, defined as an act that involved unwanted, nonconsensual, forced, or coerced touching of sexual body parts or sexual intercourse, a figure that most certainly underestimates the true prevalence of sexual assault among this population.[10] Service members have cited sexual assault as a cause of unintended pregnancy and a contributing factor for seeking abortion.[9] Although abortion care should be available to service members who experience pregnancy as a result of rape, many survivors of sexual assault in the military do not report the assault or seek follow-up care because of stigma, shame, confidentiality concerns, fears of retaliation, or lack of knowledge about services.[11]

Service Member Constraints on Abortion Care

Insurance and funding. Service members face a constellation of unique constraints when attempting to access abortion services. Although most health care is covered by TRICARE (military health insurance), federal law under US Code 1093 prohibits the use of TRICARE funding for abortion services and military treatment facilities from providing abortion services with few exceptions.[12]

Obtaining approval for abortion services under the exceptions permitted in the military statute can be burdensome and bureaucratic, which can cause delayed care.[13] The majority of service members who do not qualify under these exceptions or who cannot wait to obtain approval must pay out of pocket for abortion care. This can be especially burdensome for younger, lower-income service members.[8] Additionally, many service members are not aware that TRICARE does not cover the cost of an abortion.[8,14] This lack of knowledge can lead to delayed care, misinformation, and a lack of referrals or support for follow-up care.[8]

Travel and movement. Military assignments determine much about the life of active-duty service members. Even for those with an active-duty spouse or partner, geographical separation is common. Frequent moves can mean that service members are stationed far from their social support system. Additionally, movement is strictly regulated in the military under all circumstances. "Mileage passes" are generally required for travel off base outside of a designated range, usually more than 250 miles. If a service member is found to be out of the designated range without permission, punitive consequences may ensue, such as restriction to their place of duty or base, forfeiture of pay, extra duties, and even loss of rank.[15] Under some circumstances, such as training periods and missions that require quick recall for unit personnel, mileage passes are never granted. Obtaining a mileage pass often requires the justification of the reason for travel, which, in the event of an unplanned pregnancy, can expose service members to shaming, judgment, and other stigmatizing consequences if those in the chain of command do not support abortion.[8]

Even when a service member receives permission to travel, the cost and logistics of traveling for abortion care may be difficult to manage, especially for younger or low-income service members, who may lack transportation options or financial reserves to cover travel expenses. Additionally, inflexible schedules and the timing of leave requests being determined at a commanders' discretion can make it challenging to schedule appointments and plan for recovery.[8] Some service members are at sea for extended periods of time, with limited or no ability to travel and limited or no pregnancy-related care. For those deployed or stationed overseas, off-base travel is often more tightly constrained, and service members may experience language barriers and country-specific legal restrictions on abortion.[9]

Privacy and confidentiality. Service members face unique concerns related to their privacy and confidentiality when making abortion decisions.[8,9] Before 2023, a service member's chain of command was automatically notified when their pregnancy status was confirmed in a military treatment facility (mandatory reporting now begins at 20 weeks gestational age). Despite the updated policy, an Army enlistee living in a state with an abortion ban with limited exceptions who participated in our study said she did not want to seek pregnancy care at a military treatment facilities in 2024 because "I felt like if I would have gone to a military doctor, then my option would have been taken away to [terminate the pregnancy] because then [the pregnancy] gets put on my profile in the system, and everybody knows." She tied this to her experience with a previous pregnancy, when, after confirming her pregnancy at a military treatment facility, news she was pregnant spread from her chain of command to her entire unit, making her feel she could no longer consider seeking an abortion for that pregnancy.

Service members may also face confidentiality concerns related to the physical demands of their jobs. Patients are typically advised to avoid strenuous activities for the first few days after an abortion,[16] but service members' jobs are often physically demanding, and avoiding strenuous activities may not be possible without disclosing the need for rest. Passing regular physical fitness tests is also a requirement for active duty. One study participant disclosed her abortion to her chain of command, despite her desire not to, because she was concerned about an upcoming fitness test during her recovery period. Service members may also have medical treatment reporting requirements, and although it is likely that many service members do not report their abortion, the requirement itself may have a chilling effect that could affect abortion decision-making. One study documented a case of a service member who chose to have a procedural abortion without anesthesia because they felt they would have had to report taking abortion medications or being given anesthesia.[8]

Abortion Access After *Dobbs*

Since the *Dobbs* decision, as many states have codified partial or total abortion bans, access to abortion care in the United States has become even more geographically stratified and complicated to navigate. Although no study has yet documented the impact of the *Dobbs* decision on access to abortion for US military service members, evidence from the civilian population may be informative. Research has shown that travel time to the nearest abortion clinic increased after the *Dobbs* decision[17] and is most pronounced for abortion seekers in states with partial or total abortion bans, forcing many of them to travel across state lines to access clinic-based abortion services. Abortion seekers residing in states with protective policies may also experience negative consequences, including delays in care, given the increase in average appointment wait time after the *Dobbs* decision that was precipitated by patients traveling from states with bans.[18] Abortion bans place greater strain on practical support organizations, such as abortion funds, that provide financial assistance and logistical support for abortion seekers. Service members with fewer resources to travel for care could avail themselves of these services; however, abortion funds have reported declining resources, with higher call volumes and decreased financial support over time.[19]

Meanwhile, utilization of telehealth for medication abortion has increased substantially and now accounts for about one quarter of all abortions provided in the United States.[18] Some telehealth providers operating in states with shield laws send abortion medication to all 50 states and to Army Post Office addresses[20]; however, remote provision of medication abortion is not preferable for or acceptable to everyone, and the legal protections of shield laws extend only to providers—leaving people who receive abortion pills by mail from shield law providers legally unprotected.

The impact of *Dobbs* on active-duty service members is further illuminated when considering state of residence. Approximately half of active-duty female service members in the continental United States are stationed in states with severely restricted or no abortion services.[21] Furthermore, given the frequent movement required by military life and training, many active-duty service members reside in states with abortion bans for some proportion of time in their careers. In addition to facing potential legal restrictions on abortion services, frequent relocation means that service members may not be familiar with local laws and policies or options for obtaining abortion care. Frequent restationing also occurs among military health care providers, who may not know how to support patients seeking off-site abortion treatment or fear legal risk if they do.

Military Abortion Policy Change After *Dobbs*

In March 2023, in response to the *Dobbs* decision, the DOD instituted several new policies addressing concerns about military readiness.[2,22] These policies enabled paid leave and reimbursement for travel expenses incurred when timely access to noncovered reproductive health care (e.g., abortion, in vitro fertilization) was not locally available. However, between June and December 2023, the policy was used only 12 times to pay for travel expenses for noncovered reproductive health services.[23] It is unknown how many, if any, of these instances were for abortion care. The limited use of these policies raises questions about how well the policies were publicized in the military and thus whether many service members were aware of the benefits.

The 2023 policies offered the potential to offset some of the challenges faced by abortion seekers in the military, as well as projected cost savings for the military, including those associated with improved physical and mental health outcomes among service members able to obtain abortion care. Nevertheless, on January 29, 2025, the DOD reversed all of the military policies that had been implemented in response to the *Dobbs* decision, threatening both the bodily autonomy of service members and the readiness of the US military.[24] In February 2025, Representative Mikie Sherrill (D, NJ) reintroduced HR 1742, the Access to Reproductive Care for Servicemembers Act, a bill that would codify the policies allowing service members to take leave and receive reimbursement for travel costs to receive reproductive health care treatment. The bill currently is with the House Armed Services Committee, which has not acted on it and seems unlikely to do so in the current political climate.[25]

DISCUSSION

Active-duty service members face unique constraints on abortion access that are directly related to their military service, including geographic location for deployment, constricted mobility, threats to privacy and confidentiality, and lack of insurance coverage. These constraints have been compounded in the wake of the *Dobbs* decision, which led to increasing numbers of state-level abortion bans and risks of criminalization for abortion seekers and those who support them. The effects of the *Dobbs* decision are, as in the civilian population, likely to be unequally distributed among service members—with the greatest barriers to care faced by service members who are younger, are more junior-ranking, have fewer financial resources, are from communities that are under heightened surveillance, and are stationed in states with abortion restrictions.

The impact of *Dobbs* on access to abortion care for service members has not been well documented, but the lived experiences of our few study participants, coupled with the existing literature, shed light on what is likely an access crisis in the military. Access to abortion and contraception is an urgent matter of policy and practice for the US military, not only because it is a matter of military readiness, retention, and morale—a chief concern for the DOD—but also because it ensures the bodily autonomy and well-being of those who serve. AJPH

ABOUT THE AUTHORS

Caila Brander and Kate Grindlay are with Ibis Reproductive Health, Cambridge, MA. Caitlin Russell is with the School of Nursing, University of Pennsylvania, Philadelphia. Elisa Cardnell is with Service Women's Action Network, Washington, DC. Caitlin Gerdts is with Ibis Reproductive Health, Oakland, CA.

CORRESPONDENCE

Correspondence should be sent to Caila Brander, 2067 Massachusetts Ave, Suite 320, Cambridge, MA 02140 (e-mail: cbrander@ibisreproductivehealth.org). Reprints can be ordered at https://www.ajph.org by clicking the "Reprints" link.

PUBLICATION INFORMATION

Full Citation: Brander C, Grindlay K, Russell C, Cardnell E, Gerdts C. Access to abortion for US military service members in 2024 after the *Dobbs v Jackson* Supreme Court decision. *Am J Public Health*. 2026;116(7):1038–1043.

Acceptance Date: December 15, 2025.

DOI: https://doi.org/10.2105/AJPH.2026.308431

ORCID iDs:

Caila Brander https://orcid.org/0000-0002-1274-1848

Kate Grindlay https://orcid.org/0000-0003-4426-3710

Caitlin Russell https://orcid.org/0009-0007-0156-7892

Caitlin Gerdts https://orcid.org/0000-0002-2488-5072

CONTRIBUTORS

C. Brander wrote the first draft of the essay, and K. Grindlay, C. Russell, E. Cardnell, and C. Gerdts provided substantive input. C. Brander and K. Grindlay designed and implemented the qualitative interviews and conducted the literature review, with expert input from C. Russell and E. Cardnell. K. Grindlay conceptualized the study and this essay.

ACKNOWLEDGMENTS

This research was made possible by general institutional funds, including support from the DeMartini Family Foundation.

CONFLICTS OF INTEREST

The authors have no conflicts of interest to disclose.

HUMAN PARTICIPANT PROTECTION

The WCG institutional review board approved this study (tracking no. 20242277). Participants provided verbal consent.

REFERENCES

1. Meadows SO, Collins RL, Schuler MS, Beckman RL, Cefalu M. The women's reproductive health survey (WRHS) of active-duty service members. September 13, 2022. Available at: https://www.rand.org/pubs/research_reports/RRA1031-1.html. Accessed November 21, 2023.
2. Secretary of Defense. Ensuring access to reproductive health care. Available at: https://media.defense.gov/2022/oct/20/2003099747/-1/-1/1/memorandum-ensuring-access-to-reproductive-health-care.pdf. Accessed November 1, 2023.
3. Zuniga C, Ragosta S, Thompson TA. Recruiting foreign-born individuals who have sought an abortion in the United States: lessons from a feasibility study. *Front Glob Womens Health*. 2023;4:1114820. https://doi.org/10.3389/fgwh.2023.1114820
4. Vargas SE, Thornton K, Norris C, et al. Sexual and reproductive health in military settings: a qualitative study. *Mil Psychol*. 2025;37(2):138–147. https://doi.org/10.1080/08995605.2024.2324644
5. Hamrick JE, Ahmed AE, Witkop CT, Manetz KE, Mancuso JD. Unintended pregnancy among US military active duty servicemembers: estimates for 2018 and trends since 2005. *Contraception*. 2023;119:109894. https://doi.org/10.1016/j.contraception.2022.09.132
6. National Center for Health Statistics. US pregnancy rates drop during last decade. 2023. Available at: https://www.cdc.gov/nchs/pressroom/nchs_press_releases/2023/20230412.htm. Accessed March 11, 2025.
7. Hunter KM, Meadows SO, Collins RL, González I. How the *Dobbs* decision could affect US national security. *Rand Health Q*. 2023;10(2):9.
8. Grindlay K, Seymour JW, Fix L, Reiger S, Keefe-Oates B, Grossman D. Abortion knowledge and experiences among US servicewomen: a qualitative study. *Perspect Sex Reprod Health*. 2017;49(4):245–252. https://doi.org/10.1363/psrh.12044
9. Fix L, Seymour JW, Grossman D, et al. Abortion need among US servicewomen: evidence from an Internet service. *Womens Health Issues*. 2020;30(3):161–166. https://doi.org/10.1016/j.whi.2019.10.006
10. Wilson LC. The prevalence of military sexual trauma: a meta-analysis. *Trauma Violence Abuse*. 2018;19(5):584–597. https://doi.org/10.1177/1524838016683459
11. Burns B, Grindlay K, Holt K, Manski R, Grossman D. Military sexual trauma among US servicewomen during deployment: a qualitative study. *Am J Public Health*. 2014;104(2):345–349. https://doi.org/10.2105/AJPH.2013.301576
12. Legal Information Institute. 10 US Code § 1093—Performance of abortions: restrictions. Available at: https://www.law.cornell.edu/uscode/text/10/1093. Accessed November 18, 2025.
13. Edwards E, Fields, R. A Coast Guard commander miscarried. She nearly died after being denied care. December 13, 2024. Available at: https://www.propublica.org/article/elizabeth-nakagawa-miscarriage-military-tricare-abortion-policy. Accessed March 12, 2025.
14. Seymour JW, Fix L, Grossman D, Grindlay K. Pregnancy and abortion: experiences and attitudes of deployed US servicewomen. *Mil Med*. 2020;185(9–10):e1390. https://doi.org/10.1093/milmed/usaa128
15. Department of the Army. Army regulation 600–8–10. Personnel–general. Leaves and passes. Available at: https://asktop.net/wp/download/3/r600_8_10.pdf. Accessed November 6, 2025.
16. American College of Obstetricians and Gynecologists. Abortion care. Available at: https://www.acog.org/womens-health/faqs/induced-abortion. Accessed March 12, 2025.
17. Rader B, Upadhyay UD, Sehgal NKR, Reis BY, Brownstein JS, Hswen Y. Estimated travel time and spatial access to abortion facilities in the US before and after the *Dobbs v Jackson Women's Health* decision. *JAMA*. 2022;328(20):2041–2047. https://doi.org/10.1001/jama.2022.20424
18. Society of Family Planning. #WeCount report, April 2022 to December 2024. Available at: https://societyfp.org/research/wecount/wecount-december-2024-data. Accessed November 6, 2025.
19. Colombini S, Nadworny E. It's harder to pay and travel for abortion care, and support funds are struggling. *Shots* blog. National Public Radio. October 3, 2024. Available at: https://www.npr.org/sections/shots-health-news/2024/10/03/nx-s1-5131573/abortion-fund-travel-state-bans-ballot-measures-national-federation-budget-cuts-repro-rights. Accessed March 12, 2025.
20. Foster AM, Mark A, Drouillard KJ, et al. "Trust women": characteristics of and learnings from patients of a shield law medication abortion practice in the United States. *Perspect Sex Reprod Health*. 2024;56(3):295–302. https://doi.org/10.1111/psrh.12287
21. Hunter KM, Meadows SO. Limiting access to reproductive health care may undermine national security. July 6, 2023. Available at: https://www.rand.org/pubs/commentary/2023/07/limiting-access-to-reproductive-health-care-may-undermine.html. Accessed March 12, 2025.

22. Gill EA, Zeng W, Lamme JS, et al. Decision and economic evaluation of abortion availability in the United States military. *Am J Obstet Gynecol.* 2025;232(3):301.e1–301.e10. https://doi.org/10.1016/j.ajog.2024.09.003
23. Lopez CT. DOD releases usage numbers for reproductive health care travel. March 26, 2024. Available at: https://www.war.gov/News/News-Stories/Article/Article/3719375/dod-releases-usage-numbers-for-reproductive-health-care-travel. Accessed March 12, 2025.
24. Department of Defense. Remove travel for non-covered reproductive health care services. January 29, 2025. Available at: https://media.defense.gov/2025/Jan/29/2003634768/-1/-1/0/utd_for_map_04-25(s)_remove-travel-for-non-covered-reproductive-health-care-services.pdf. Accessed March 12, 2025.
25. Rep. M. Sherrill [D N 11]. H.R. 1742—119th Congress (2025–2026): Access to Reproductive Care for Servicemembers Act. February 27, 2025. Available at: https://www.congress.gov/bill/119th-congress/house-bill/1742. Accessed November 5, 2025.

Keeping Sight of Albay: Vitamin A Blindness, Randomized Controlled Trials, and Cold War Foreign Aid Policy

Rajiv M. Sastry, AM

Physicians have long known that vitamin A deficiency causes pediatric blindness. However, in 1986, Johns Hopkins researchers examining the impact of vitamin A supplementation on overall child mortality in Albay, Philippines, encountered strong local opposition, forcing the study's termination. Drawing on internal documents, interviews, and archival correspondence, this article uses the Albay study's collapse as a case study to examine how Cold War–era cultural, geopolitical, and social forces shaped the public health knowledge production process. This history offers insights into how policymakers might develop effective modern foreign aid projects, especially as funding priorities continue to evolve. (*Am J Public Health*. 2026;116(7):1044–1052. https://doi.org/10.2105/AJPH.2026.308447)

AJPH July 2026, Vol. 116, No. 7

By November 1986, Keith West and Alfred Sommer's research in the Philippines had hit an unusual roadblock. After weeks of threats against the study's staff, the leader of a local medical advocacy group informed West that their study was going to be shut down, with force if necessary. West gathered his research colleagues: "I don't mind giving our careers to vitamin A, [but] we're not going to give our lives to vitamin A." That night, they packed whatever data they could, drove 15 hours to Manila, and flew back to the United States.[1]

West, then a graduate student at Johns Hopkins University, and Sommer, an ophthalmologist at the Johns Hopkins Wilmer Eye Institute, had been attempting a field trial in the rural province of Albay. Physicians had long known that supplementing malnourished children with vitamin A helped prevent nutritional blindness diseases such as xerophthalmia, which is caused by vitamin A deficiency (VAD).[2] Beyond saving vision, however, Sommer and West believed that four cents' worth of vitamin A capsules could also reduce childhood mortality risk by more than 30%.[3] If true, this hypothesis had the potential to significantly shift international nutrition priorities.

Sommer and West faced strong pushback and skepticism within academia, further raising the stakes for this follow-up randomized controlled trial in the Philippines. But the strongest opposition they faced came from the Albay community itself. After more than two dozen children enrolled in the vitamin A supplementation (VAS) study fell ill in August 1986, some in Albay, instigated by local radio personalities, physicians, and communist dissenters, branded the study's staff as cruel experimenters, pharmaceutical profiteers, and spies affiliated with the US government.

From the 1950s onward, the US government implemented international development projects as a means of building soft power in regions vulnerable to undesirable political influences. Organized through the US Agency for International Development (AID), the Central Intelligence Agency (CIA), and private organizations, these projects were intended as low-cost solutions to regional challenges. Certain populations, however, received these projects poorly, especially when initiatives were considered pretexts for surveillance.[4] The Johns Hopkins team's project was a research endeavor and a pivotal career moment, but a closer analysis shows that its funding and philosophy partially mirrored past public health modernization efforts undertaken in the Philippines.[5]

Sommer and his team's VAS research accomplishments have been discussed in materials written by Richard Semba.[6] Semba's writing draws on strong primary sources, but it carries the risk of bias, as he is Sommer's colleague at the Wilmer Eye Institute.[7] Other accounts, drawing on interview material collected long after the research itself took place, risk portraying VAS in a triumphalist manner—occluding challenges that arose along the way. Although Sarah Wallace has discussed opposition that one VAS project sparked in India, that incident took place in 2001 as part of a community health care project, rather than a research study. It also occurred well after the VAD–mortality link had become widely accepted in the medical community.[8]

The 1986 Albay study has seldom been discussed in existing scholarship. Semba has argued that the study collapsed chiefly because its organizers miscalculated community support for the study and underestimated the impact of regional political instability. But he stopped short of contextualizing the incident within broader histories of international health and development, and his analysis did not examine the study's technical documents and internal reports.

Using Albay as a case study, this essay aims to illuminate how Cold War geopolitical, methodological, and ideological forces shaped knowledge production in late 20th century public health research. I argue that the same characteristics that made the Johns Hopkins team's project a strategic Cold War science effort—based in an area of previous intelligence activity, measurable through randomized controlled trials, and centered around an apparent magic bullet solution—incited resistance in a region where past foreign development attempts were considered to be serving outside interests.

A region's history, culture, and political context are important considerations when designing public health initiatives abroad.[9] But examining how domestic priorities within aid-giving nations shaped past outcomes offers insight into the design, ethics, and effectiveness of interventions. Especially as shifting policy frameworks continually impact the landscape of American foreign aid, these insights may help optimize resources and inform funding priorities.

EARLY US INTERNATIONAL DEVELOPMENT STRATEGY

In the early 20th century, US efforts to improve health in international contexts focused primarily on its territories. Projects aimed to stop the spread of diseases that threatened military interests and endangered the health of American management personnel. It was only in the 1950s, in response to Asian and African colonies gaining independence, that American policymakers reoriented these projects away from territory management and toward fostering democratic ideals.

The United States' early 20th century disease regulation methods in its territories were characteristic of what Randall Packard termed the "disease-campaign approach to public health."[10] After the Spanish–American War ended in 1898, Spain ceded Cuba and the Philippines to the United States; both were considered strategic assets for military and economic interests. Soon after, the United States began to address yellow fever outbreaks in Cuba, which had spread to the continental American South. Officials ordered "meticulous reporting and surveillance" of disease spread, as well as home fumigations and insecticide sprayings.[11] As Mariola Espinosa's research showed, American prosperity was the clear priority of these efforts, and any benefits for Cubans were secondary.[12]

Similar efforts took place in the Philippines. Among the most extensive projects implemented by American staff concerned Filipino human excrement infrastructure, which was thought to be a public health concern. One American physician wrote that the culture of "promiscuous defecation is dangerous and should be discontinued," a reference to the lack of Western-style indoor plumbing and certain hygiene practices perceived as substandard.[13] Warwick Anderson has concluded that beyond quality-of-life improvement for American expatriates, these efforts held little benefit for native populations.[14]

Many experts in Philippine studies have chronicled parallel narratives. Reynaldo Ileto and Gideon Lasco have written histories regarding invasive cholera management efforts and infantilizing stature comparison, respectively.[15] Alfred McCoy's work has examined the surveillance networks and information collection methods developed to monitor individuals deemed politically destabilizing.[16] Vicente Rafael has detailed census-taking efforts that rendered each person "essentialized, regulated, and therefore retrievable."[17] These strategies were used to further justify American authority during this period, despite sustained, organized resistance from Filipinos.

Scholars have observed a distinct shift in the United States' post–World War II approach to foreign aid and development strategy, with some projects serving as pretexts to influence politics in young or unstable nations. In 1955, the US State Department consolidated a series of smaller aid divisions into the International Cooperation Agency, which eventually became an independent organization—known as AID—under the Kennedy Administration in 1961.[18] As one author wrote in *AJPH* in 1955, public health could "combat communism at its most vulnerable point[s]."[19] Projects operated worldwide, spanning from health systems development in postindependence India to malaria eradication efforts in Mexico.[20]

The CIA used similar development projects to facilitate anticommunism campaigns in many Asian and African nations.[21] Daniel Immerwahr has argued that the CIA considered community development investment "a form of counterinsurgency" in rural areas of the Philippines that could be susceptible to ideological influences like communism. These projects centered on easily quantifiable outcomes, like infrastructure and technology improvement, rather than socioeconomic interventions or policy reform.[22] The long pattern of multi-intentioned aid interventions in the Philippines—especially in rural areas—set the stage for the opposition that the Johns Hopkins team faced in 1986.

EARLY VITAMIN A DEFICIENCY DEVELOPMENT PROJECTS

In 1972, about 15 years before the Albay study, the mass distribution of vitamin A capsules by the Indian government to child refugees helped attract American international development organizations to VAD. Soon after the Bangladesh Liberation War erupted in March 1971, migrants crossed the Indian border and were placed in temporary camps just north of Calcutta, where it became apparent that many children were suffering from VAD-induced blindness.[23] In January 1972, through the logistical support of the Indian government and several nongovernmental organizations (NGOs), 300 000 high-dose vitamin A capsules were delivered to Calcutta, which were then distributed over the next few months.[24] As the final report of one of the NGOs concluded, the project was considered broadly successful.[25]

This campaign directed the United Nations Children's Fund (UNICEF) and the World Health Organization (WHO) to examine VAD. In March 1972, WHO representatives and UNICEF's Executive Board held a meeting concerning VAD, noting that it was the "largest single cause of preventable blindness in many developing countries." Attendees noted the economic impact of blindness was "staggering," of which the cost of VAS was "a small fraction."[26] UNICEF's 1972 annual report also suggests that the instability in South Asia had triggered this new interest: it noted that in 1971, "controlled distribution of vitamin A was begun in . . . Bangladesh."[27]

By 1973, the United States had also taken interest in VAD. That year, AID compiled a three-volume manual—a substantial investment—that surveyed VAD's impact and treatment options.[28] From a cost-optimization perspective, the authors concluded capsule supplementation was the most inexpensive option to address VAD and particularly ideal for short-term interventions. Food fortification with vitamin A was "the best long range practice" but far more difficult to implement because of high manufacturing and research costs.[29]

Sommer, meanwhile, had conducted research in Indonesia from 1976 to 1979 that suggested VAD and pediatric mortality were linked, and to confirm this hypothesis, he and his team organized a rigorous follow-up study.[30] Their April 1986 proposal to AID, which requested $950 000 in funding, outlined a clear, measurable objective and an efficient timeline: the team aimed

> to compare the efficacy of high dose . . . versus low dose . . . vitamin A supplementation of children six months through five years of age on a thrice yearly basis in reducing overall mortality by at least 25%.[31]

A quantifiable mortality reduction target and the possibility that this inexpensive intervention could save lives in addition to preventing blindness was a promising enough combination to secure AID's support.

ALBAY'S ENTANGLEMENTS IN DEVELOPMENT AND INTELLIGENCE LEGACIES

Known as the Albay Mother and Child Health Project, the study was a partnership between Johns Hopkins, the Philippines Ministry of Health, and Helen Keller International (an NGO focused on blindness prevention). The team's rationale for selecting the Philippines as the study site focused on logistics and stability. Sommer wrote that "the Philippines provide a unique environment" because "it is a country with Government, health profession, and development infrastructures sufficient to support a large scale intervention trial."[32]

Although this infrastructure was helpful for executing a well-run study, scholars such as Latham, Immerwahr, and Anderson would eventually argue that much of it was installed through American development projects that some local populations considered unwelcome or suspicious. Through this lens—admittedly, a lens of hindsight—I posit that aspects of the Albay community's response to the VAS study may have been grounded in collective memory of these past interventions.

Though the study began smoothly, on August 21, 1986, radio broadcaster Nelson Arao alleged "two dozen children . . . had fallen ill with nausea, vomiting, and diarrhea" after receiving

VAS.[33] Even though these symptoms were well-known side effects of VAS, Arao's allegations stirred community unrest. As reported in *The Manila Times* and *The Manila Bulletin*, physician Francis Burgos rallied the public around claims that "American researchers were using the children of Albay . . . 'as guinea pigs.'"[34]

Among the issues Burgos publicized, he considered the "double-blind" aspect of the research especially troublesome, in addition to his perception that most of the study's field staff were "nonhealth graduates."[35] In response, the Philippines Ministry of Health then held a press conference, where local journalists questioned "why the project was being funded by the U.S. government." Some even theorized that the study aimed to establish Filipino dependence on capsules for the American pharmaceutical industry's future profit.[36]

The recurrent themes of autonomy, experimentation, and financial motivations broadly encompassed in these concerns align with examples of past intelligence projects in the Philippines, which sometimes doubled as development initiatives. CIA-run projects in the 1950s often employed creative methods to sideline opponent leaders and promote figures considered friendly to America. As Immerwahr detailed, using a community civics development organization, CIA officer Edward Lansdale "drummed up campaign donations . . . from U.S. corporations such as Coca-Cola" to help American ally Ramon Magsaysay win the 1953 presidential election.[37] Lansdale also galvanized his cover by "befriending and eventually marrying a Filipina" who he already knew was an affiliate of the communist rebel group Lansdale was working to dismantle.[38]

Returning to 1986, when fieldworkers tried to continue the VAS study, they were "branded 'anti-Philippine' and 'puppets of the Americans,'" and in one incident, a team was "intercepted, interrogated, and ordered to quit the project" by members of the Philippine Communist Party.[39] Despite negotiation with Burgos, in November 1986, Sommer and West concluded that the study could not continue. A year later, one of the study's Filipina collaborators, Thiele Lunas, contacted West to inform him that they had made the right choice. By her account, most of the barangays (villages) had become "totally infiltrated by communists," and fieldworker lives would have been "endangered had the project continued"[40] (Figure 1).

To be clear, the Albay study was not linked to any US intelligence projects, and by all accounts, Sommer and his

AJPH July 2026, Vol. 116, No. 7

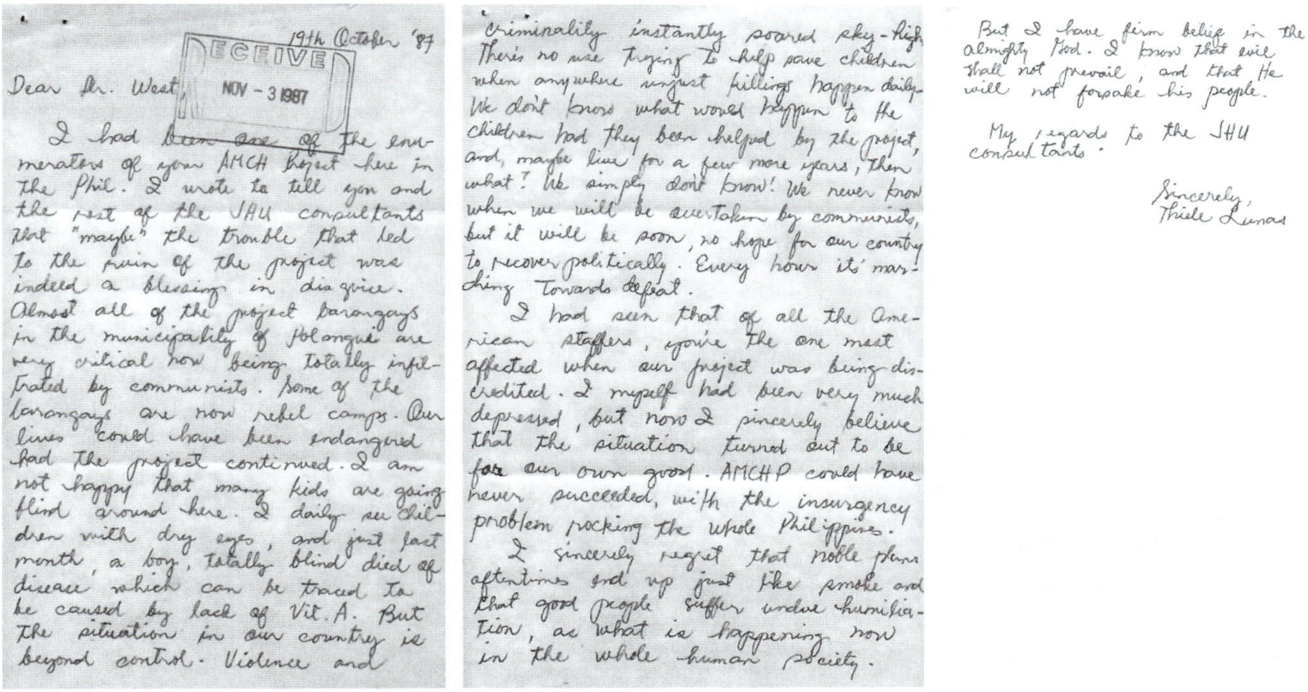

19th October '87

RECEIVED NOV - 3 1987

Dear Mr. West,

I had been one of the enumerators of your AMCH Project here in the Phil. I wrote to tell you and the rest of the JHU consultants that "maybe" the trouble that led to the ruin of the project was indeed a blessing in disguise. Almost all of the project barangays in the municipality of Polangui are very critical now being totally infiltrated by communists. Some of the barangays are now rebel camps. Our lives could have been endangered had the project continued. I am not happy that many kids are going blind around here. I daily see children with dry eyes, and just last month, a boy, totally blind died of disease which can be traced to be caused by lack of Vit. A. But the situation in our country is beyond control. Violence and criminality instantly soared sky-high. There's no use trying to help save children when anywhere unjust killings happen daily. We don't know what would happen to the children had they been helped by the project, and, maybe live for a few more years, then what? We simply don't know! We never know when we will be overtaken by communists, but it will be soon, no hope for our country to recover politically. Every hour it's marching towards defeat.

I had seen that of all the American staffers, you're the one most affected when our project was being discredited. I myself had been very much depressed, but now I sincerely believe that the situation turned out to be for our own good. AMCHP could have never succeeded, with the insurgency problem rocking the whole Philippines.

I sincerely regret that noble plans oftentimes end up just like smoke and that good people suffer undue humiliation, as what is happening now in the whole human society.

But I have firm belief in the almighty God. I know that evil shall not prevail, and that He will not forsake his people.

My regards to the JHU consultants.

Sincerely,
Thiele Lunas

FIGURE 1— Letter From Thiele Lunas to Keith West, October 19, 1987

Source. Alfred Sommer Collection, Box AS2–4, Johns Hopkins University, Alan Mason Chesney Medical Archives.

collaborators were ethical researchers and implemented a protocol that had been vetted by the Johns Hopkins University and the Philippines Ministry of Health. But less than 10 years earlier, the CIA had attempted to fund nutrition research abroad. In 1978, professors at Cornell University received a letter from the CIA soliciting study proposals to investigate nutritional diseases in Mexico, Cuba, Brazil, Nigeria, and the Philippines. The CIA was especially interested in deficiencies that could cause "debilitation and crippling diseases in the labor force."[41]

One of the professors, Michael C. Latham, recalled that from 1967 to perhaps 1975, the "No. 2 man at USAID in the Philippines, Joe Whelton, was the No. 1 CIA man."[42] According to Whelton's obituary, he completed AID service in 1975 as assistant director of the Manila office, and previously worked as an "information officer and program officer" in Washington, Vietnam, and Cambodia.[43] Latham recalled that Whelton "held sway in [their] nutrition programs" and "veto[ed]" ideas.[44]

In 1979, the CIA's letter was also leaked in *CounterSpy*, a magazine that exposed US intelligence programs and identified undercover CIA personnel abroad.[45] While it is difficult to determine what came of these particular CIA objectives—and if populations abroad learned of them—that the letter appeared in a globally circulated outlet indicates that some programs lost their covert status.

COLD WAR RATIONALITY AND RANDOMIZED CONTROLLED TRIALS

Examining how the Albay study's design was influenced by new standards of Cold War scientific knowledge production offers further insight into the suspicion expressed in Albay. The study methodology Sommer and his team used—the randomized controlled trial—emerged within an intellectual climate that Paul Erickson et al. have termed "Cold War rationality."[46] Cold War rationality championed rigid methodological focus on quantitative objectivity that was "sometimes not only in competition with but in downright opposition to reason, reasonableness, and common sense."[47]

Developed out of methods originated by early 20th century scientists to reduce experimental bias, the randomized controlled trial did not initially receive widespread acclaim when it was introduced in the 1940s.[48] As Jeremy Greene has written, "generalizing between experimental knowledge and clinical experience" had already inspired myriad experimental methodologies dating back to the early modern period.[49] But beginning in the early Cold War years, new technology and treatments had influenced medical culture and practice such that the randomized controlled trial's utility became more apparent.

At universities, engineers and physicians experimented with using computers for clinical diagnoses. Prototype devices that used Bayesian logic and early machine learning drew only on patient data, rather than direct examination. Some physicians cautiously celebrated this technology—which operationalized patients as anonymous and numerical—as a means of standardizing care and reducing errors.[50]

Similarly, the randomized controlled trial allowed regulatory bodies to systematize the assessment of the many pharmaceuticals that had emerged after World War II. Government organizations such as the National Institutes of Health and the UK Medical Research Council were among the earliest and most enthusiastic adopters of the randomized controlled trial. Rather than accept drug manufacturers' results and testimony, the randomized controlled trial presented a fixed methodology to verify drug safety, especially useful after the thalidomide tragedy in 1961.[51] Through widespread use across disciplines since the 1950s, the randomized controlled trial eventually gained a reputation as the "gold standard" study methodology. It is unsurprising that some epidemiologists would later celebrate randomized controlled trials as "the best means to make medicine more rational."[52]

Randomized controlled trials, however, were challenging to implement in certain fields. As David S. Jones has argued, factors unique to the surgical field, like standardizing surgeon skill or the ethics of surgical placebo, meant that strict adherence to the gold standard was not always the most practical or informative means of assessing a therapy.[53] Jones would go on to note that these and other tensions have bedeviled the use of randomized controlled trials in surgery for more than 50 years.[54]

Randomized controlled trials were similarly vexing in public health field trials. These studies often took place in environments where external factors and human behavior were difficult to control for. In fact, part of the impetus for the Albay project came from methodological criticism levied against Sommer's original VAD–mortality research, especially concerning apparent discrepancies in the participants' demographic characteristics.[55] Accordingly, in designing the new study, Sommer and his collaborators attempted to minimize any sources of data irregularity.[56]

Given the political shifts in the Philippines in the months before the Albay study was to start, some residents may have misinterpreted these accuracy efforts as attempts to manage local populations. In February 1986, after nearly two decades in office, US-backed president Ferdinand Marcos was overthrown.[57] The fact that Marcos—a dictator associated with decades of torture, disappearances, and other human rights abuses—had just been granted asylum in the United States after absconding with billions likely underlaid Filipinos' mistrust of an American research project being launched at this volatile political moment.[58]

Regardless, nearly 30 000 households had agreed to participate in the study, constituting 40 000 preschool-aged children across 250 villages. Handling this cohort required solutions that could be implemented in a low-resource setting.[59] In this spirit, the team hired a blacksmith to make metal plates engraved with each family's study ID number, which were then affixed outside each home.[60] Fieldworkers also created detailed village maps so they could cross-reference plate numbers when collecting data and administering VAS. Once opposition emerged, however, these plates became a visible representation of community distrust and sentiments of dehumanization. As Semba noted, "fieldworkers began to find . . . the plates they had posted torn down, tacked to conspicuous coconut palms, and marked with graffiti: R.I.P."[61]

Families may have also become suspicious because some of the study's data collection questions extended to areas that seemed less relevant to a public health project. One form instructed fieldworkers to ask families if they owned agricultural land and if they had a TV or radio at home, in addition to querying household income and the source of the household's drinking water. The form also instructed staff to ask families, "Do you use any toilet?" and, if yes, "Is it public or private?"[62]

These questions were likely intended to help the research team better understand upstream public health factors. Under different circumstances, however, some of this information—ranging from communication outlets to basic necessities for survival—could have been useful for anticipating and managing grassroots movements. This background may better explain why local opponents theorized the study "could have doubled as an anti-insurgency plot of the government in collusion with American intelligence."[63]

ALBAY AT THE CENTER OF DIVERGING COLD WAR HEALTH FRAMEWORKS

Even before this on-the-ground resistance, the Albay study was poised to mediate a core ideological tension in international health during the late Cold War, from the 1970s onward.[64] As Sommer's original mortality findings from Indonesia spread, critics questioned both his proposed mortality link and the long-term value of capsule VAS, positioning it as an example of a "magic bullet" approach. In their eyes, Sommer's research risked oversimplifying pediatric mortality into a problem that could be solved through a two-cent capsule; the Albay study had the potential to further lead funding bodies to this conclusion.

Latham—one of the Cornell professors contacted by the CIA—argued it would be unwise for international health advocates to make "alterations in health and nutrition priorities . . . in the belief [that vitamin A capsules] reduce childhood mortality." Instead, he advocated increasing the production and consumption of vitamin A–rich foods in developing nations, including through food fortification, which AID had considered in 1973.[65] Latham believed capsule supplementation disincentivized policy-level reform, which required more commitment, but may have held greater long-run potential to alleviate nutritional disease.[66]

Conversely, West has argued that it "takes decades to create . . . a reliable food system," let alone one in which "children who are poor get vitamin A in their diets."[67] Soon after the Albay study collapsed, Sommer emphasized that until widespread primary care became cost-feasible, "we'll have to employ quick fixes if we're going to help people now."[68] Especially considering these limitations, both considered capsule VAS a miracle therapy that could save a child's vision and life for just four cents per year.[69]

Latham and the Johns Hopkins team's opposing perspectives reflected a fissure in 1980s international health policy. Broadly speaking, this debate focused on ideal versus pragmatic interventions, with the latter aligning more closely with American Cold War priorities.[70] The landmark 1978 Alma Ata declaration, for instance, set the goal of implementing worldwide, universal primary care by 2000.[71] American physicians argued in response that spot-treatment—like "measles and diphtheria-pertussis-tetanus vaccination, treatment of febrile malaria and oral hydration for diarrhea in children"—was a more pragmatic approach. These physicians predicted future decades would be an "age of diminishing resources," and flexible and low-cost interventions needed to be prioritized when addressing international health concerns.[72] In this context, the Albay study was an opportunity to show funding bodies that capsule VAS fit squarely within this framework. Indeed, despite the challenges in Albay, AID continued to support the Johns Hopkins team's research, including the confirmatory 1991 Nepal study that helped spur UNICEF to implement mass capsule VAS programs in dozens of developing nations beginning in 1992.[73]

CONCLUSIONS

Until now, the Albay study has been considered an aberration within the successful narrative of VAS research. Despite this incident and the ensuing research delay, the Johns Hopkins team's research—and their persistence in the face of opposition—has been credited with saving the vision and lives of millions of children worldwide.[74] Despite pushback, UNICEF continues to operate international VAS programs.[75] This success hinged on the knowledge production process that established VAS could significantly reduce childhood mortality. Examining the Albay study within the intertwined histories of the Cold War and American involvement in the Philippines helps reveal the causes and broader meanings of the opposition researchers faced in 1986.

Throughout the 20th century, the United States undertook efforts to shape the Philippines' public health infrastructure and politics. The earliest attempts, which focused on hygiene, primarily aimed to improve quality of life for Americans living in the Philippines. After World War II, postindependence American development projects attempted to prevent communist rebellions from gaining traction in rural regions. Concurrently, Cold War science culture elevated research tools like the randomized controlled trial and prioritized public health interventions that were quantitatively measurable, short-term, and cost-efficient. The Albay study's collapse demonstrates how these particular domestic objectives, even as reflected by projects as innocuous as nutrition research, sometimes prompted the very resistance they aimed to quell.

Despite the challenges it highlights, this case study should not be interpreted as a justification for completely shuttering American public health efforts in other nations, nor for casting doubt on the stated intent of ongoing research. Rather, it reveals that cultural memory of past American projects—particularly those that facilitated policy and ideological objectives—can collide with modern-day research and humanitarian goals. Examining these legacies more carefully may assist policymakers to develop projects that can provide genuine public health benefits for global populations while advancing American interests and values abroad. **AJPH**

ABOUT THE AUTHOR

Rajiv M. Sastry is with the Department of the History of Science, Harvard University, Cambridge, MA; the Department of Global Health and Social Medicine, Harvard Medical School, Boston, MA; and the Department of Ophthalmology, Massachusetts Eye and Ear and Harvard Medical School, Boston.

CORRESPONDENCE

Correspondence should be sent to Rajiv M. Sastry, Department of the History of Science, Harvard University, 1 Oxford St #371, Cambridge, MA 02138 (e-mail: rsastry@alumni.harvard.edu). Reprints can be ordered at https://www.ajph.org by clicking the "Reprints" link.

PUBLICATION INFORMATION

Full Citation: Sastry RM. Keeping sight of Albay: vitamin A blindness, randomized controlled trials, and Cold War foreign aid policy. *Am J Public Health*. 2026;116(7):1044–1052.

Acceptance Date: January 8, 2026.

DOI: https://doi.org/10.2105/AJPH.2026.308447

ORCID iD:
Rajiv M. Sastry https://orcid.org/0000-0002-5810-0229

ACKNOWLEDGMENTS

I would like to especially thank David S. Jones, who advised my undergraduate thesis and encouraged me to adapt a portion of it into this essay. I am also deeply grateful to Allan Brandt, Ben Wilson, Salmaan Keshavjee, and Luke Messac for their generous advice and mentorship. Finally, I extend my thanks to Al Sommer, Keith West, and Joanne Katz, and to the archivists at the Johns Hopkins Chesney Medical Archives, Harvard Business School Special Collections and Archives, and Cornell University Division of Rare and Manuscript Collections.

CONFLICTS OF INTEREST

The author reports no conflicts of interest.

ENDNOTES

1. Conversation with Keith West, November 25, 2023.
2. W. A. Evans, "How to Keep Well: Sore Eyes and Vitamin A," *Chicago Daily Tribune (1923–1963)*, June 27, 1933.
3. Alfred Sommer et al., "Impact of Vitamin A Supplementation on Childhood Mortality: A Randomised Controlled Community Trial," *The Lancet*, originally published as volume 1, issue 8491, 327 (May 24, 1986): 1169–1173, https://doi.org/10.1016/S0140-6736(86)91157-8; definitionally, pediatric mortality refers to "the probability a newborn would die before reaching exactly 5 year of age," World Health Organization, "Under-Five Mortality Rate," https://www.who.int/data/nutrition/nlis/info/under-five-mortality-rate (accessed February 25, 2024).
4. Daniel Immerwahr, *Thinking Small: The United States and the Lure of Community Development* (Cambridge, MA: Harvard University Press, 2014), https://doi.org/10.4159/harvard.9780674735835
5. Alfred Sommer and Michael B. Amey, "Impact of Vitamin A Supplementation on the Reduction of Childhood Mortality in The Philippines; Proposal to: Office of Nutrition, Bureau of Science and Technology, United States Agency for International Development, From: The International Center for Epidemiologic and Preventive Ophthalmology, The Johns Hopkins University in Collaboration with the Ministry of Health, Republic of the Philippines, and Helen Keller International, Inc.," April 22, 1986, Alfred Sommer Collection, Box AS2-2, Johns Hopkins University, Alan Mason Chesney Medical Archives.
6. Richard D. Semba, *The Vitamin A Story: Lifting the Shadow of Death* (Basel, Switzerland: Karger Medical and Scientific Publishers, 2012).
7. Johns Hopkins University, "Richard D. Semba, M.D., M.A., M.P.H., Professor of Ophthalmology," *Johns Hopkins Medicine*, https://www.hopkinsmedicine.org/profiles/details/richard-semba (accessed February 29, 2024).
8. Sarah K. Wallace, "Global Health in Conflict Understanding Opposition to Vitamin A Supplementation in India," *American Journal of Public Health* 102, no. 7 (2012): 1286–1297, https://doi.org/10.2105/AJPH.2012.300759; for a similar case examining local pushback encountered by the global Smallpox Eradication Program, see Erez Manela, "A Pox on Your Narrative: Writing Disease Control Into Cold War History," *Diplomatic History* 34, no. 2 (2010): 315–318.

9. For examples, see Paul Farmer, *AIDS and Accusation: Haiti and the Geography of Blame* (Berkeley, CA: University of California Press, 1992); Salmaan Keshavjee, *Blind Spot: How Neoliberalism Infiltrated Global Health* (Berkeley, CA: University of California Press, 2014); Luke Messac, *No More to Spend: Neglect and the Construction of Scarcity in Malawi's History of Health Care* (New York, NY: Oxford University Press, 2020).
10. Randall M. Packard, *A History of Global Health: Interventions Into the Lives of Other Peoples* (Baltimore, MD: Johns Hopkins University Press, 2016), 22.
11. Ibid., 20.
12. Mariola Espinosa, *Epidemic Invasions: Yellow Fever and the Limits of Cuban Independence, 1878–1930* (Chicago, IL: University of Chicago Press, 2019), 5.
13. Thomas R. Marshall, "Asiatic Cholera in the Philippine Islands," Manila, Philippines: Bureau of Public Printing, 1904, 9, quoted in Warwick Anderson, "Excremental Colonialism: Public Health and the Poetics of Pollution," *Critical Inquiry* 21, no. 3 (1995): 642, https://doi.org/10.1086/448767
14. Warwick Anderson, *Colonial Pathologies: American Tropical Medicine, Race, and Hygiene in the Philippines* (Durham, NC: Duke University Press, 2006).
15. Reynaldo C. Ileto, "Cholera and the Origins of the American Sanitary Order in the Philippines," in Arnold D, ed., *Imperial Medicine and Indigenous Societies* (Manchester, UK: Manchester University Press, 2017); Paul Gideon Dionela Lasco, *Height Matters: The Making, Meanings, and Materialities of Human Stature in the Philippines* (Manila, Philippines: University of the Philippines Press, 2023).
16. Alfred W. McCoy, *Policing America's Empire: The United States, the Philippines, and the Rise of the Surveillance State* (Madison, WI: University of Wisconsin Press, 2009).
17. Vicente L. Rafael, *White Love and Other Events in Filipino History* (Durham, NC: Duke University Press, 2021), 31.
18. Elizabeth Fee, Marcos Cueto, and Theodore M. Brown, eds., "The Cold War and Eradication," in *The World Health Organization: A History, Global Health Histories* (Cambridge, UK: Cambridge University Press, 2019), 90, https://doi.org/10.1017/9781108692878.005
19. John A. Logan, "Counteracting Communism Through Foreign Assistance Programs in Public Health," *American Journal of Public Health* 45, no. 8 (1955): 1020, quoted in Shirish Kavadi, "The Cold War, Non-Alignment, and Medicine in India: The Case of Medical Education and Pharmaceutical Self-Sufficiency, 1947–57," in Neelakantan V, ed., *The Geopolitics of Health in South and Southeast Asia* (Abingdon, UK: Routledge, 2023), 59.
20. Kavadi, "The Cold War, Non-Alignment, and Medicine in India"; Marcos Cueto, *Cold War, Deadly Fevers* (Baltimore, MD: Johns Hopkins University Press, 2007).
21. Michael E. Latham, *Modernization as Ideology: American Social Science and "Nation Building" in the Kennedy Era* (Chapel Hill, NC: University of North Carolina Press, 2000); Immerwahr, Thinking Small.
22. Immerwahr, *Thinking Small*, 100, 120. Some scholars, like Nick Cullather, have framed the 1960s' US Agency for International Development–organized agricultural "Green Revolution" in the Philippines as another example of this type of project. For more, see Nick Cullather, *The Hungry World: America's Cold War Battle Against Poverty in Asia* (Cambridge, MA: Harvard University Press, 2013), 159–79, https://doi.org/10.4159/9780674262881
23. Julian Francis, "When India Recognized Bangladesh," *Dhaka Tribune*, December 6, 2019, https://www.dhakatribune.com/opinion/op-ed/195273/when-india-recognized-bangladesh (accessed December 21, 2023); Pierce Gardner, Jon E. Rohde, and M.B. Majumdar, "Health Priorities Among Bangladesh Refugees," *The Lancet (British Edition)* 299, no. 7755 (1972): 834–836, https://doi.org/10.1016/S0140-6736(72)90813-6
24. Charles Stenberg, "Letter from Charles Stenberg to Dr. Vulimiri Ramalingaswami, Col. Pran Luthra, and Dr. Jon Rohde," January 3, 1972, James E. Austin Papers, 1965–2006, Carton 94, Folder 2, Harvard Business School, Baker Library Special Collections and Archives; U. G. Patel, "Invoice from Roche Products Limited to The International Rescue Committee," January 10, 1972, James E. Austin Papers, 1965–2006, Carton 94, Folder 2, Harvard Business School, Baker Library Special Collections and Archives.
25. A. J. Zerfas, Mass Distribution of Vitamin A Programme for Refugee Children in India—Jan-Feb 1972 (International Union for Child Welfare, February 1972), James E. Austin Papers, 1965–2006, Carton 94, Folder 2, Harvard Business School, Baker Library Special Collections and Archives.
26. United Nations Children's Fund Executive Board, Draft Report of a Meeting under the Auspices of the World Health Organization on Prevention of Xerophthalmia, 27–29 March 1972, National Institute of Nutrition, Hyderabad, India (Hyderabad, India, March 27, 1972), 1, James E. Austin Papers, 1965–2006, Carton 94, Folder 2, Harvard Business School, Baker Library Special Collections and Archives.
27. UNICEF, "UNICEF Annual Report 1972," June 30, 1972, 4, https://digitallibrary.un.org/record/4042666?v=pdf (accessed February 21, 2024).
28. Wadie Kamel, *Volume I: A Global Survey of Mass Vitamin A Programs, Vitamin A, Xerophtalmia, and Blindness: A Status Report in Three Volumes* (Chicago, IL: University of Illinois Medical Center, Office of Nutrition, Technical Assistance Bureau, Agency for International Development, US Department of State; July 1973), James E. Austin Papers, 1965–2006, Carton 93, Folder 42, Harvard Business School, Baker Library Special Collections and Archives; Andre G. van Veen and Marjorie Scott van Veen, *Volume II: Vitamin A Problems With Special Reference to Less Developed Countries, Vitamin A, Xerophtalmia, and Blindness: A Status Report in Three Volumes* (Office of Nutrition, Technical Assistance Bureau, Agency for International Development, US Department of State, July 1973), James E. Austin Papers, 1965–2006, Carton 93, Folder 47, Harvard Business School, Baker Library Special Collections and Archives; J. C. Baurenfeind, *Volume III: Vitamin A Technology, Vitamin A, Xerophtalmia, and Blindness: A Status Report in Three Volumes* (Nutley, NJ: Hoffman La Roche Inc, July 1973), James E. Austin Papers, 1965–2006, Carton 94, Folder 1, Harvard Business School, Baker Library Special Collections and Archives.
29. Baurenfeind, *Volume III: Vitamin A Technology*, 83.
30. Sommer et al., "Impact of Vitamin A Supplementation on Childhood Mortality."
31. Ibid., 13.
32. Ibid., 12.
33. Semba, *The Vitamin A Story*, 173.
34. "Stop Albay Research Project, Gov't Urged," *The Manila Times*, August 28, 1986, and "Albay Project Stirs Row," *The Manila Bulletin*, August 30, 1986, Michael Latham papers, 1950–2010, Box 29, Folder Florentino Solon, Cornell University Rare and Manuscript Collections.
35. "Stop Albay Research Project, Gov't Urged."
36. Semba, *The Vitamin A Story*, 174.
37. Immerwahr, *Thinking Small*, 110.
38. Ibid., 107.
39. Semba, *The Vitamin A Story*, 174.
40. Thiele Lunas, "Letter from Thiele Lunas to Keith West," October 19, 1987, Alfred Sommer Collection, Box AS2-4, Johns Hopkins University, Alan Mason Chesney Medical Archives.
41. Central Intelligence Agency, "Letter from the Central Intelligence Agency to the Department of Nutrition, Cornell University," April 28, 1978, Michael Latham papers, 1950–2010, Box 29, Folder 16, Cornell University Rare and Manuscript Collections. For another example of CIA attempts to gain information from academics conducting research abroad, see this account by cardiologist Henry Blackburn, "'If It Isn't Fun.'—Undercover for the CIA Heart Attack Prevention," November 4, 1958, http://www.epi.umn.edu/cvdepi/essay/if-it-isnt-fun-undercover-for-the-cia (accessed April 24, 2025).
42. Michael C. Latham, "Memorandum from M.C. Latham to M.C. Nesheim RE: CIA Request for Proposals for Nutrition Research," May 5, 1978, Michael Latham papers, 1950–2010, Box 29, Folder 16, Cornell University Rare and Manuscript Collections.
43. "Joseph M. Whelton," *The Washington Post*, November 28, 1992, https://www.washingtonpost.com/archive/local/1992/11/28/ralph-r-reed-dies-at-65/0920a953-9a4e-48c8-8e18-b0b9bba60e16 (accessed August 2, 2025).
44. Latham, "Memorandum from M.C. Latham to M.C. Nesheim."
45. Unknown, "CIA: Plowshares Into Swords?," *CounterSpy* 4, no. 1 (1979): 19–22; "Counterspy; Catalogue of the National Library of Australia," https://catalogue.nla.gov.au/catalog/1106695 (accessed April 16, 2025).
46. Paul Erickson et al., *How Reason Almost Lost Its Mind: The Strange Career of Cold War Rationality* (Chicago, IL: University of Chicago Press, 2015).
47. Ibid., 2.
48. Laura E. Bothwell et al., "Assessing the Gold Standard—Lessons From the History of RCTs," *New England Journal of Medicine* 374, no. 22 (June 2, 2016): 2175–2181, https://doi.org/10.1056/NEJMms1604593
49. Jeremy A. Greene, "Therapeutic Proofs and Medical Truths: The Enduring Legacy of Early Modern Drug Trials," *Bulletin of the History of Medicine* 91, no. 2 (2017): 424.
50. Jeremy A. Greene and Andrew S. Lea, "Digital Futures Past—The Long Arc of Big Data in Medicine," *New England Journal of Medicine* 381, no. 5 (August 1, 2019): 480–485, https://doi.org/10.1056/NEJMms1817674
51. Bothwell et al., "Assessing the Gold Standard," 2175.
52. Ibid., 2176.
53. David S. Jones, "Visions of a Cure. Visualization, Clinical Trials, and Controversies in Cardiac Therapeutics, 1968–1998," *Isis; an International Review Devoted to the History of Science and Its Cultural*

Influences 91, no. 3 (2000): 504–541, https://doi.org/10.1086/384853

54. Laura E. Bothwell and David S. Jones, "Innovation and Tribulation in the History of Randomized Controlled Trials in Surgery," *Annals of Surgery* 274, no. 6 (2021): e616–24, https://doi.org/10.1097/SLA.0000000000003631
55. Anthony Costello and Ronald Gray, "Vitamin A Supplementation and Childhood Mortality," *The Lancet* 328, no. 8499 (1986): 161–162, https://doi.org/10.1016/S0140-6736(86)91971-9
56. For more on the criticism of randomized controlled trials that later emerged in the social sciences and allied fields, see Martin Ravallion, "Should the Randomistas Rule?," *The Economists' Voice* 6, no. 2 (2009), https://doi.org/10.2202/1553-3832.1368; Kevin P. Donovan, "The Rise of the Randomistas: On the Experimental Turn in International Aid," *Economy and Society* 47, no. 1 (2018): 27–58, https://doi.org/10.1080/03085147.2018.1432153
57. Pamela Constable, "Marcos Era Ends in Philippines; Aquino Presides; Longtime Leader Flees to Guam: [Third Edition]," *Boston Globe* (Pre-1997 Fulltext), sec. National/Foreign, February 26, 1986.
58. University of the Philippines College of Law, "Martial Law Revisionism and the Fight for History," September 22, 2020, https://law.upd.edu.ph/martial-law-revisionism-and-the-fight-for-history (accessed December 26, 2025).
59. Semba, *The Vitamin A Story*, 172.
60. Kate Burns, quoted in *The Vitamin A Story*, 172.
61. Semba, *The Vitamin A Story*, 175.
62. "Department of Health VAD Control Project, Household Questionnaire (VAD Form 5)," July 1987, Alfred Sommer Collection, Box AS2-3, Johns Hopkins University, Alan Mason Chesney Medical Archives.
63. M. Cuezon, "Albay Vitamin A Research Project Questioned," *The Drug Monitor*, No. 7 (1986): 1–6; quoted in Semba, *The Vitamin A Story*, 174.
64. For more on Cold War periodization, see Odd Arne Westad, *The Global Cold War: Third World Interventions and the Making of Our Times* (Cambridge, UK: Cambridge University Press, 2016), 4.
65. Michael Latham, Homero Martinez, and Meera Shekar, "Vitamin A Supplementation and Child Mortality," *The Lancet* 328, no. 8504 (1986): 451–452, https://doi.org/10.1016/S0140-6736(86)92149-5
66. Ibid.
67. Conversation with Keith West, November 25, 2023.
68. Paul Icamina, "Not Seeing Eye to Eye: Vitamin A Suffers a Setback," Development International, April 1987, Alfred Sommer Collection, Box AS2-4, Johns Hopkins University, Alan Mason Chesney Medical Archives.
69. Two cents per pill, with a recommended dosage of two pills per child each year, equates to four cents per child, per year.
70. For more on these tensions, see Matthew Basilico et al., "Health for All? Competing Theories and Geopolitics," in *Reimagining Global Health: An Introduction*, ed. Paul Farmer et al. (Berkeley, CA: University of California Press, 2019), 74–110.
71. World Health Organization, "Declaration of Alma-Ata," in Declaration of Alma-Ata, 1978, https://pesquisa.bvsalud.org/portal/resource/pt/who-347879 (accessed April 22, 2025).
72. J. A. Walsh and K. S. Warren, "Selective Primary Health Care: An Interim Strategy for Disease Control in Developing Countries," *The New England Journal of Medicine* 301, no. 18 (1979): 967, https://doi.org/10.1056/NEJM197911013011804
73. For the landmark study, see K. P. West et al., "Efficacy of Vitamin A in Reducing Preschool Child Mortality in Nepal," *The Lancet*, originally published as volume 2, issue 8759, 338, (July 13, 1991): 70, https://doi.org/10.1016/0140-6736(91)90070-6. For the conference that engendered widespread support for capsule vitamin A supplementation, see Alfred Sommer, "Conference: Vitamin A Deficiency and Childhood Mortality," *The Lancet (British Edition)* 339, no. 8797 (1992): 864; For information showing when mass supplementation started, see UNICEF, "UNICEF Annual Report 1993," 1993, https://digitallibrary.un.org/record/174445 (accessed February 25, 2024).
74. Mark Hofschneider, "Alfred Sommer: Discovering a Two-Cent Remedy That Saves Children's Lives," Lasker Foundation, April 6, 2020, https://laskerfoundation.org/alfred-sommer-discovering-a-two-cent-remedy-that-saves-childrens-lives (accessed May 2, 2023); Mark Hofschneider, "Vitamin A Therapy for Preventing Infections and Blindness," Lasker Foundation, https://laskerfoundation.org/winners/vitamin-a-therapy-for-preventing-infections-and-blindness (accessed July 9, 2023); "Rx for Survival. Global Health Champions. Alfred Sommer, MD, MHS. PBS," https://www.pbs.org/wgbh/rxforsurvival/series/champions/alfred_sommer.html (accessed February 8, 2023); Christine Grillo, "Al Sommer on Better Science: Data Versus Beliefs," Center for a Livable Future, December 2, 2020, https://clf.jhsph.edu/viewpoints/al-sommer-better-science-data-versus-beliefs (accessed April 23, 2025).
75. For Latham's final argument against vitamin A supplementation, see Michael Latham, "The Great Vitamin A Fiasco," *World Nutrition* 1, no. 1 (2010), https://www.worldnutritionjournal.org/index.php/wn/article/download/570/513 (accessed February 26, 2024). For one example of contemporary pushback, see Shally Awasthi et al., "Vitamin A Supplementation Every 6 Months With Retinol in 1 Million Pre-School Children in North India: DEVTA, a Cluster-Randomised Trial," *The Lancet* 381, no. 9876 (2013): 1469–1477. For evidence of continued vitamin A supplementation projects, see "UNICEF's Vitamin A Supplementation Programme Achieved 100% Coverage Reaching Vulnerable Children Aged 6-59 Months Living in Hard-to-Reach (HTR) Areas Across Bangladesh: United Nations in Bangladesh," July 3, 2024, https://bangladesh.un.org/en/273027-unicef%E2%80%99s-vitamin-supplementation-programme-achieved-100-coverage-reaching-vulnerable (accessed April 23, 2025).

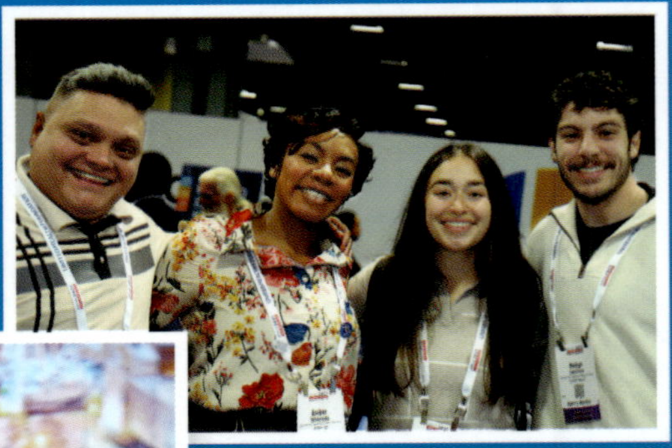

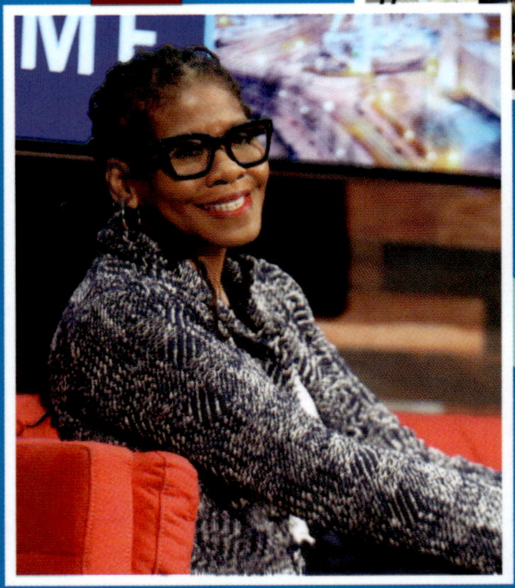

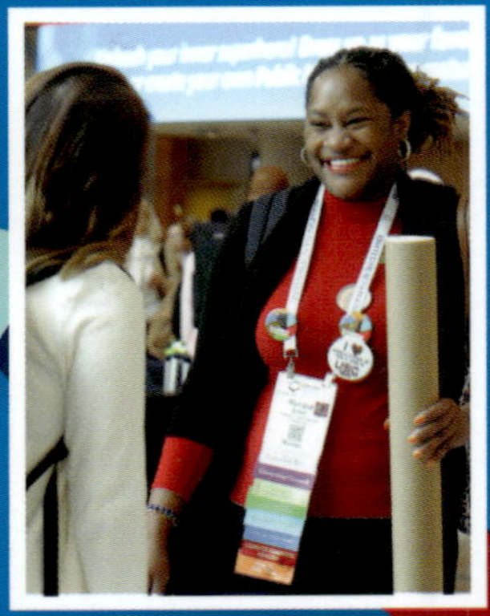